Tumors of the skull base

Tumors of the skull base

Extra- and intracranial surgery of skull base tumors

Editors
H. Scheunemann · K. Schürmann · J. Helms

W DE G
Walter de Gruyter
Berlin · New York 1986

Prof. Dr. med. Dr. med. dent. Horst Scheunemann
Direktor der Klinik für Mund-Kiefer-Gesichtschirurgie
Klinikum der Johannes-Gutenberg-Universität Mainz
Langenbeckstr. 1 · D-6500 Mainz

Prof. Dr. med. Dr. med. h.c. Kurt Schürmann
Direktor der Neurochirurgischen Klinik
Klinikum der Johannes-Gutenberg-Universität Mainz
Langenbeckstr. 1 · D-6500 Mainz

Prof. Dr. med. Jan Helms
Direktor der Hals-Nasen-Ohren-Klinik
Klinikum der Johannes-Gutenberg-Universität Mainz
Langenbeckstr. 1 · D-6500 Mainz

This book contains 34 illustrations and 110 tables.

CIP-Kurztitelaufnahme der Deutschen Bibliothek

Tomors of the skull base : extra- and intracranial surgery of skull base tumors ; [based on papers presented at the 2. internat. meeting of the Skull Base Study Group, held June 21-23. 1984 in Mainz, Germany] / ed. H. Scheunemann ... - Berlin ; New York : de Gruyter, 1986.
ISBN 3-11-010299-4 (Berlin)
ISBN 0-89925-116-1 (New York)
NE: Scheunemann, Horst [Hrsg.]; Skull Base Study Group

Library of Congress Cataloging in Publication Data

Tumors of the skull base.
Based on papers presented at the Second International Meeting of the Skull Base Study Group, held June 21-23, 1984 in Mainz, Germany.
Includes bibliographies and indexes.
1. Basicranium-Tumors-Surgery-Congresses.
I. Scheunemann, Horst. II. Schürmann, K. III. Helms, J. (Jan), 1937- .
IV. Skull Base Study Group. International Congress (2nd : 1984 : Mainz, Rhineland-Palatinate, Germany) [DNLM: 1. Brain Neoplasms-congresses. 2. Neurosurgery-congresses. 3. Skull Neoplasms-congresses.
WE 705 T925 1984]
RD662.5.T86 1986 616.99'4715 86-8942
ISBN 0-89925-116-1 (U.S.)

Typesetting: Appl, Wemding. - Printing: Gerike GmbH, Berlin. - Binding: Lüderitz & Bauer GmbH, Berlin. Cover design: Rudolf Hübler, Berlin.

Preface

Unfortunately there is no existing specialist in the medical field today who deals with the skull base. Aspects such as extracranial and intracranial areas have in the past been dealt with by various other surgical disciplines. Since the early seventies however, skull base surgery has reached a new dimension, not only through the application of new microsurgical techniques and the availability of LASER and CUSA equipment but also, more significantly, by a new level of understanding in many problems concerning the skull base. Neurosurgeons, otorhinolaryngologists, maxillofacial as well as plastic and reconstructive surgeons, opthalmologists and neuroradiologists have found new methods through close cooperation which have opened new perspectives for lowering risks and raising effectiveness in skull base surgery, particularly in tumors affecting both the intracranial and extracranial space.

This past experience led to the foundation of the Skull Base Study Group in 1973 whose aim was to bring together experts from different fields to achieve greater interdisciplinary consultation and jointly performed surgery. It is thanks to these recent developments that skull base surgery has made such progress in the last few years.

The results of the Second International Meeting of the Skull Base Study Group are recorded in this volume where specialists from various fields exchange their experiences and views on the subject. It is hoped that a multidisciplinary approach to our problems may be encouraged which will assist in preparing the next step forward and therefore contribute towards further development of this specialist field.

The text shows the effectiveness of such interdisciplinary teamwork together with a presentation of an exchange of ideas between colleagues who approach the same problem from different points of view. In a condensed form, it contains a great deal of information on the topic of skull base tumors which is normally only available in articles which are widely dispersed throughout various journals.

Articles from various experts (anatomists, pathologists, radiologists, neuroradiologists, neurosurgeons, ENT-surgeons, maxillofacial surgeons, plastic and reconstructive surgeons) who have made substantial contributions to this field, have been compiled in the form of this unique volume providing the reader with an unusual survey of surgery of skull base tumors and also presenting the possibilities and limits of this remarkable field.

If this book serves our colleagues and benefits in particular our patients, then it will have achieved its purpose.

We should like to thank Professor Horst Scheunemann and his co-editors as well as de Gruyter Publishers for their kind co-operation who have enabled this volume to be presented in short time and good design.

Mainz, December 1985 KURT SCHÜRMANN

President of the Skull Base Study Group

Contents

I Anatomy and neuroradiology of the skull base related to tumor surgery

Topographical anatomy of the skull base and adjacent tissues

J. Lang

Orbital and optic nerve tumors, anatomy

The maximum height of the orbital opening in neonates is about 23 mm and in adults 35 mm. The height of the orbit is greatest about 3.5–4 mm behind the opening, mainly because the roof rises about 3.5–4 mm. A coronal section behind the orbital rim in the adult is approximately circular, but in the neonate it resembles an elongated oval with its blunt end pointing upwards and outwards. In the interior of the orbit we distinguish the zones lying along the walls from the rectus cone. The cone is marked off from the other zones by the four rectus muscles and their fascial sheaths (which are thin at the back of the orbit, but thick in the front). The recti are usually only 1–2 mm away from the orbital walls (4–6 mm at the most) and, like the longitudinal part of the superior oblique muscle, they run parallel to them. The optic nerve does not lie in the center of the rectus cone, but in a zone enclosed by the medial borders of the levator palpebrae superioris and the superior and inferior rectus muscles. Also running within the cone is the ophthalmic artery, which usually crosses above the optic nerve to its medial side. Ophthalmic veins, the nerves supplying the extrinsic ocular muscles, and, in the posterolateral part, the roots of the ciliary ganglion, the ciliary ganglion itself, and the ciliary nerves emerging from the front of the ganglion are also situated inside the cone. Contained within the rectus cone is the cushion of retrobulbar fat which allows frictionless movements of the vessels and nerves and also prevents recession of the eyeball (fig. 1).

Approaches

The lateral approach to the orbit (Krönlein-Berke operation) is through relatively thin skin and a variable depth of fatty connective tissue containing branches of the facial, lacrimal and zygomaticotemporal nerves. With the lateral approach to the orbit the frontal and zygomatic branches of the facial nerve could be severed. According to Hamby [7], Welti [28] described a pterional approach to the orbit and the anterior and middle cranial fossae. Hamby [7] reflected the temporal muscle and exposed the pterion (suture between the frontal, parietal, temporal and sphenoid bone). Welti [28] described three trepanations, one of them through the lowest part of the frontal bone, another to the middle cranial fossa and one anterior and

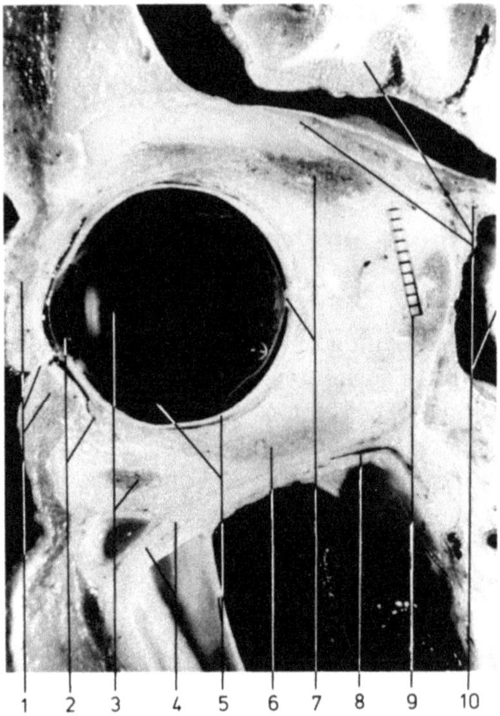

Fig. 1 Paramedian section through the orbit, viewed from medially.
1 = Orbicularis oculi muscle, palpebral part and palpebral rim; 2 = Cornea and lower fornix of the conjungtival sac; 3 = Posterior pole of the lens and inferior oblique muscle; 4 = Infraorbital nerve, inside its canal; 5 = Retina, sclera and small septum of the maxillary sinus; 6 = Inferior rectus muscle; 7 = Superior rectus and levator muscles and papilla n. optici; 8 = Infraorbital artery, cut; 9 = Lateral rectus muscle, mm-paper; 10 = Frontal lobe, orbital roof and temporal pole.

downwards through the lateral orbit wall. In this way it is possible to expose the periorbita and the dura mater of the lesser sphenoidal wing. The latter can be removed, and the roof of the orbit and the lateral orbit wall exposed. An approach to the roof of the optic canal is possible.

The approach to the lateral wall of the orbit is via the anterior (orbital) part of the temporal fossa. Here the fossa is occupied by the anterior part of the temporal muscle and by veins, which may be large, including the middle and deep temporal veins. The most anterior part of the fossa contains an accumulation of fatty tissue. (For further details see Lang [10].)

Lateral wall of the orbit

The posterior part of the lateral wall of the orbit is bounded above by the superior orbital fissure and the roof of the orbit and below by the inferior orbital fissure. Between these, the greater wing of the sphenoid makes up the largest part of the lateral wall.

It is generally assumed that the lateral wall of the orbit makes an angle of about 45° with the median plane. In our specimens the mean angle made with the median plane by the junction between the roof and the lateral wall (from the lateral extremity of the superior orbital fissure to the fronto-zygomatic suture) was 35.58° on the right side and 34.67° on the left. There is normally an outward concavity about 4 mm deep.

The angle between a tangent from the dacryon to the fronto-zygomatic suture and a sagittal plane through the dacryon we found to measure 79.92 ± 4.5 (70.0–90.0)° on the right and 80.35 ± 4.24 (72.0–90.0)° on the left.

It should be noted that the average distance from the dacryon to the median sagittal plane is 12.3 mm on the right and 11.8 mm on the left. The average distance between the lateral orbit edge in the area of the fronto-zygomatic suture and a coronal plane through the nasion is 17.57 ± 2.79 (11.0–24.0) mm on the right side and 16.54 ± 2.73 (11.0–23.0) mm on the left. We found this distance to be greater on the right in 63.6% of our cases, equal on both sides in 21.2% and greater on the left in 15.2%. Also the distance between the lateral margin of the orbit (covered by skin)

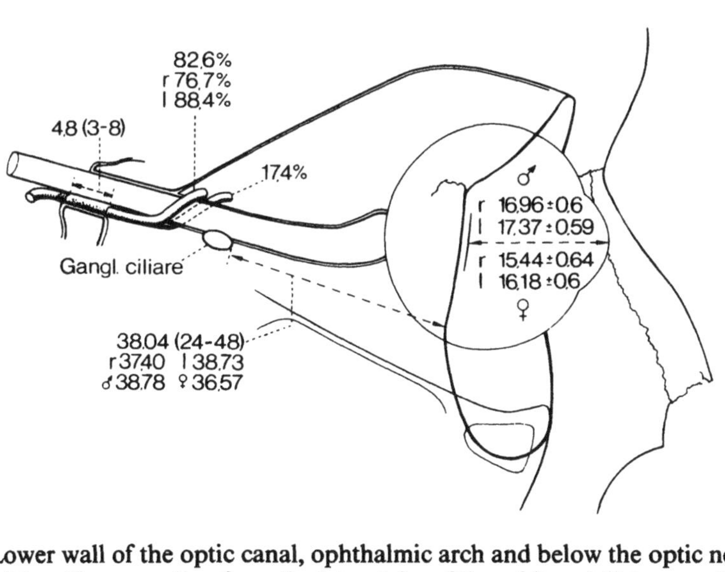

Fig. 2 Lower wall of the optic canal, ophthalmic arch and below the optic nerve, distance of the ciliary ganglion from the lateral rim of the orbit and distances of the cornea to the lateral orbital wall (with skin). Given are right-left and sex-differences.

is greater on the left (e.g. in men 17.34 mm) than on the right (16.96 mm). This difference between the sides should be taken into account during ophthalmometric measurements (fig. 2).

Common tendinous ring

At the apex of the orbit are the origins of the rectus, levator palpebrae superioris and superior oblique muscles. These arise from a ring of fibrous tissue known as the tendinous ring. The ring divides the superior orbital fissure into three parts, one above and lateral to it, one enclosed by it, and the other below it. The lateral part outside the ring transmits (in order from inferomedial to superolateral) the trochlear nerve, frontal nerve, superior ophthalmic vein, lacrimal nerve and, most laterally, an branch of the middle meningeal artery which anastomoses with the lacrimal artery and occasionally replaces the ophthalmic artery. Within the ring (in order from above down) are the superior ramus of the oculomotor nerve, the nasociliary nerve, the inferior ramus of the oculomotor nerve with the abducent nerve to its lateral side and, rarely, the superior ophthalmic vein as well. Posteromedially, still within the common tendinous ring, the optic nerve and ophthalmic artery enter the orbit through the optic canal. The part of the superior orbital fissure below the tendinous ring sometimes accommodates an additional superior ophthalmic vein which opens into the cavernous sinus.

The superior ophthalmic vein usually emerges from the rectus cone at the back of the orbit between the superior and lateral recti and then curves sharply down and round the lateral side of the nerves to the ocular muscles (except for the sixth nerve). It then curves sharply back into the sagittal plane and travels on the lateral side of the tendinous ring to enter the inferolateral corner of the cavernous sinus after a 2-3 mm long course under cover of the merging periorbita and dura mater. In the vertical part of its course it usually receives several tributaries which are often known collectively as the inferior ophthalmic vein. Occasionally the inferior ophthalmic vein travels back under the tendinous ring and then up towards the cavernous sinus. Fibers of the orbitalis muscle always run along the lateral side of the ophthalmic vein and strengthen the anterior part of the lateral wall of the cavernous sinus. The superior ophthalmic vein has no valves, but the inferior ophthalmic vein may have a valve where it enters the superior ophthalmic vein (and so may its small tributary veins).

At the apex of the orbit is the ciliary ganglion, lying on the medial side of the lateral rectus muscle (which is entered in its posterior third by the abducent nerve) and on the lateral side of the optic nerve (usually a little below it). The ganglion has a height of rather more than 2 mm and its mean length is 2.88 (1.5-4.5) mm in the right orbit and 3.19 (1.5-5.0) mm in the left. Its mean distance from the back of the eyeball is 17.13 (13.5-21.0) mm in the right orbit and 18.93 (16.0-26.5) mm in the left. The distance between the ganglion and the lateral rim of the orbit is 38 (24–48) mm. The sensory root of the ciliary ganglion comes from the nasociliary nerve and usually leaves it behind the superior orbital fissure while still part of the ophthalmic nerve. The oculomotor root, often double or even triple, is derived from the inferior ramus of the oculomotor nerve or one of its motor branches. The extremely fine sympathetic root comes either from the sympathetic plexus of the cavernous sinus or from the pterygopalatine ganglion and passes through the orbitalis muscle.

Between three and six ciliary nerves emerge from the anterior border and lateral and medial surfaces of the ciliary ganglion and travel forwards to the eyeball along the perimeter of the optic nerve while still dividing further. Some enter the sclera about 2 mm away from the point where the dural sheath of the optic nerve merges with it. Only the long posterior ciliary arteries and nerves enter the sclera as far as 4 mm away from the optic nerve. The distances between the lateral margin of the orbit and the ciliary ganglion and the course of the ophthalmic artery and its right-left differences are given in figure 2.

Course of the ethmoidal canals

Ethmoidal canals

The anterior, posterior and third ethmoidal canals usually run parallel to the Frankfurt horizontal plane, but some descend at angles of up to 20° to it and some rise at angles of up to 30° to it.

Anterior ethmoidal canal

The anterior ethmoidal canal ist usually oval, with mean major and minor diameters of 2.5 mm and 1.3 mm. Towards the middle of the canal the diameter decreases to 65% of its inital value. The intracranial and orbital openings are expanded. There is close correlation between the diameters of the anterior ethmoidal arteries and those of the canals. The mean diameter of the artery at the entrance to the canal (0.60 mm) is significantly greater than that at the middle (0.49 mm). The diameter of the artery increases near the intracranial end of the canal (on average by 0.5 mm). On average, the artery gives off 4.6 branches while in the canal; Their mean diameter is 0,08 mm. Most of these supply the contents of the canal. Others, mostly larger, leave the canal in their own branch canals and help to supply the anterior ethmoidal air cells and the frontal sinus.

The anterior ethmoidal nerve does not change in size while in the canal; it is usually about 0.33 mm in diameter. In 54% of instances it consists of two to four fasciculi. Numerous other nerve filaments, mostly unmedullated, travel in the anterior ethmoidal canal; the average number is ten (1-23) and the average diameter ist usually 0.04 mm or less.

Posterior ethmoidal canal

The posterior ethmoidal canal, like the anterior, is usually oval in cross-section and narrower in its middle part than at either end. The mean major diameter is 2.05 mm in the first part of the canal, decreases to 1.56 mm in the middle part and increases to 1.94 mm at the intracranial end. The minor diameter is 1.04 mm in the orbital part and 0.84 mm in the middle part of the canal, after which it remains the same. An artery passes through the posterior ethmoidal canal and is peculiar in 26% of instances in that its orbital diameter is less than its intracranial. Mean diameters of the artery are: 0.45 mm on entering the posterior canal from the orbit, 0.39 mm in the middle part of the canal and 0.38 mm from there to the intracranial end. The mean number of branches given off by the posterior ethmoidal artery inside the canal is 3.6 (0-9); their mean diameter is 0.09 (0.02-0.28) mm. Some branches run back into the orbit and supply muscles there. The mean number of nerve filaments running in the posterior ethmoidal canal is 6 (1-10); their mean diameter is 0.05 mm. In our opinion most of these are autonomic fibers derived from the pterygopalatine ganglion [12]. It is rare to find a nerve which resembles a somatic nerve histologically; the mean diameter of such nerves is 0.1 mm.

Third ethmoidal canal

When third ethmoidal canals have been observed, they have also been oval in cross-section, with the major diameter steadily decreasing from the orbital end (mean: 1.39 mm) to the intracranial end (mean: 1.22 mm), but with the minor diameter remaining unchanged. An artery was found in 83% of canals; the mean diameter of these vessels was 0.24 mm, decreasing slightly during passage through the canal. We have once found a third ethmoidal artery replacing a missing anterior ethmoidal artery. The mean number of very fine branches of the artery was 1.2 (0-5); their mean diameter was 0.09 mm. The proportion with no branches was 50%. In our opinion, the only nerve fibers in the third ethmoidal canal (like the posterior one) are autonomic; the mean number found was 4.2 (1-13); their mean diameter was 0.05 mm [12].

The fourth canal, it present, contained a few small nerves and veins.

Ethmoidal veins

The ethmoidal canals also transmit the ethmoidal veins. If the various diameters of these veins are interpreted to indicate direction of flow, the main drainage appears to be to the anterior cranial fossa. The smallest diameters are found in the middle parts of the posterior ethmoidal canal. About 40% of the veins drain into the anterior cranial fossa. A preponderance of flow towards the ethmoidal air cells is the least frequently found (in 16% of anterior ethmoidal canals and 12% of posterior ethmoidal canals). The ethmoidal veins are of importance in transorbital infections from the paranasal sinuses.

Olfactory fibers

Passage of the olfactory fibers through the cribriform plate. The anterior fibers run rostrally, the posterior fibers dorsally and the middle fibers straight downwards to reach to medial and lateral marginal zones of the olfactory fossa. They pass through the latter and end on the medial and lateral walls of the nose in the olfactory region. These fibers, known as the olfactory fascicles, are bundles of the central process of the olfactory cells and in their passage through the openings in the dura they are accompanied by arachnoidal sheaths. The olfactory bulb and tract are supplied by branches of the anterior cerebral artery in particular from the medial frontobasal artery, the ethmoidal arteries and the long central artery, which usually crosses the posterior portion of the olfactory tract. The olfactory tract runs dorsally within a small cistern, which it pierces posteriorly and is then related below to the continuation of the cisterna valleculae. Venous drainage from this region is carried by the orbital veins of the orbital surface of the frontal lobe to the anterior cerebral vein, to the superior sagittal sinus and also through the cribriform plate to the nasal cavity. (For further details see Lanz/Wachsmuth, Praktische Anatomie, Vol. I, 1 B.)

Optic canal: general

Optic canal: form

During postnatal growth the canal assumes the shape of a cylinder drawn out at one side and flattened at the intracranial end. The orbital cross-section, however, retains its elongated oval shape. Up to 20 years of age the lower wall of the canal grows by an average of only 20.7%, but the upper wall increases by 91% reaching an average length of 9.8 mm. Most of this growth takes place in the first two years but there is a further growth spurt between 8 and 9 years. Adult dimensions are

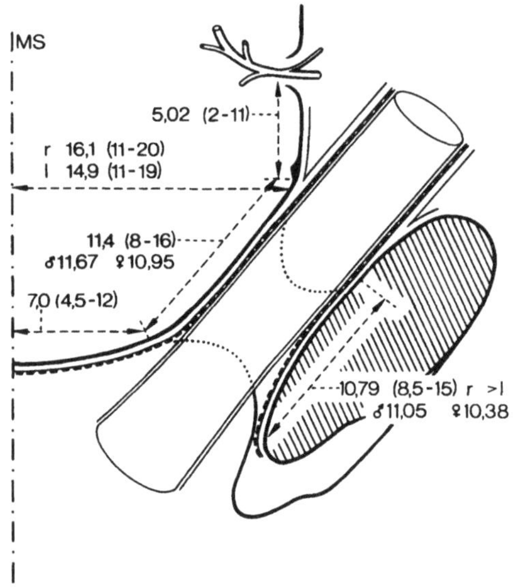

Fig. 3 Medial and lateral wall of the optic canal and distance to the posterior ethmoideal canal and artery. All measurements in mm (extremals), right-left-differences and sex-differences.

reached by 11 years. The overall growth in the roof is more than 4 times greater than the growth of the floor which has a length of 4.8 mm. The length of the medial and lateral wall is given in figure 3. During surgical operations in the vicinity of the apex of the orbit it is occasionally necessary to unroof the superior orbital fissure. The lesser wing of the sphenoid has a dural layer up to 3 mm thick which covers it posteriorly together with the sphenoparietal sinus. The ramus communicans between the lacrimal artery and the frontal branch of the middle meningeal artery is woven into the dural layer. Above the common tendinous ring the trochlear nerve runs medially and forwards over the tendinous origins of the m. levator palpebrae superioris.

Arising from the frontal branch of the middle meningeal artery, the communicating branch with the lacrimal artery runs in the lateral angle of the superior orbital fissure or even through the greater wing of the sphenoid and as a rule anastomoses with the lacrimal artery immediately after the latter has arisen from the ophthalmic artery. In occasional instances this branch may be absent or very small. Singh and Dass [22, 23] found that the communicating branch with the lacrimal artery replaced the entire ophthalmic artery in approximately 2%. In some 1% of subjects [8] the entire lacrimal artery arises from the frontal branch of the middle meningeal artery. Not infrequently a branch arising from the anastomotic region of the ophthalmic artery runs backwards through the superior orbital fissure and takes part in the blood supply of nerves, bone and dura in the cavernous sinus.

In order to unroof the optic canal its superior wall is removed. During postnatal life there is significant thinning of the posterior segment of the superior wall of the canal. In the newborn its average thickness is 2.23 mm measured at a point 2 mm rostral to the intracranial aperture of the optic canal, while in adults the mean thickness is 0.75 (0.2–2.2) mm. The lateral and inferior wall of the optic canal merges dorsally into the anterior clinoid process. The thickness of this zone is of some importance to the surgeon engaged in unroofing the canal.

Optic nerve

Because the axis of the optic canal shifts as age advances, the optic nerves in newborn infants and young children deviate further laterally and downwards than in adults.

At its interior end the dura mater cerebri merges directly with the dural periosteum which lines the canal. At the orbital aperture of the optic canal the two layers again diverge. The parietal or periosteal layers are continuous with the periorbital lining. The visceral layer envelops the optic nerve as the dura mater of the optic nerve. The optic nerve itself is accompanied by the pia mater of the optic nerve, a relatively thick layer, even in its course through the optic canal. The pia is firmly attached to the nerve by numerous connective tissue septa which radiate into the nerve. The arachnoid sheath can also be traced throughout the entire length of the canal and

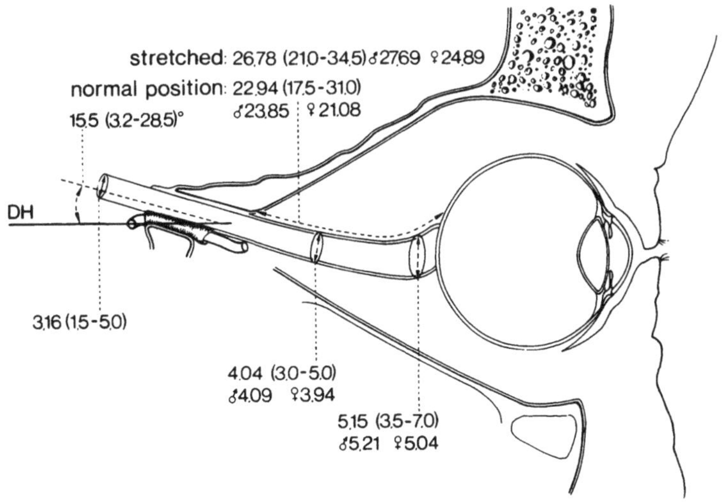

Fig. 4 Angle of the optic canal to the Frankfurt-plane in degrees (extremals), vertical diameter of the optic nerve, orbital part of the optic nerve, stretched and in normal position, diameters of the optic nerve with its sheaths at different zones. All these measurements in mm (extremals) and sex-differences.

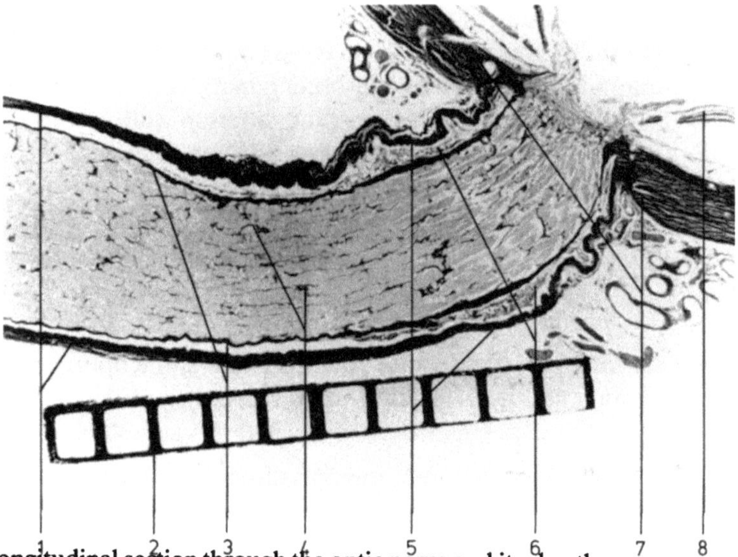

Fig. 5 Longitudinal section through the optic nerve and its sheaths.
1 = Dura mater of the optic nerve; 2 = mm-paper; 3 = Pia mater of the optic nerve; 4 = Connective tissue septa inside the optic nerve; 5 = Thinned dura mater behind the bulb; 6 = Arachnoideal angle; 7 = Sclera; 8 = Retina, dislocated.

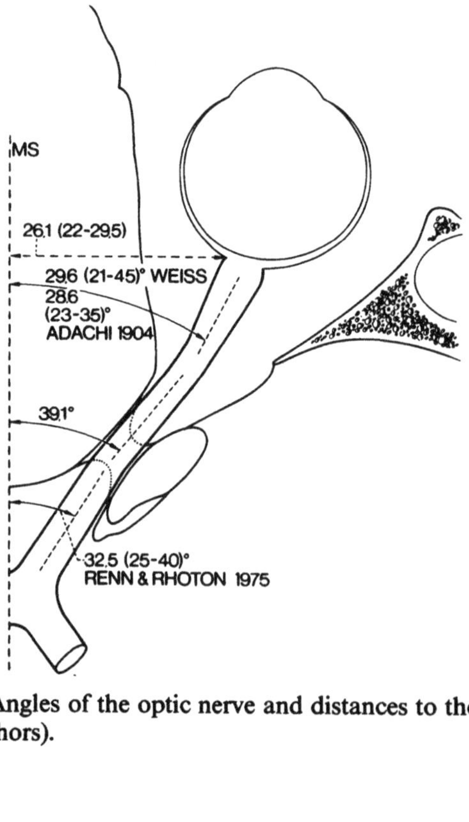

Fig. 6 Angles of the optic nerve and distances to the median sagittal plane (different authors).

in the orbital part of the optic nerve. In adults, however, there are numerous connective tissue strands between the arachnoid and the pia of the optic nerve as it passes through the canal. These bind the nerve firmly together and narrow the subarachnoid fluid spaces in this zone.

In adults the intraorbital portion of the optic nerve has an average length on its upper surface of about 23 (17.5–31) mm and if it is stretched 26.8 (21–34.5) mm. The thickness with sheaths is different usually in the posterior and anterior part. In the anterior part the circular fibers of the dural sheath are almost absent and this causes a dilatation (figs. 4 and 5). Other measurements are seen in figure 6. It usually follows a somewhat sinuous course (reserve length) as it runs forward to the eyeball. In newborn infants the optic nerve is 2.7 mm thick and approximately 24 mm in total length [20]. The angle of the optic nerve with the sagittal plane is about 29 (21–45)°.

Oculomotor nerve

The oculomotor nerve divides, usually in the anterior part of the cavernous sinus, into the superior ramus and the inferior ramus, the latter being somewhat thicker. The two rami are usually separate when they enter the superior orbital fissure. The superior ramus runs upwards and enters the superior rectus muscle from below at the junction of the posterior and middle third. The branch to the levator surrounds the medial border of the superior rectus in 83%, in the remaining cases it pierces totally or partly the muscle to reach the levator.

The somewhat larger inferior ramus of the oculomotor nerve runs downwards and then forwards on the lateral or lower side (7.1%) of the inferior rectus muscle. It crosses the posterior border of the inferior oblique muscle at its midzone, divides into two or three branches and pierces the upper or posterior surface of the muscle.

The parasympathetic branch to the ciliary ganglion is known as the oculomotor root. One, two or three short twigs branch off from the posterior segment of the inferior ramus of the oculomotor nerve and enter the ganglion, which is usually situated lateral to the nerve, from below.

The branch for the medial rectus muscle usually leaves the inferior ramus near the apex of the orbit and enters the muscle in its posterior third.

Abducent nerve

The abducent nerve passes through the common tendinous ring. At first it usually lies between the upper and lower oculomotor rami, then laterally and between the two. After a short distance it enters the medial surface of the lateral rectus muscle with 6.4 (3–10) twigs. The area nervosa is situated 28 (18–44) mm behind the lateral margin of the orbit.

Nasociliary nerve

The nasociliary nerve usually branches off from the ophthalmic nerve within the cavernous sinus, its origin being situated in the medial and lower part of the latter. It runs at first in the lateral wall of the cavernous sinus and passes through the common tendinous ring between the superior and inferior rami of the oculomotor nerve into the orbit. Within the posterior part of the muscle cone the nerve usually runs at first below the nerve to the inferior oblique muscle and then (like the ophthalmic artery) passes medially across the optic nerve. During this part of its course it gives off 1–3 long ciliary nerves which pass to the posterior surface of the eyeball. Near the medial border of the superior rectus muscle the nasociliary nerve gives off the anterior ethmoidal nerve and the infratrochlear nerve. Occasionally the infratrochlear nerve is absent and is then replaced by the supratrochlear nerve derived from the frontal nerve. It should be emphasized that the posterior ethmoidal nerve does not originate from the nasociliary nerve, but is derived from fine autonomic fibers which gain access to the orbit with the ophthalmic artery and through the orbitalis muscle.

Ramus communicans with ciliary ganglion

Near the apex of the orbit, either just at or before the superior orbital fissure, the nasociliary nerve gives off a branch 0.6–1.25 cm long and approximately 250 μm thick. This runs along the lateral side of the optic nerve and enters the upper or posterior part of the ciliary ganglion, to which it carries predominantly sensory fibers.

Ophthalmic artery (fig. 7)

The ophthalmic artery is between 1.0 and 1.5 mm in diameter. According to Singh and Dass [22, 23], in 96% of subjects it arises from the internal carotid artery, but in 4% its chief blood supply comes from the middle meningeal artery via the anastomotic branch with the lacrimal artery. These authors state that the ophthalmic artery runs in the subdural cleft on the dorsal surface of the canal in approximately 90%. In our material [4] the artery enters the optic canal at the medial border of the optic nerve in 41.4%, exactly in the middle and below the optic nerve in 32.7%, and lateral to the optic nerve in 25.9%. In one case of our material the ophthalmic ar-

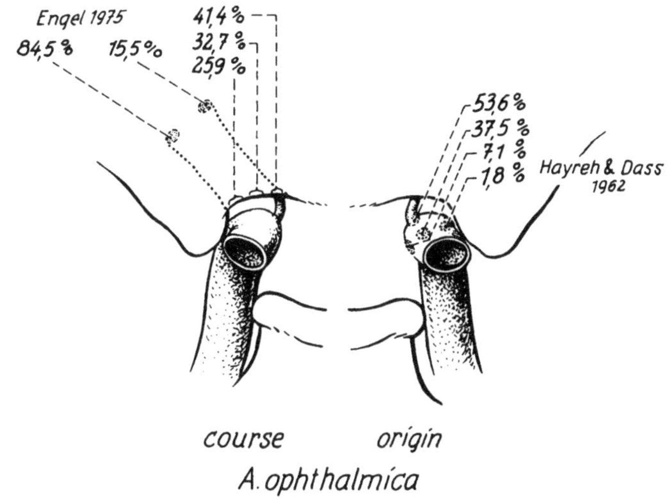

Fig. 7 Ophthalmic artery, origin and course to the intracranial opening of the optic canal and on the intraorbital aperture.

tery was a branch of the cavernous part of the internal carotid artery and was running through the superior orbital fissure. At the orbital aperture of the optic canal the ophthalmic artery is situated medial to the nerve in 15.5% and lateral to it in 84.5%. Within the optic canal there is a boundary zone between the areas of blood supply to the optic nerve. The intracranial portion is supplied by various branches of the internal carotid artery (for further details see Pituitary region), while the intraorbital portion is supplied by branches from the corresponding segment of the ophthalmic artery, some of which run backwards into the optic canal.

As a rule, small branches to the dura mater of the optic nerve arise from the first part of the ophthalmic artery and run beneath the optic nerve. They may even run into the optic canal. It then usually gives off the posterior ciliary arteries, the central retinal artery and also the lacrimal artery, which also run below the optic nerve.

Ophthalmic foramen

In approximately 1% of cases the ophthalmic artery enters a short foramen of its own below the optic canal. This ophthalmic foramen opens into the middle or anterior part of the optic canal [14]. Other investigators [1] found such foramina more frequently.

Ophthalmic arch

In its further course the ophthalmic artery runs medially towards the optic nerve. In our material it crosses above the nerve in 82,6% (left side in 88,4%, right side in 76,7%) and then continues medially; in 17,4% the artery passes below the nerve [18, 30]. According to Adachi [1] in Japanese subjects the artery crosses above the nerve in 93.5%, and in 6.5% it crosses below the nerve, running forwards and medially. Our results are given in figure 2.

Variation

In one dissection by Meyer [18] the ophthalmic artery ran above the superior oblique muscle.

Sequence of branches

Whereas the central retinal artery and the ciliary arteries usually run on the underside of the optic nerve, the lacrimal artery frequently arises at the point where the ophthalmic artery curves into its arch and runs along the lateral side of the optic nerve. The ophthalmic artery then gives off a superior lateral muscular branch, which supplies the lateral muscles of the orbit and which may alternatively arise from the lacrimal artery. Exactly in the middle above the optic nerve is the vessel usually known as the supraorbital artery, which gives off the other orbital branches. It then gives off the narrow posterior ethmoidal artery, which in about 82% overlies the superior oblique muscle and supplies a few muscle branches to the levator palpebrae superioris and the longitudinal portion of the superior oblique muscle. It also contributes to the blood supply of the orbital periosteum. This artery then passes into the posterior ethmoidal foramen. Occasionally a number of posterior ciliary arteries (superior) arise from this segment. The artery then passes below the superior oblique muscle, in adults forming several sinuous curves, and runs forwards and medially giving off the inferior medial muscular branches, from which the anterior ciliary arteries also arise. The main trunk of the supraorbital artery runs further anteriorly. At a point rostral to the anterior ethmoidal foramen it usually gives off the anterior ethmoidal artery, which runs backwards to the anterior ethmoidal foramen, passing beneath the superior oblique muscle in 98% [15].

External sheath of the optic nerve

The dura mater of the optic nerve is now termed the vagina externa nervi optici (Nomina Anatomica). This layer of the sheath commences at the orbital aperture of the optic canal, where it is formed from the duroperiosteal lining, and envelops the nerve as far as its entry into the sclera of the eye. Three to five millimeters behind the sclera there is usually an expansion of the optic sheaths which is known as the bulb of the optic nerve sheath. The dural sheath is 0.3-0.5 mm thick. It consists of collagen fibers and a few elastic fibers - longitudinal in the outer layer, oblique in the intermediate zone and circular in the inner layer. The circular fibers are fewer or absent behind the bulbus oculi (see fig. 5).

Internal sheath of the optic nerve

The internal sheaths of the optic nerve are the arachnoid and the pia mater. The arachnoid is closely apposed to the inner layer of the dura of the optic nerve and is anchored to the latter by numerous trabeculae which traverse a cleft comparable to the subdural cleft. On the outer surface of the arachnoid there are villi 200-300 μm broad and 150 μm high, projecting into the subdural space. In certain zones they come in contact with the dura mater of the optic nerve or may even (like the arachnoid villi) project into it. At those points they occasionally abut upon veins belonging to the external sheath.

Another component of the internal sheath is the pia mater of the optic nerve. It is closely attached to the surface of the nerve and gives off numerous connective tissue septa which pass into it. Between the arachnoid and the pia there is a space which contains cerebrospinal fluid and which communicates with the subarachnoid cavity of the skull. In children this space is usually of some width but in adults it is partially or wholly obliterated. In cases of elevated intracranial pressure the optic nerve (or its sheaths) appears to undergo thickening demonstrable by computer tomography [2].

Vascular supply to the optic nerve

The main vessel of the intraorbital portion of the optic nerve is the central artery of the retina, which is approximately 200 μm in diameter. The intracranial portion of the optic nerve is supplied from the internal carotid, anterior cerebral, anterior communicating and ophthalmic arteries. There is an arterial "watershed" in the optic canal.

The optic chiasma is perfused directly from the internal carotid artery, the superior hypophyseal artery and also from the anterior cerebral and posterior communicating arteries; less frequently it derives some blood from the anterior communicating artery, the middle cerebral artery and the anterior choroidal artery.

Origin of the central retinal artery

This artery most commonly arises from the curved portion of the ophthalmic artery and runs medially. Less commonly it arises proximal or distal to the curve. According to Singh and Dass [22, 23] it is usually the first branch of the ophthalmic artery. It occasionally originates as a branch from the medial or lateral posterior ciliary artery or some other small artery in the orbit.

Its entry takes place most commonly on the inferior or medial side of the optic nerve, less frequently on the inferolateral side and least commonly on the lateral side. Once within the optic nerve the artery at first runs upwards in approximately 90% of cases (pars verticalis). When it reaches the middle of the optic nerve it turns forwards and continues as the pars horizontalis as far as the anterior termination of the nerve.

Besides the central retinal artery there are usually several other small arteries which enter the nerve (accessory arteries of the optic nerve). Within the optic nerve the retinal artery regularly gives off a few twigs which run backwards to other parts of the nerve. The central retinal vein runs in close proximity to the central artery and emerges from the lower surface of the optic nerve somewhat posterior to the latter. The postcentral vein is the name given to a tributary of the central retinal vein which continues further dorsally in the direction of the optic canal.

Internal carotid artery and anterior cerebral artery - optic nerve (fig. 8)

After the emergence of the internal carotid artery from the cavernous sinus its upper surface abuts against the inferolateral surface of the optic nerve. The vessel then runs laterally and backwards, dividing into the middle and anterior cerebral arteries. In this part of its course it comes into contact with the inferolateral surface of the optic chiasma. The anterior cerebral artery runs medially, passing either above part of the optic chiasma (in the case of a long internal carotid artery, the subarachnoid part) or above the optic nerve. The optic nerve may therefore be compressed between the two arteries (in the event of raised pressure in the cranial fossa or of atheromatous degeneration or of a dolichomegaly of the arteries) [5, 24, 26].

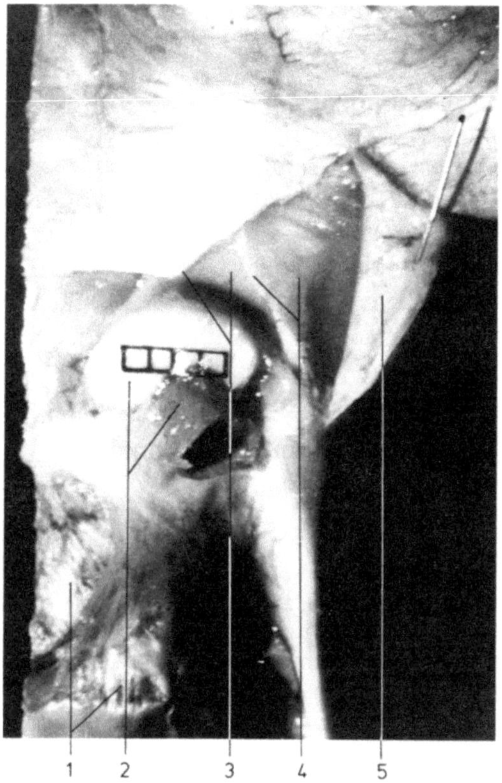

Fig. 8 Optic nerve compressed by raised intracranial pressure (tumor).
1 = Diaphragma sellae and proc. clin. post; 2 = N. opticus, involved from the internal carotid artery; 3 = N. opticus and canalis opticus membranaceus; 4 = Thinned osseous roof of the optic canal; 5 = Dura mater, retracted laterally.

Middle cranial fossa

In cases with tumors the foramina of the middle cranial fossa are often widened. Neumann [19] was the first specifically to describe the occurrence of neural metastases of the head and neck. Larson et al. [7] have emphasised that tumors growth along nerves is a result of extension along tissue planes of least resistance: perineurium and endoneurium. These spaces extend from the smallest ramifications of a nerve to the central subarachnoid spaces.

Willis [29] has proposed three basic criteria requisite for the establishment of the diagnosis: (1) that extension of the primary growth be present about the peripheral nerves up to their entry at the bony foramina; (2) that the nerve roots and ganglia exhibit similar changes within the spinal canal or skull; and (3) that secondary growths in the brain or spinal cord be absent or unlikely to yield meningeal metastases.

Intracranially the tumors tend to involve the meninges spreading in a sheetlike fashion through the subarachnoid space.

The second and third divisions of the fifth nerve are the most amenable to radiographic exploration. The maxillary or second division leaves the middle fossa through the foramen rotundum. It then traverses the pterygopalatine (sphenomaxillary, pterygomaxillary) fossa and enters the orbital cavity by way of the inferior orbital fissure. In the orbit, it occupies the infraorbital groove and canal and emerges anteriorly through the infraorbital foramen to supply a portion of the face. The third or mandibular division leaves the skull via the foramen ovale and divides into lingual and inferior alveolar nerves. The latter enters the mandibular canal and its largest branch leaves through the mental foramen. The other major branches are the auriculotemporal and the marticatory muscle branches.

Dodd et al. [3] found these metastases coming through the foramina in over 40% of cases of squamous carcinoma of the head.

Foramen rotundum

In our material the internal aperture of the foramen rotundum was most frequently transverse oval, approximately 3.4 (2.1-5.2) mm wide and somewhat over 2.7 (1.4-5.5) mm high [27]. The distance between the foramen rotundum and the median sagittal plane averages 16.47 (6.2-25.4) mm on the right and 17.36 (12.3-27.3) mm on the left. The distance between the two foramina rotunda averages 34.29 (25.3-43.5) mm [27]. In our material the distance from the lateral wall of the skull (at the middle of the upper edge of the zygomatic process) in the vicinity of the articular tubercle averaged 20.17 mm on the right and 19.67 mm on the left, these figures being measured in neonates. In adults the averages were 43.88 (32.50-53.00) mm on the right and 43.11 (35.0-53.00) mm on the left side [13].

Foramen ovale

In our material the foramen ovale had an average length of 7.26 (4.2-9.9) mm on the right and 7.15 (3.2-9.7) mm on the left. Its width averaged 3.65 (2.2-6.5) mm on the right and 3.77 (1.7-5.9) mm on the left. The long axis of the foramen ovale is normally orientated obliquely, running from anteromedial to posterolateral. The average distance from the medial border of the foramen ovale to the median sagittal plane was 20.9 (15.5-25.7) mm on the right and 22.49 (17.0-30.0) mm on the left.

Distances of the foramen ovale from the lateral skull wall

In adults the average distance between the foramen ovale and the external acoustic meatus was 36.19 (30.2-43.4) mm on the right and 36.67 (28.7-42.8) mm on the left. The distance between the two foramina ovalia averaged 44.84 (36.0-52.8) mm. In females the distance between the two foramina is relatively greater than in males.

In newborn infants the distance between the lateral border of the foramen ovale and the upper edge of the zygomatic process in the vicinity of the articular tubercle averages 15.50 (15.0-16.0) mm on the right and 14.67 (13.0-16.5) mm on the left. It adults this measurement averages 34.36 mm on the right and 34.30 mm on the left. The limits range between 29.0 and 40.0 on the right and between 27.0 and 40.5 mm on the left.

Foramen lacerum externum (fig. 9)

In cases of tumor metastases are found coming through the foramen lacerum. The jagged gap on the external surface of the skull base between the sphenoid bone in front and the basilar part of the occipital bone behind and medially was named the

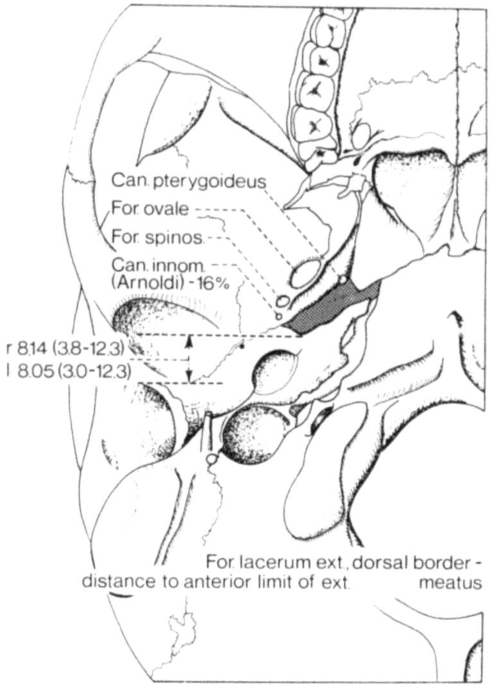

Fig. 9 Posterior border of the external aperture of foramen lacerum, distances to the anterior limit of the external auditory meatus.

foramen lacerum anterius. It averages 9.4 (3-16) mm and its major width 7.5 (2.5-16) mm. The gap is filled by fibrocartilage and forms the floor of the last part of the carotid canal.

Small or larger veins pierce the foramen lacerum internum

Our findings [16] indicate that the foramen lacerum internum is covered by a sheet of connective tissue. In its lateral part its orientation is mainly transverse and in its medial part mainly sagittal. It is termed the inferior sphenopetrosal ligament.

The transverse part of this ligament separates the rostral and lateral wall of the internal carotid artery, the adjacent internal carotid venous plexus and the sympathetic carotid nerves and its branches from the trigeminal ganglion and its pars triangularis. The lateral part of the wall is usually narrow while the medial part is broader and is attached to the borders of the foramen lacerum internum (the posteromedial) border of the greater wing of the sphenoid and the anterior inferior border of the anterior surface of the petrosal part). If the foramen lacerum internum is very small the gaps are filled with connective tissue fibers. The foramen lacerum internum was totally absent in two out of 43 dissections [25].

Venous portals of the cavernous sinus

Superior orbital fissure

As a rule, the superior ophthalmic vein runs lateral to the nerve group and lateral to the common tendinous ring and enters the cavernous sinus from below.

Foramen rotundum

Below the medial end of the superior orbital fissure there are small veins and arteries which pass through the "canalis rotundus" (approx. 6 mm long) together with the maxillary nerve. They form communications between the pterygopalatine fossa and the cavernous sinus.

Foramen ovale

Besides the mandibular nerve, the foramen ovale occasionally carries the accessory meningeal branch from the middle meningeal artery and the meningeal branch of the mandibular nerve. Also within it is the wide caliber venous plexus of the foramen ovale. This plexus is connected with the cavernous sinus and usually with the middle meningeal vein, though less commonly with a paracavernous sinus (ophthalmopetrosal sinus - HYRTL). The plexus usually extends upwards as far as the region of the trigeminal ganglion (in 68%) and constantly reaches the proximal part of the maxillary nerve and the anterior, upper half of the intracranial part of the mandibular nerve [21].

Basilar plexus

The basilar plexus varies greatly in its degree of development. It arises medial to the trigeminal pore from a widely varying range of sources. It develops between the two dural layers on the clivus and is traversed by numerous connective tissue septa and trabeculae. Within its venous blood space run the clivus branches, covered in parts by endothelium.

Inferior petrosal sinus (fig. 10)

The inferior petrosal sinus enters the posterior cranial fossa 2–6 mm medial to the trigeminal pore (Dorello's canal). The actual portal is situated below the superior sphenopetrosal ligament and also contains the abducent nerve in its lateral angle.

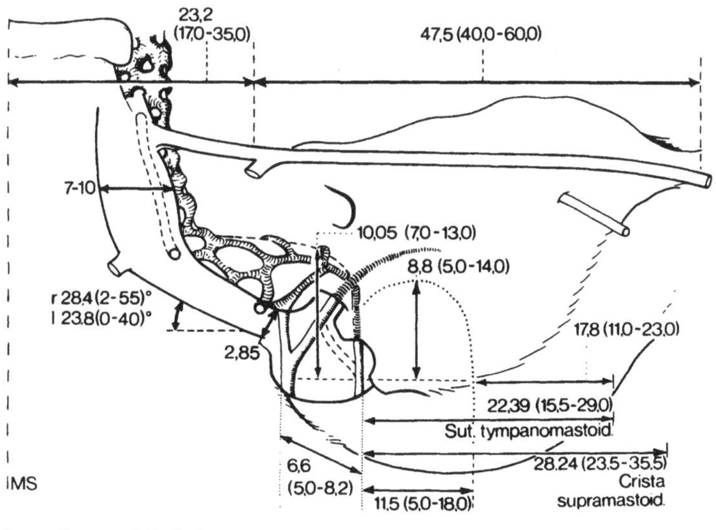

Fig. 10 Superior and inferior petrosal sinus and jugular foramen, viewed from dorsally. The connections of the venous network in the carotid canal and the medial and lateral intrapetrosal veins are given. The height of the jugular bulb above the terminal sigmoid crest in the length of the ascending part of the internal carotid artery. Distances from landmarks on the outer skull base to these canals are also mentioned. All measurements in mm (extremals) and right-left-differences. The angle of the last part of the inferior petrosal sinus with the horizontal plane is given in degrees.

In its longitudinal part the sinus is 7-10 mm wide, and in its transverse part it is 2.85 (0.5-5.0) mm wide.

Internal carotid venous plexus (see fig. 10)

The internal carotid artery is enveloped by a plexus of veins which runs through the canal together with the artery, the sympathetic nerves and the tissues of the arterial sheath. At the external aperture of the carotid canal there are usually two longitudinal veins which originate near the bend of the internal carotid artery. The initial part of the internal carotid plexus communicates with the inferior petrosal sinus via a medial intrapetrosal vein in approx. 46% and via a lateral intrapetrosal vein in approx. 50%. The medial intrapetrosal vein terminates at an average of 11 mm above the jugular foramen, while the lateral intrapetrosal vein terminates in the vicinity of the foramen.

Foramen venosum (of Vesalius)

In our material the foramen venosum (of Vesalius) was present in approx. 40%. It was most commonly situated medial to and between the foramen rotundum and the foramen ovale. It may be up to 2 mm in diameter. This portal carries transbasal veins from the cavernous sinus to the exterior of the skull.

Jugular foramen

Passage of nerves and vessels

Contrary to what is stated in most of the textbooks, the ninth, tenth and eleventh cranial nerves do not traverse the medial and anterior part of the jugular foramen, but run inside a connective tissue septum set obliquely at a variable angle in this major vascular portal of the posterior cranial fossa. Furthermore, a posterior meningeal artery regularly runs from the ascending pharyngeal artery through the jugular foramen to the floor of the posterior cranial fossa. As a rule, small twigs of this posterior meningeal branch can be seen through the thin endothelium of the jugular foramen and the sigmoid sinus (and other sinuses).

In our material (48 specimens [11]) there was only one instance in which the meningeal branch of the ascending pharyngeal artery was not to be found (approx. 2%). In 50% there was one meningeal artery, in 37.5% there were two meningeal branches and in 10.5% three meningeal branches from the ascending pharyngeal artery running into the jugular foramen. The average number of twigs arising from this vessel and supplying the bone and dura of the posterior cranial fossa is hence 1.52. The mean diameter of the vessels is 0.63 (0.2–1.1) mm, and the diameter most frequently found (in 20.6%) was 0.4 mm. As their diameter increases, so the number of posterior meningeal branches from the ascending pharyngeal artery decreases. Right-left differences in the numbers and diameters of these vessels are common. In most instances (40%) the vessels arise from the ascending pharyngeal artery close to the base of the skull; an origin from a more proximal segment is much less common. In two out of the 48 specimens, twigs from the occipital artery to the jugular foramen were demonstrated. The ascending supplies pharyngeal artery primarily the glomus jugulare and tympanicum and tumors of these organs.

Condylar emissary vein and jugular foramen

A condylar emissary vein is developed in 64% on the right and in 68% on the left side. In 38.46% the condylar emissary vein communicates with the jugular vein lateral to the intrajugular process of the petrous temporal; in 25% the communication is situated exactly at the margo sigmoidea terminales, in 7.69% the vein joins the terminal segment of the sigmoid sinus lateral to the margo terminalis sigmoidea, in 3.84% it joins the hypoglossal venous plexus in its canal medial to the jugular foramen and in a further 3.84% - the so-called low confluence - it joins the internal jugular vein below the actual jugular foramen. If the roof of the emissary canal is rarefied, the vein may even run on the floor of the posterior cranial fossa.

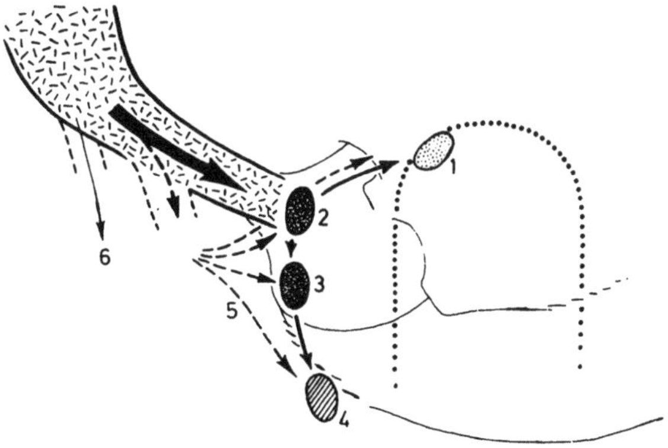

Fig. 11 Inferior petrosal sinus, height of orifice in relation to the internal jugular vein. 1 = Upper level of the bulb, right 11.53%, left 5.76%; 2 = upper level of the jugular foramen, right 9.61%, left 13.46%; 3 = opening in the transitional zone between the bulb of the jugular vein and the vein itself, right 15.38%, left 17.3%; 4 = opening of the sinus below the skull in the internal jugular vein, right 11.53%, left 9.61%; 5 = additional connection of the inferior petrosal sinus through small canals of the cranial skull base, right 10%, left 7.3%; 6 = the inferior petrosal sinus, pierces the skull base, right 1.92% left 3.84% in its own canal (J. Lang, M. Weigel, 1983).

Termination of the inferior petrosal sinus (fig. 11)

In 23.07% the inferior petrosal sinus runs into the middle plane of the jugular foramen, and in 32.69% into the lower zone of the foramen. In 21.15% the inferior petrosal sinus terminates extracranially in the internal jugular vein, and in 17.3% in the jugular bulb. In approx. 7% there was no demonstrable connexion between the inferior petrosal sinus and the jugular foramen or jugular bulb (= low confluence into the internal jugular vein); in 24% arrangements of this kind were present in addition to the main outflow.

Height of the bulb of the jugular vein above the margo terminalis sigmoidea (see fig. 10)

The margo terminalis sigmoidea marks the transition between the sigmoid sinus and the bulb of the jugular vein. On the right side this transition forms an average angle of 76 (51–110)° with the median sagittal plane, the corresponding angle on the left side being 72 (40–100)°.

In our material the dome of the bulb of the jugular vein was situated an average of 8.8 (5–14) mm above the margo terminalis sigmoidea on the right side, and 8.2 (5–13) mm on the left. The bulb of the jugular vein has an average diameter of 11.5 (5–18) mm, while according to Gabrielsen et al. [6] the average diameter of the internal jugular vein below the bulb is 9.5 (6–16) on the right side and 8.0 (5–13) mm on the left. The highest point of the jugular fossa in our material is situated laterally from the median plane 33.4 (27–40) mm to the right and 32.1 (26–38) mm to the left.

Jugular foramen and venous plexus of the hypoglossal canal

In 34.61% the hypoglossal venous plexus communicates with the inferior petrosal sinus and in the same percentage with the marginal plexus of the foramen magnum and the basilar plexus. In 13.46% it communicates with the terminal segment of the sigmoid sinus and in 11.53% with the bulb of the jugular vein. In 5.76% of our specimens it had an extracranial communication with the vertebral vein via a "veine prévertébrale".

References

[1] Adachi, B.: Das Arteriensystem der Japaner. Bd. I, II. Verlag der Kaiserlich-Japanischen Universität, Kyoto 1928.

[2] Ambrose, E., D. H. Mistry, J. Stephen: Optical and Scanning Electron Microscopy of Human Carcinomas. J. Microscopie Biol. Cell. **25** (1976) 173-180.

[3] Dodd, G. D., P. A. Dolan, A. J. Ballantyne et al.: The dissemination of tumors of the head and neck via the cranial nerves. Radiologic Clinics of North America **8** (1970) 445-461.

[4] Engel, A.: Ursprungs- und Verlaufsvariationen der ersten Ophthalmica-Strecke. Med. Diss. Würzburg 1975.

[5] Fuchs, E.: Textbook of ophthalmology. 8th edn. J. B. Lippincott, Philadelphia 1924.

[6] Gabrielsen, T. O., J. J. Bookstein: Jugular venography by catheter approach from the arm. Radiology **91** (1968) 378-379.

[7] Hamby, W. B.: Carotid-cavernous fistula. Report of 32 surgically treated cases and suggestions for definitive operation. J. Neurosurg. (Chicago) **21** (1964) 859-866.

[8] Jazuta, K. S.: Zur Anatomie der A. meningea media des Menschen und der Säugetiere. Eine vergleichend-anatomische Untersuchung (in Russisch). Inaug. Diss. St. Petersburg 1905.

[9] Lang, J.: Praktische Anatomie: e. Lehr- u. Hilfsbuch d. anat. Grundlagen ärztl. Handelns/begr. von T. von Lanz, W. Wachsmuth. Fortgef. u. hersg. von J. Lang, W. Wachsmuth. NE: Lang, J. (Hrsg.) Lanz, T. von (Begr.) Teil 1: Bd. 1 Kopf. Teil B Gehirn- und Augenschädel/von J. Lang. In Zsarb. mit K.-A. Bushe, W. Buschmann und D. Linnert. Springer, Berlin-Heidelberg-New York 1979.

[10] Lang, J.: Clinical Anatomy of the Head. Neurocranium - Orbit - Craniocervical Regions (translated by R. R. Wilson and D. P. Winstanley). Springer, Berlin-Heidelberg-New York 1983.

[11] Lang, J., E. Heilek: Anatomisch-klinische Befunde zur A. pharyngea ascendens. Anat. Anz., Jena **156** (1984) 177-207.

[12] Lang, J., Th. Horn, U. von den Eichen: Über die äußeren Augenmuskeln und ihre Ansatzzonen. Gegenbaurs morphol. Jahrb. **126** (1980) 817-840.

[13] Lang, J., R. Maier, O. Schafhauser: Über die postnatale Vergrößerung der Foramina rotundum, ovale et spinosum und deren Lageveränderungen. Anat. Anz., Jena **156** (1984) 351-387.

[14] Lang, J., G. Oehmann: Formenentwicklung des Canalis opticus, seine Maße und Einstellung zu den Schädelebenen. Verh. Anat. Ges. **70** (1976) 567-574.

[15] Lang, J., K. Schäfer: Arteriae ethmoidales: Ursprung, Verlauf, Versorgungsgebiete und Anastomosen. Acta Anat. (Basel) **104** (1979) 183-197.

[16] Lang, J., F. Strobel: Über den Einbau des Ganglion trigeminale. Verh. Anat. Ges. **72** (1978) 437-439.

[17] Larson, D. L., A. E. Rodin, D. K. Roberts et al.: Perineural lymphatics: Myth or fact. Amer. J. Surg. **112** (1966) 488-492.

[18] Meyer, Fr.: Zur Anatomie der Orbitalarterien. Gegenbaurs morphol. Jahrb. **12** (1887) 414ff.

[19] Neumann, E.: Secondare cancroid-Infiltration des Nervus mentalis bei einem Fall von Lippen-cancroid. Virchows Arch. **24** (1862) 201.

[20] Scammon, R., E. L. Armstrong: On the growth of the human eyeball and optic nerve. J. Comp. Neurol. **38** (1925) 165-219.

[21] Simoes, S.: Relacoes Anatomicas do seio emiŝario do forame oval e suas implicacoes clinico-cirurgicas. Arq. Neuro-Psiquiatr. **31** (1973) 31.

[22] Singh, S., R. Dass: The central artery of the retina. I. Origin and course. Brit. J. Ophthalmol. **44** (1960) 193-212.
[23] Singh, S., R. Dass: The central artery of the retina. II. A study of its distribution and anastomoses. Brit. J. Ophthalmol. **44** (1960) 280-299.
[24] Smith, E.: A note on nervous lesions produced mechanically by atheromatous arteries. Rev. Neurol. Psychiat. **3** (1905) 182.
[25] Strobel, F. J.: Über Lagebeziehungen des Ganglion trigeminale. Med. Diss. Würzburg 1980.
[26] Sunderland, S.: Neurovascular relations and anomalies at the base of the brain. J. Neurol. Neurosurg. Psychiatry **11** (1948) 243-257.
[27] Tisch-Rottensteiner, K. F.: Öffnungen und Varietäten der mittleren Schädelgrube. Med. Diss. Würzburg 1975.
[28] Welti (1943), quoted in W. B. Hamby (1964).
[29] Willis, R. A.: The Spread of Tumors in the Human Body. 2nd ed. C. V. Mosby Co., St. Louis 1952.
[30] Zuckerkandl, E.: Zur Anatomie der Orbitalarterien. Med. Jahrb. (Wien) **3** (1876) 343.

Tumors of the skull base. The role of the diagnostic and therapeutic angiography

K. Ter Brugge, P. Lasjaunias

Introduction

Lesions along the base of the skull represent a diagnostic and therapeutic challenge. Because of the topography of such lesions it requires a multidisciplinary approach and often the radiologist forms the necessary link between the different specialties such as neurosurgery, head and neck surgery and otolaryngology.

It is, therefore, mandatory that the radiologist understands the clinical questions which will be raised and conducts the investigations with these questions in mind. After all the tests have been performed, there must be a clear understanding about the extent of the lesion, the blood supply of the lesion and the adjacent healthy tissues, as well as the possible post-therapeutic effects on the blood supply towards and away from the central nervous system.

In order to evaluate these lesions properly, complete knowledge of the bony and soft tissue anatomy along the base of the skull is essential, including the blood supply and its variations. It is also of great practical importance to analyse the vascularization of the dura, the base of the skull and the cranial nerves which may give crucial information with regard to future decisions about treatment.

Diagnostic radiology (non-invasive)

The diagnostic imaging tools which are available to the radiologist are the plain skull films, conventional tomography, computed tomography, magnetic resonance and angiography [1, 3, 9].

The role of plain skull films is limited to the demonstration of bony erosion and destruction, soft tissue calcification and the demonstration of nasopharyngeal soft tissue masses. Interpretation of these skull films, however, represents a challenge to the radiologist and much too often the abnormal findings are missed or wrongly interpreted. Frequently, no abnormality can be identified on skull films even in the presence of extensive pathology. Although skull films often represent the first step in the diagnostic process, their role should be questioned and qualified.

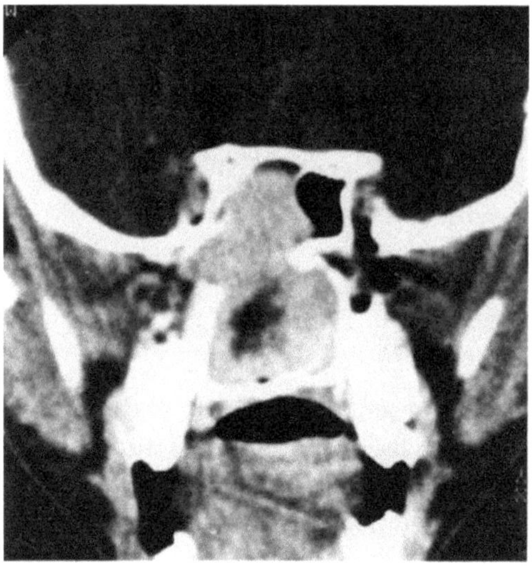

Fig. 1 Juvenile angiofibroma in a 14-year-old male. Coronal CT section. Note the invasion of the sphenoidal sinus by the tumor. Contrast enhancement helped in differentiating reactive sinusitis adjacent to the tumor from true extension into the sinus.

Conventional complex motion tomography represented in the 70's the second diagnostic step in the evaluation of the base of the skull. If performed properly, it may add further detailed information with regard to the bony structures. Tomography is of course unable to show the extension of a lesion into the adjacent soft tissues and therefore its role in that respect is limited.

CT has added significant information when used for the diagnosis of lesions along the base of the skull [2, 8, 10]. It allows for excellent visualization of the bony and soft tissue structures (fig. 1). Although not specific, it represents a very sensitive method for diagnosing soft tissue and bony lesions along the skull base. However, lesions can be missed on CT, in particular when small and adjacent to the skull base since the usual trans-axial acquisition mode tends to volume average bone and adjacent soft tissues. Lesions adjacent to the skull base may only be demonstrated if acquisition is done in the coronal plane (fig. 2). Intravenous contrast enhancement is recommended to characterize the lesion further. Clinical information is crucial in order to conduct and interpret the CT findings properly.

Magnetic resonance has recently been added to the diagnostic instrumentarium. Field strength and acquisition techniques appear to have a great impact on the accuracy of this method. Although initially perceived to be of limited use in the evaluation of bony structures, recent advances have shown great potential in tissue characterization of neoplastic disease affecting the bony skeleton. The experience of magnetic resonance visualization of lesions along the base of the skull is still anecdotal and no definite conclusions can be drawn at the present time. Tissue

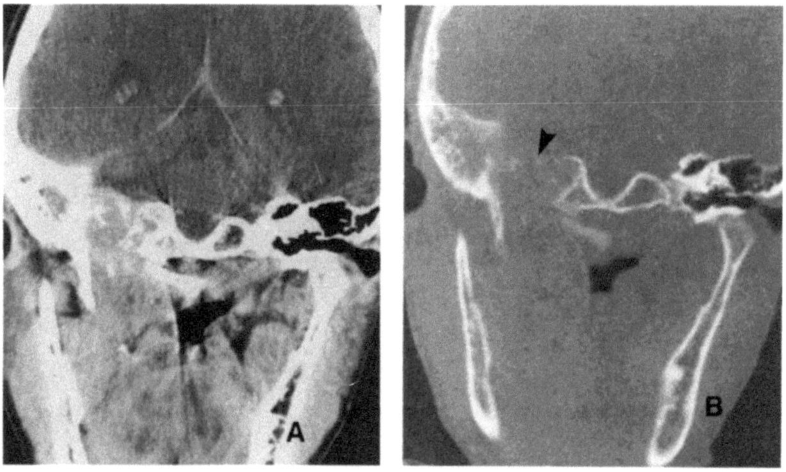

Fig. 2 Jugulo-tympanic paraganglioma in a 79-year-old female. Coronal CT section, after injection of contrast; (A) soft tissue study, (B) bone tissue study. This tumor thought to be non-surgical has been previously embolized (two years before this examination). Lower cranial nerve paresis has regressed, and the pulsatile tinnitus disappeared. Note the absence of contrast enhancement at the level of the "tumor" bed, and the presence of the radiopaque emboli in situ (arrow head): Polyvinyl alcohol foam, 160 micron.

characterization (spectroscopy) may represent an important tool which might enable us to diagnose neoplastic disease at an earlier stage before morphological changes occur.

Angiography

Angiography is obligatory in the investigation and treatment planning of lesions along the base of the skull. Clinical information and topographic data obtained by CT and NMR are necessary to build the proper angiographic protocol. Although digital subtraction angiography has made some progress in the past few years, it still compares unfavourably with the quality of conventional magnification subtraction techniques. Tumor blushes however may be more easily seen with this new method.

Routine superselective catheterization of secondary or tertiary branches of the external carotid artery is now possible using the femoral approach and small size catheters (4 F or less) and in well trained teams this diagnostic procedure is without risk [6].

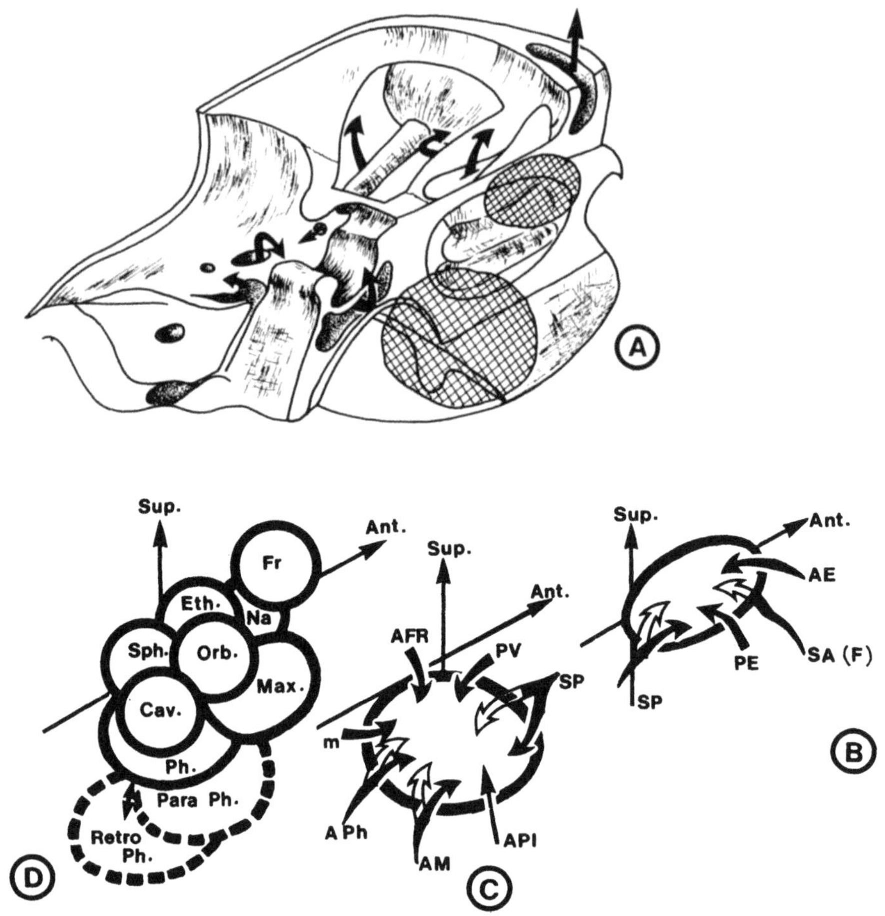

Fig. 3 Tumors invading the anterior cranial fossa, orbit, middle cranial fossa and adjacent sinus cavities. Supero-lateral view of the base of the skull. (A) Two tumors have been represented in the right nasal fossa and in the right choana. The arrows illustrate the different course followed by the tumor tissue to invade the structures in the base of the skull. (B) Schema of the arterial supply of the nasal fossa tumour. AE and PE = anterior and posterior ethmoidal arteries; SA (F) = septal branch of the facial artery; SP = sphenoidal artery. The plain arrows are located on the midline and indicate the superior and anterior directions. (C) Schematic arterial supply of the choanal tumor. AFR = artery of the foramen rotundum; m = mandibular artery; PV = pterygo-vaginal artery; SP = sphenopalatine artery; AP = ascending palatine artery; AM = accessory meningeal artery; APh = ascending pharyngeal artery. The plain arrows are located as on (B) (D) Pattern of invasion of tumors developed in the nasopharynx. Fr = frontal sinus; Na = nasal fossa; Eth = ethmoidal cells; Orb = orbit; Max = maxillary sinus; Sph = sphenoidal sinus; Cav = cavernous region; Ph = pharyngeal cavity. Both parapharyngeal (Para Ph) and retro-pharyngeal (Retro Ph) regions correspond to passage extension towards the posterior base of the skull and the carotid region. The plain arrows are located as in (B) and (C). Each of the extensions of tumor illustrated can be identified specifically during angiography.

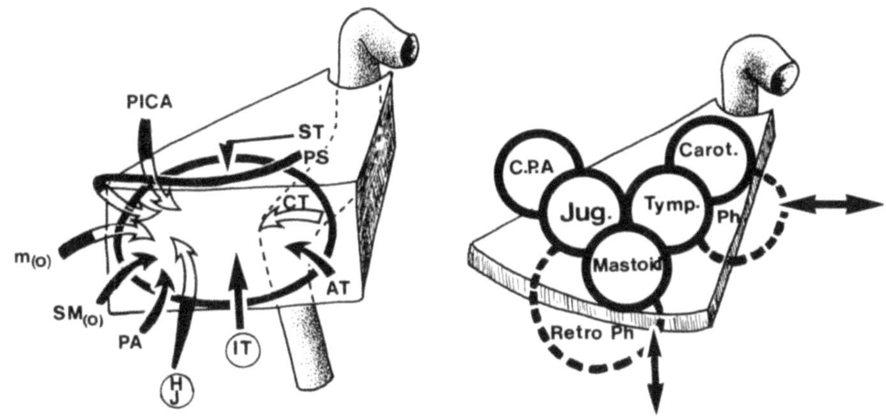

Fig. 4 Lateral view of the temporal pyramid with schematic representation of a jugulo-tympanic paraganglioma. The possible feeders of the tumors are indicated (A) as well as the territories identifiable during angiography (B). PICA = posterior inferior cerebellar artery; ST = superior tympanic (middle meningeal artery); PS = petro-squamous (middle meningeal artery); CT = carotico-tympanic artery; AT = anterior tympanic artery; IT = inferior tympanic artery (ascending pharyngeal artery); HJ = Hypoglossal and jugular branches (ascending pharyngeal artery); PA = posterior auricular artery; SM = stylo-mastoid artery (occipital artery); m = mastoid artery (occipital artery); CPA = cerebello-pontine angle; Jug = jugular foramen; Carot = carotid canal; Para Ph = parapharyngeal space; Retro Ph = retropharyngeal space. Note the passage territories with the cavum and carotid regions.

The territorial blood supply can then be analysed in order to build a three dimensional puzzle of the area involved where each piece of the puzzle is a vascular territory and corresponds to a potential area of tumor invasion (figs. 3–6) [7].

Since the accurate discrimination of the territories depends on the super-selectivity achieved, the information gained from angiography will depend on the skill and expertise of the angiographer. Only when angiography is done superselectively can it represent the most accurate method for detecting the presence and extent of a tumor, otherwise CT will still be the best method for giving this information but usually at a later stage.

Many lesions in the base of the skull, although benign, are locally invasive and they tend to recur if not removed completely (juvenile angiofibromas, paragangliomas and basal meningiomas). Because of technical difficulties related to the close proximity of major blood vessels as well as the cranial nerves, many of these benign lesions are not operated upon, but are being radiated.

In some centres in Europe and for the past seven years, presurgical *embolization* performed routinely has resulted in complete *surgical removal* and a low recur-

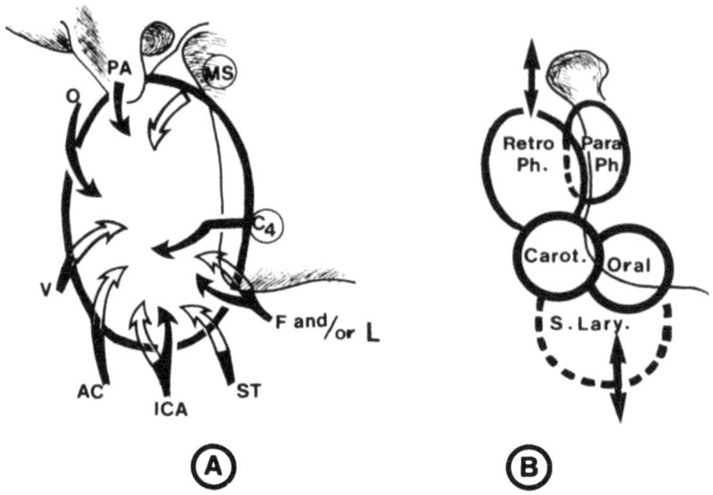

Fig. 5 Lateral view of the carotid region with schematic representation of a cervical paraganglioma (vagal or carotid body) and the arterial feeders involved (A). PA = posterior auricular artery; MS = Musculo-spinal branch (ascending pharyngeal artery); C4 = C-4 collateral (external carotid artery); F-L = facial or lingual arteries; ST = superior thyroidal artery; ICA = internal carotid artery; AC = Ascending cervical artery; O = occipital artery; Retro Ph = retropharyngeal area; Carot = carotid bifurcation region; Oral = oral cavity; Para Ph = para-pharyngeal region. The territorial extension of the tumours are shown (B) on the lateral view of the neck at the level of the vertical ramus of the mandible.

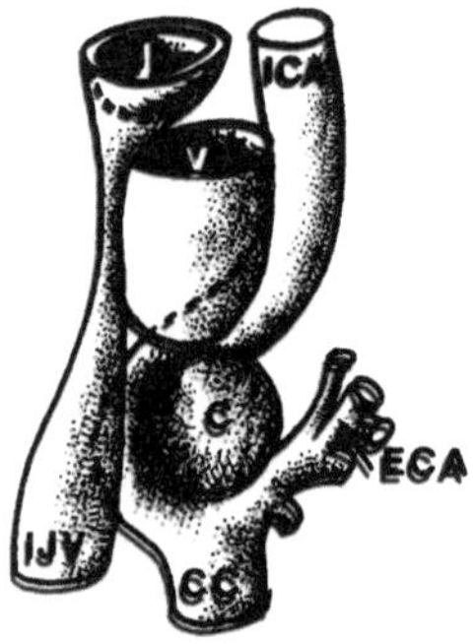

Fig. 6 Schematic representation of the cervical arterio-venous relationships with the various types of paragangliomas. J = jugular paraganglioma; V = vagal paraganglioma; C = carotid body paraganglioma; ICA = internal carotid artery; ECA = external carotid artery; CC = common carotid artery; IJV = internal jugular vein.

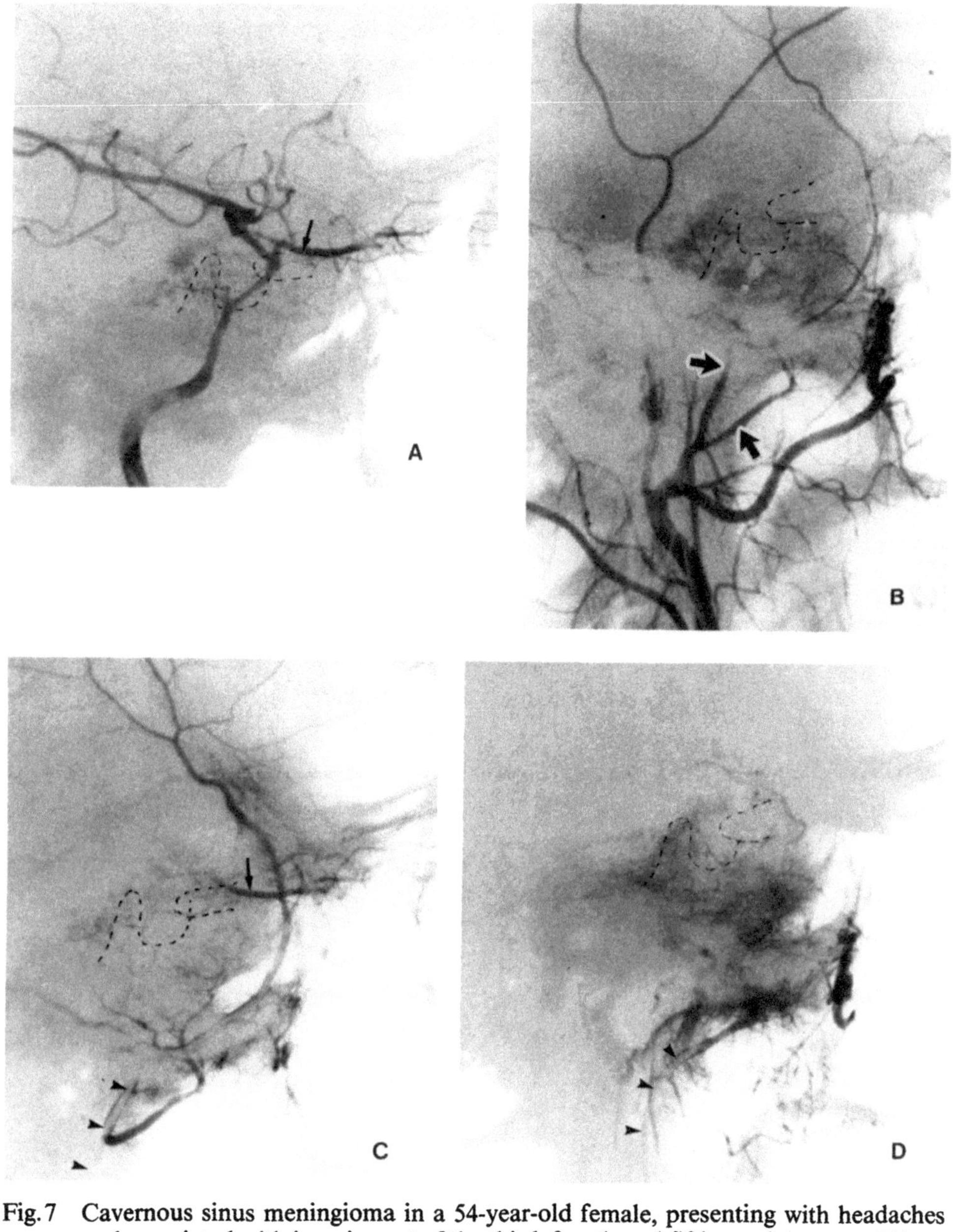

Fig. 7 Cavernous sinus meningioma in a 54-year-old female, presenting with headaches and associated with impairment of the third, fourth and fifth cranial nerves. (A) selective angiography of the internal carotid artery. The arrow points to the ophthalmic artery. (B) "Global" external carotid injection. Note the pattern of the tumor parenchyma and the middle and accessory meningeal arteries (arrow).

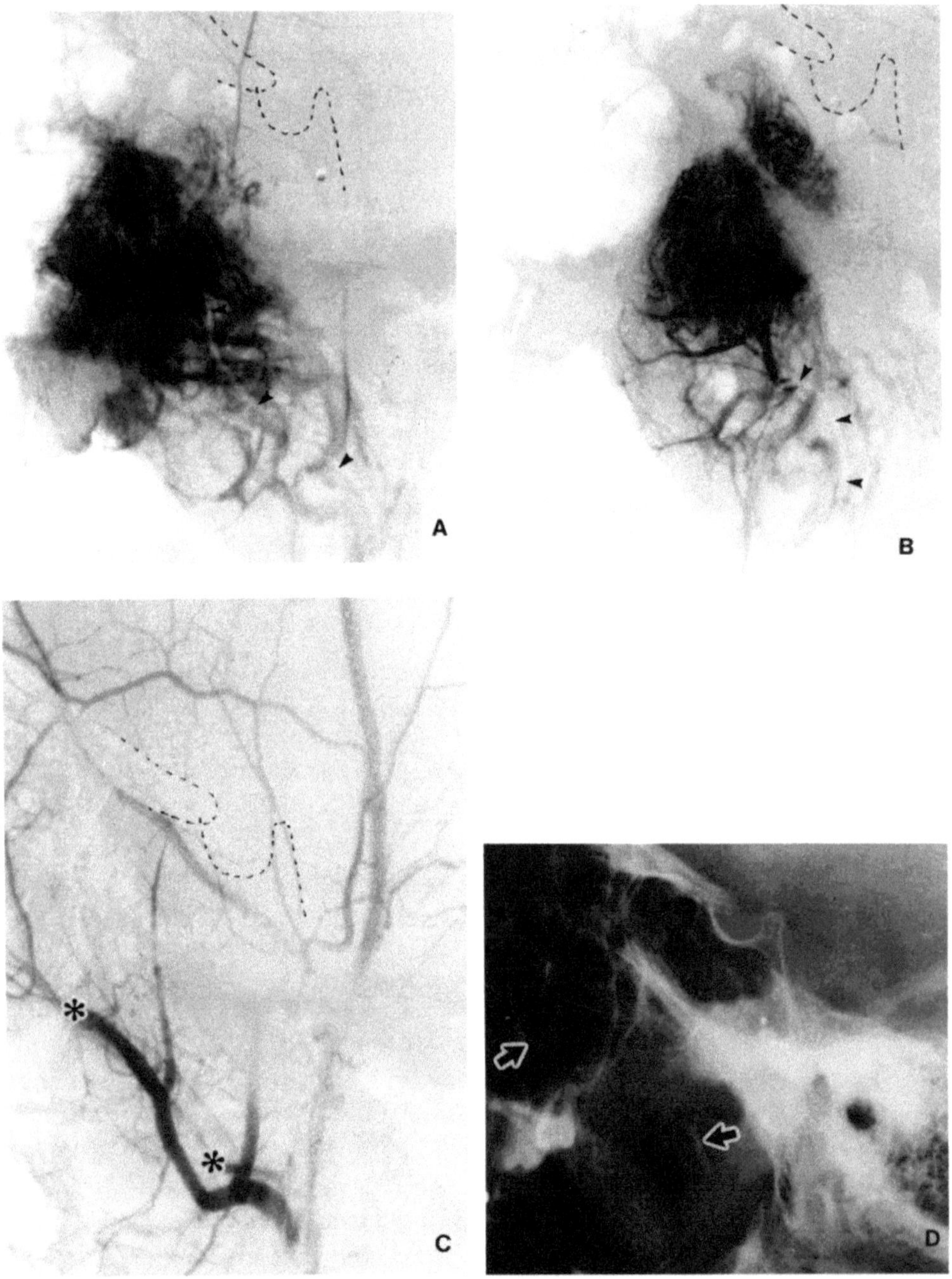

Fig. 8 Juvenile angiofibroma in a 15-year old male. (The arrow-heads point to the catheter.) (A) Superselective injection of the distal internal maxillary artery. (B) Superselective injection of the accessory meningeal artery. (C) Angiographic control following embolization (asterisks) of (A) and (B). Note that all the maxillary arteries are patent. (D) Plain skull film after embolization of A and B, showing stagnation of contrast in both tumor pedicles.

rence rate (less than 10%) of benign tumors of the base of the skull [4, 5]. No definite complications related to the endovascular procedures have been noted.

Some lesions previously thought to be inoperable became *operable after embolization,* while others which previously would have been considered for radiation treatment can now be *embolized* successfully, as *a unique therapeutic attempt* (cavernous sinus meningiomas, temporal bone paragangliomas) (fig. 7).

From this experience, combining skill and anatomical knowledge, therapeutic angiography has reached a favourable position to add to the management of these lesions at this time. Tumor feeders can be catheterized (fig. 8) and/or the blood supply to a tumor can be rerouted. The former allows the use of *hyperactive cytotoxic* drugs (absolute alcohol), while the latter can *increase the response* of the entire tumour to *in situ* infusion of chemotherapy. However, in malignant tumors the objective of endovascular treatment is still limited to the improvement of the quality of survival rather than to accomplishing a cure. Embolization in these patients may diminish pain by decreasing the mass effect of the tumor or it can be used to control hemorrhage, sometimes resulting from arterial ulceration or post-radiation necrosis.

Conclusion

Lesions of the base of the skull require a multidisciplinary approach in order to provide the most appropriate treatment for each patient. Superselective catheterization techniques have made it possible to demonstrate significant diagnostic information upon which a proper plan of treatment can be built. Endovascular embolization techniques, although dependent on the skill and experience of the angiographer, should be considered as a form of presurgical treatment and an alternative measure for non-operable benign lesions.

References

[1] Bergeron, R. T., A. G. Osborn, P. M. Som: Head and neck imaging, excluding the brain. Mosby Company, St. Louis 1984.
[2] Bohman, L., A. Mancuso, J. Thompson et al.: CT approach to benign nasopharyngeal masses. AJR **136** (1981) 173-180.
[3] Bryan, R. N., R. B. Sessions, B. L. Horowitz: Radiographic management of juvenile angiofibromas. AJNR **2** (1981) 157-166.
[4] Lasjaunias, P., L. Picard, C. Manelfe et al.: Juvenile angiofibroma, review of 53 cases embolized. J. Neuroradiology **7** (1980) 73-95.

[5] Lasjaunias, P.: Branchial paragangliomas; review of 40 cases embolized between 1977 and 1984 (in French). J. Français d'orc (in press).
[6] Lasjaunias, P.: Cranio-facial and upper cervical arteries: Anatomy, normal angiographic aspects. Williams and Wilkins Edt., Baltimore 1981.
[7] Lasjaunias. P.: Cranio-facial and upper cervical arteries: collateral circulation and angiographic protocol. Williams and Wilkins Edt., Baltimore 1983.
[8] Leekham, R., K. G. Ter Brugge, M. C. Chiu: Computed tomography of the pterygopalatine fossa. Journal of the Canadian Association of Radiologists **32** (1981) 97-100.
[9] Osborn, A. G.: Radiology of the pterygoid plates and pterygopalatine fossa. AJR **132** (1979) 389-394.
[10] Valavanis, A., U. Fisch: The contribution of computed tomography to the management of glomus tumours of the temporal bone. Revue de Laryngologie **104** (1983) 411-415.

Echographical diagnosis of orbital tumors

A. Nover, R. Rochels

Introduction

Standardized A-scan sonography [5, 6] enables us to detect orbital lesions in almost 100 per cent of cases; furthermore they can be localized, measured and differentiated into nearly 60 different diseases with an accuracy of 80 per cent. Orbital inflammation, cysts, vascular and metastatic tumors, neoplasms of the lacrimal system, subperiosteal, bony and periorbital tumors, the group of lymphoma-sarcoma-pseudotumors as well as disorders of the optic nerve and the extra-ocular muscles and traumatic lesions are the main conditions that can accurately be differentiated with standardized A-scan sonography [7, 9, 10].

The A-scan provides a reliable evaluation of the structure, reflectivity, consistency and vascularity of an orbital lesion, whereas B-scan indicates its location, topography and shape [1–3, 8].

The indications for orbital echography are unilateral and bilateral exophthalmos, enophthalmos, symptoms suggesting a lesion of the optic nerve or the extra-ocular muscles, unexplained lid swelling, chemosis, congestion and paresis [5] as well as inflammatory and neoplastic lesions of the paranasal sinuses where orbital involvement is suspected.

Methods

The echographical A-scan examination of the orbit comprises several steps:

1. *Quantitative echography* is performed to evaluate the structure (regular/irregular), the reflectivity (low/high) and the sound attenuation (slight/strong) of an orbital lesion.
2. *Topographic echography* estimates its borders (diffuse/cystic), bony defects (single and large/multiple and irregular), location and shape.
3. *Kinetic echography* is then used to detect blood flow in an orbital tumor as well as to evaluate its consistency (soft/hard) and mobility (mobile/immobile) [5, 6].

Standardized A-scan sonography is performed with the Kretz-Technik 7200 MA machine using a small probe with a working frequency of 8 MHz, allowing a good

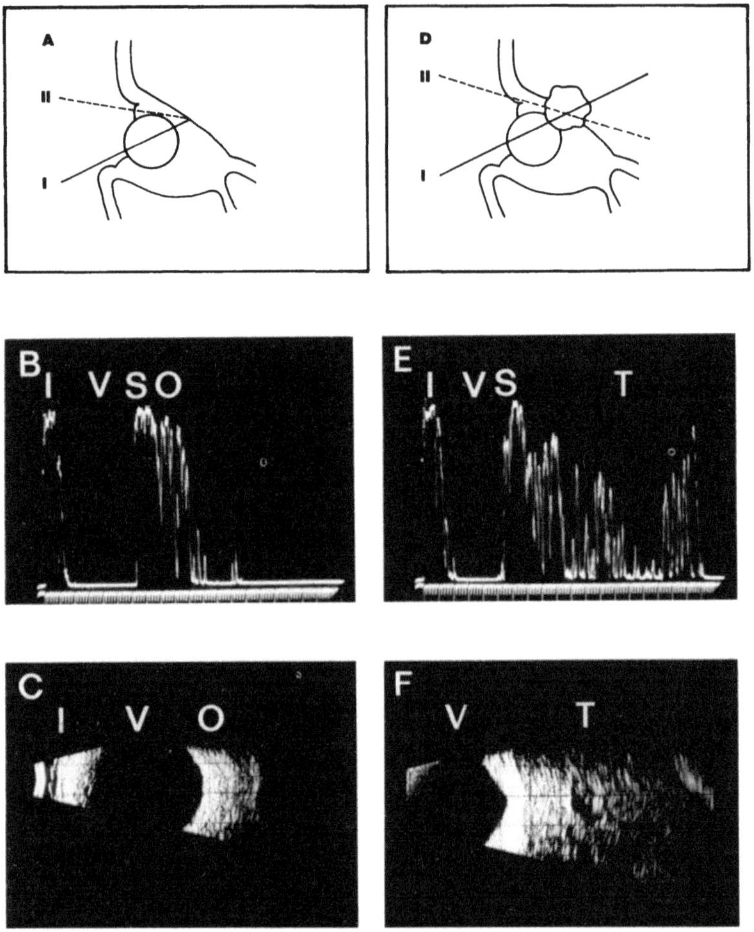

Fig. 1 Normal and pathological A- and B-scan pictures of the orbit (transocular examination). A = Schematic drawing of the orbit demonstrating the transocular (I) and paraocular (II) examination; B = Normal A-scan picture of the orbit (transocular examination): I = initial spikes; V = echo-free vitreous, S = high scleral spike, O = highly reflective orbital pattern; C = Normal B-scan picture of the orbit (transocular examination): the orbital pattern (O) is sharply outlined; I = initial echo, V = echo-free vitreous; D = Schematic drawing of an orbital tumor invading the anterior skull base. I = transocular, II = paraocular examination; E = A-scan picture of an orbital carcinoma invading the anterior skull base (transocular examination). Compared to fig. 1 B the orbital echo pattern is broadened by the tumor (T) and irregular; F = B-scan picture of the same patient (transocular examination): the orbital echogram is heterogeneous, the tumor (T) is poorly outlined.

compromise between resolution and sound penetration into the tissues. B-scan is done with the Ocuscan 400 at 10 MHz.

There are two possibilities in examining the orbital structures (fig. 1 A): the sound beam can either be directed through the globe (transocular examination; figs. 1 A I, B, C) or through the lids, avoiding the eyeball (paraocular examination; fig. 1 A II; figs. 2 A, B).

Along with further B-scan findings and additional clinical criteria a definite pre-operative diagnosis can almost always be achieved.

Clinical findings

The *normal orbital tissue* shows a highly reflective A-scan pattern, sharply outlined by the bony walls. The B-scan of the orbit is homogeneous, whereas the optic nerve and the extraocular muscles can be detected as non-echogenic structures.

Cavernous hemangiomas are usually located within the muscle cone. A-scan echography shows a regularly structured, highly reflective lesion of regular shape, hard consistency and medium sound attenuation produced by the mixture of blood-filled spaces and numerous septa.

Lymphangiomas on the other hand, are irregularly outlined and soft; because of the vascular spaces filled with homogeneous fluid, there is a mixture of high spikes and echo-free areas.

Orbital dermoids are characterized by regular structure, low reflectivity, regular borders, soft to hard consistency and low sound attenuation in the A-scan.

Meningiomas of the sphenoidal wings have irregular structure, reflectivity, shape and borders. Bony defects can sometimes be demonstrated. The consistency is extremely hard, and there is of course no mobility.

Lymphomas, sarcomas and pseudotumors of the orbit are characterized by regular internal structure, low reflectivity, regular shape, hard consistency and slight sound attenuation, thus reflecting the homogeneous histological picture of these tumors.

Carcinomas and metastases of the orbit are highly reflective, regularly structured but poorly outlined, thus reflecting the infiltrative growth of such a lesion, that in addition is immobile and hard.

Rhabdomyosarcomas on the contrary are characterized by low reflectivity, irregular shape and borders as well as hard consistency. The low reflectivity can be explained by the very homogeneous and regular histological picture of this tumor.

Optic nerve tumors can easily be recognized with A-scan sonography because they lead to a thickening of the optic nerve; sometimes it is even possible to distinguish between glioma and meningioma of the nerve.

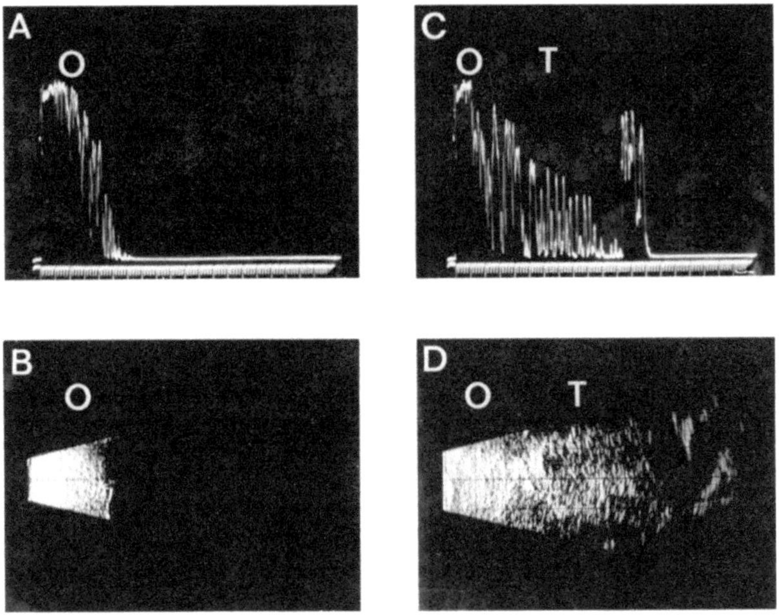

Fig. 2 Normal and pathological A- and B-scan pictures of the orbit (paraocular examination). A = Normal, highly reflective orbital (O) echogram in paraocular examination (compare with Fig. 1 A II) (A-scan); B = Normal, homogeneous, well-outlined orbital (O) echo pattern in paraocular examination (B-scan); C = Paraocular A-scan picture (compare with fig. 1 D II) of an orbital carcinoma invading the anterior skull base: the tumor (T) has caused a broadening of the echo-pattern of the orbit (O); D = Paraocular B-scan picture of an orbital carcinoma invading the anterior skull base: the tumor (T) is characterized by a diffuse, heterogeneous and poorly outlined echo pattern of the orbit (O).

Tumors invading the orbit (periorbital malignancy). The A-scan pattern of the orbital tissue is always well outlined because of the bony walls, reflecting the sound beam totally. Tumors of the paranasal sinuses or of the anterior skull base can invade the orbit by destroying the bony walls (fig. 1 D). If the sound beam is directed through such defects, it can penetrate into the tumor, the paranasal sinuses or the cranial cavity. The transocular A-scan (fig. 1 E) shows a widening of the echo-chain; the spikes are very irregular and of varying height. In B-scan (fig. 1 F) these tumors are characterized by a heterogeneous echo-pattern and poorly outlined borders. The paraocular scans (figs. 2 C, D) are similar. The bony defects can also be demonstrated; invading tumors always cause multiple and irregularly shaped defects in contrast to mucoceles which lead to a single, large, and well outlined bony defect.

Periorbital malignancy can be diagnosed if the following criteria are present: irregular structure, reflectivity, borders and shape as well as sound attenuation, multiple bony defects, hard consistency, immobility and extraorbital localization. Tissue differentiation of such a tumor is possible if the intraorbital portion is large enough to be evaluated according to the criteria described under "Methods".

Discussion

Standardized A-scan sonography [5-7] is a reliable and reproducible method for examining the orbit in order to detect, localize, measure and - above all - differentiate orbital tumors. More than 60 different lesions can be diagnosed because of their pathognomonic A-scan picture, that must be analyzed according to the criteria of structure, reflectivity, sound attenuation, shape, borders and location as well as consistency and mobility. The accuracy of the echographic diagnosis is in the range of 80 to 90 per cent [4, 7] underlining the importance of standardized A-scan sonography in the pre-operative examination of orbital tumors. Along with further advantages such as avoidance of radiation exposure and absolute painlessness it is a method that should always be used as a very useful screening test in detecting and differentiating orbital tumors.

Summary

Standardized A-scan sonography has proved to be a very reliable method in detecting, localizing, measuring and differentiating orbital tumors. According to the special criteria such as structure, reflectivity, sound attenuation, shape, borders, location, consistency and mobility more than 60 different orbital lesions can be diagnosed with an accuracy of 80-90 per cent. In this paper characteristic examples of primary orbital tumors and those invading the orbit are demonstrated and discussed.

References

[1] Bronson, N. R., Y. L. Fisher, N. C. Pickering et al.: Ophthalmic contact B-scan ultrasonography for the clinician. Intercontinental Publications, Westport 1976.
[2] Coleman, D. J., F. L. Lizzi, R. L. Jack: Ultrasonography of the eye and orbit. Lea & Febiger, Philadelphia 1977.
[3] Hassani, S. N.: Real time ophthalmic ultrasonography. Springer, New York 1978.
[4] Nover, A., R. Rochels, C. Tuch: Ergebnisse der A-Bild-Echographie bei Erkrankungen der Orbita. Klin. Mbl. Augenheilk. **184** (1984) 168-170.

[5] Ossoinig, K. C.: Echography of the eye, orbit, and periorbital region. In: Orbit roentgenology (P. H. Arger, ed.), pp. 224-269. Wiley & Sons, New York 1977.
[6] Ossoinig, K. C.: Standardized echography: basic principles, clinical applications, and results. In: Ophthalmic ultrasonography: comparative techniques (R. L. Dallow, ed.), pp. 127-210. Little, Brown and Comp., Boston 1979.
[7] Ossoinig, K. C.: Advances in diagnostic ultrasound. In: Acta: XXIVth International Congress of Ophthalmology (P. Henkind, ed.), pp. 89-114. Lippincott, Philadelphia 1983.
[8] Poujol, J.: Echographie en ophtalmologie. Masson, Paris 1981.
[9] Rochels, R.: Ultraschalldiagnostik in der Augenheilkunde - Lehrbuch und Atlas. Ecomed, Landsberg, 1986.
[10] Shammas, H. J.: Atlas of ophthalmic ultrasonography and biometry. Mosby, St. Louis 1984.

II Anterior skull base tumors

Orbital tumors involving the skull base

J. P. A. Gillissen

In the last 10 years the orbital center of the University of Amsterdam registered 1200 patients with orbital disorders. In the present review, endocrine ophthalmopathy, trauma, congenital malformations, inflammations, cosmetic and lacrimal surgery are excluded. The remaining group of 574 patients with oncologic disorders will be discussed.

This group is divided into three groups: The first group consists of those orbital tumors that were seen most frequently. Meningioma ranks first, then pseudolymphoma, non-Hodgkin tumors, mucoceles, dermoid cysts, basal carcinoma and neurogenic tumors (tab. 1).

The second group is about a quarter of the patients and the last group consists of very rare disorders and ends with histiocytosis X, chordoma and hemangiopericytoma (tab. 2).

The third group (25,9% of the patients) is presented in table 3.

Table 1 Orbital tumors (n = 574)

Meningioma	84 = 14.6%
Pseudolymphoma	74 = 12.8%
Non-Hodgkin tumors	58 = 10.0%
Mucoceles	52 = 9.0%
Dermoid cysts	44 = 7.5%
Basal cell carcinoma	41 = 7.0%
Neurofibroma	40 = 6.9%
	393 = 68.4%

1200 patients with orbital disorders.

Table 2

Blastoma	11
Mucocystic carcinoma	9
Chocolate cysts	6
Hemangiopericytoma	2
Histiocytosis X	2
Chordoma	2
	32 = 5.5%

Table 3

Metastases	32 = 5.5%
Squamous cell carcinoma	22 = 3.8%
Rhabdomyosarcoma	22 = 3.8%
Sarcoma	17 = 2.9%
Glioma	15 = 2.6%
Osteoma	15 = 2.6%
Fibrous dysplasia	14 = 2.6%
Wegener's disease	12 = 2.1%
	149 = 25.9%

In the study of orbital lesions it is know that intra-orbital pain and a relatively rapid development of exophthalmos, diplopia, loss of vision or loss of ocular movement favor the diagnosis of a malignant tumor. Long standing proptosis with normal ocular movements is often associated with benign lesions.

In this short paper it is impossible to discuss all orbital tumors, and I will restrict myself to orbital tumors involving the base of skull.

Meningioma

Meningioma of the sphenoid bone and the base of skull is the most frequent tumor in our series. There were 84 cases admitted to our center since 1974, mostly middle-aged females. In many cases it was difficult to reach a consensus as regards the treatment. In general, it has to be palliative treatment and it is seldom possible to remove the lesion completely.

In 6 cases where we thought the tumor was removed completely a meningioma developed elsewhere in the skull. In three patients a neurinoma of the acoustic nerve was diagnosed later. In one patient this neuronima was bilateral. We often had discussions as to whether operation can stimulate the growth of the lesion or not. For that reason we are very conservative. We have a rule that meningiomas are only operated on when vision is threatened or for severe cosmetic reasons. On the other hand if one can predict such complications, operation should be discussed anyhow.

A typical example is this 27-year-old man who presented to us with an eye which had been blind since he was 7 years old. He had an exophtalmos, optic atrophy, vocal cord pareses and an atrophy of the quadriceps femoris muscle on the left side. An orbital exenteration was carried out and a meningioma behind the orbit was removed. After this operation a large recurrence was removed two years later, but since 1978 the process has been stable and recently a reconstruction of the orbit was performed. This is one of our most interesting patients because multiple meningioma occurs in many members of his family.

Lymphogenetic tumors

Pseudolymphoma and non-Hodgkin tumors of the orbit never gave rise to cranial involvement in our series, so they are not discussed here.

Mucoceles

Mucoceles occur in all ages, but most frequently, in patients of over 45 years of age. We have treated 52 patients. The majority of these cysts arise in the frontal and ethmoid sinus. It is a slow growing lesion and it is often at an advanced stage when discovered. Typical for the diagnosis is the palpation of the tumor which gives the feeling of a table-tennis ball. The X-rays and the CT-scan are characteristic. There is an expansion of the border of the orbit and occasionally, invasion of the anterior cranial fossa.

In about one quarter of our patients a defect in the dura was discovered. As we knew this before operation leakage of CSF. complicated the operation in only 2 cases, without any subsequent ill effects however.

When a mucocele becomes infected, vision and even life can be in danger. For that reason a mucocele should always be treated without any delay. The therapy consists of surgical exenteration of the sinus involved and the establishment of a satisfactory drainage to the nose.

Two of our patients came to us in such a state and they lost vision pre-operatively as a result of this infection. Of the 52 non-infected patients we operated on, only 4 had a recurrence which had to be removed.

Basal cell carcinoma

Basal cell carcinoma accounts for more than 90% of malignant tumors of the lid and at this site is more common than squamous cell carcinoma, by a ratio of 40:1.

In our series we have 41 basal carcinomas and 22 squamous carcinomas. Our ratio is 2:1. The reason that our ratio is so different is because basal cell carcinoma is in most cases treated effectively by operation and radiotherapy in general hospitals and there is no need to send them to our center.

The patients presented to us are mostly the bad cases where treatment had failed. If there is an orbital invasion the earliest symptom is diplopia on extreme gaze.

Pain occurs when the orbital nerves are involved. If the tumor invades the orbital roof one has to exenterate the orbit and subsequently to remove the affected bone. We followed this procedure in 4 cases.

If possible, radiotherapy is given after operation, but in most cases this is impossible because the patient has already received irradiation.

Neurogenic tumors

Neurogenic tumors represent nearly 7% of the orbital tumors, but we did not encounter one patient in which the base of skull was affected. Even in severe cases the orbital roof was intact.

Squamous cell carcinoma

Squamous cell carcinoma was seen in 22 patients. The majority are more than 50 years of age. Clinically it presents as a white, roughened, irregular exophytic mass, that may be adherent to the globe. Squamous carcinoma grows superficially and diffusely and can involve the orbit. Operation combined with subsequent radiotherapy is effective in most cases.

Our most dramatic patient was a 44-year-old printer who had such a tumor in both eyelids. Despite repeated radical excisions and despite radiotherapy, both orbits were invaded and both eyes had to be exenterated. After exenteration there was a defect left in the orbital roof because of the tumor invasion. Recently this patient had another recurrence.

Rhabdomyosarcoma

Embryonal rhabdomyosarcoma is a rare malignancy but is, on the other hand, the most common primary orbital tumor in childhood. In the last 10 years we have treated 22 children with this tumor. Rhabdomyosarcoma usually presents itself as a rapidly growing exophthalmos, but it may also present itself as a palpable subconjunctival mass. The treatment of choice is chemotherapy. It is amazing to see how a marked degree of exophthalmos is reduced to virtually nothing after two weeks of a chemotherapeutic regime. This treatment is not without danger. We lost two patients as a results of chemotherapy, and consequently we now tend to stop the medical treatment 6 months after chemotherapy was started, by removal of the residue of the tumor. Radiotherapy was used 10 years ago with no very apparent success. Radiation gives severe malformation of the orbit and face as it stops the growth of the radiated area. In 2 radiated patients there was invasion of the cranial cavity. One patient died from invasion of the brain by tumor.

Adenoid cystic carcinoma

Lacrimal tumors include mixed tumors, adenoid cystic carcinoma and other carcinomas.

Benign mixed tumors account for approximately 50% of lacrimal tumors and the malignant adenoid cystic carcinoma for 27%. Swelling of the upper lid or a palpable mass in the superior temporal portion of the orbit in association with abnormal position on primary gaze is virtually diagnostic for both types. NMR scanning can differentiate this tumor from other lesions in this region. A cholesterol granuloma is like a tumor on the CT-scan, but the resonance is the same as that of orbital fat. Adenoid cystic carcinoma is the most dramatic group of our series because of its invasive growth. In spite of a very extensive operation where large parts of the orbital roof were removed, the tumor is seldom removed radically. Radiotherapy seems of little value.

We have treated 9 patients; 6 died within 18 months, two are doing well and one patient who was operated recently is undergoing radiotherapy at the moment.

Osteoma

Osteomas were treated in 15 patients. These arise most often in the frontal and ethmoidal sinus. The sphenoidal sinus is the least frequently involved.

An osteoma has to be removed totally. In one patient we encountered a severe recurrence because we were unable to remove the osteoma completely on account of its involvement in the skull-base.

Wegener's disease

In our series we have 12 patients with Wegener's disease in the orbit. In 2 of our cases the orbital roof was involved. Before the possibility of treatment with corticosteroids and cyclophosphamide, the prognosis was very poor. Death occurred in 50% of the cases within one to five months after the onset of glomerulonephritis.

A typical example was a 22-year-old female who had a proptosis of the right eye, edema of the upper lid and reduced vision. Her painful proptosis did not respond to prednisone and high doses of analgesics. The orbit was decompressed transcranially. A thickened peri-orbita was found and the orbital roof and the lateral wall were removed. Locally, an inflammatory infiltrate was seen. After treatment with prednisone and cyclophosphamide the proptosis disappeared and she was without pain. This lasted for two years. Recently the lesion flared up again and exenteration was necessary.

The tumors discussed are the main orbital tumors which can involve the base of skull.

Esthesioneuroblastoma

M. Samii, H. J. Löblich, W. Draf

The olfactory nerve tumors, also known as esthesio-neuromas are uncommon. Blockmanis, in his review of world literature in 1972 [1] mentioned only 40 cases which had been hitherto reported. The five year survival rate in Skolnik's series [5] was a mere 52%. Both these authors have reported on local recurrences in half of the cases, whereas metastases into the regional lymph nodes and to the lung occurred in about 20% of all patients. Thus, even though the tumor histology may seem to deny it, its clinical behaviour does suggest frank malignancy.

Although opinions with regard to their therapy have been somewhat controversial and Caballes [2] and Tringwald [6] considered them to be radiosensitive, radiotherapy alone does not cure them. On account of its propensity to manifest malignant biological behaviour it is imperative that these tumors are radically excised; this appears to be the only way to ensure removal of the tumor matrix [3]. The following case report upholds this belief and exemplifies its operative management.

A 29-year-old Yugoslavian male complained of difficulty in breathing through his nose. A large reddish-grey tumor occupied the entire left nasal vestibule and bled

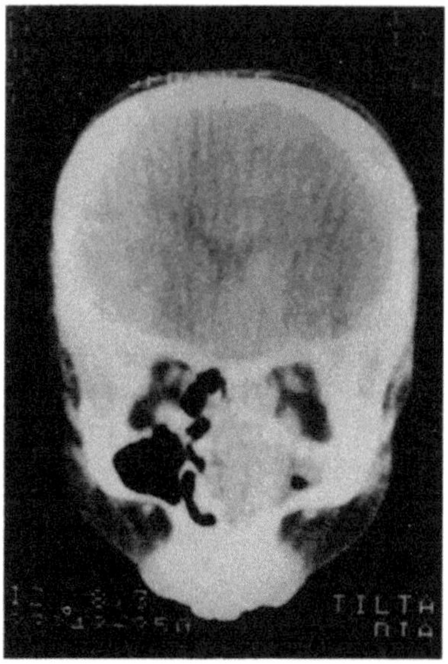

Fig. 1 CT scan of a 29-year-old patient with a large tumor of the left nasal cavity and partial involvement of the adjacent paranasal sinuses. Histological examination revealed an olfactory "neurocytoma".

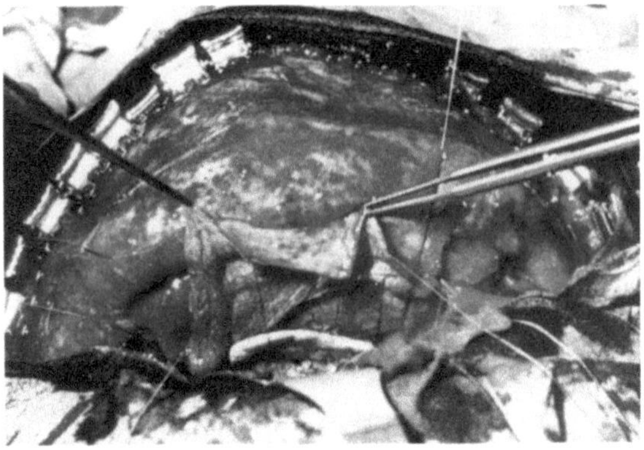

Fig. 2 Operative photograph of patient whose scan appears in fig. 1: After resection of the dura protecting the lamina cribrosa, the ethmoid roof and the anterior part of the planum sphenoidale, the crista galli was removed. The skull base was reconstructed, as shown above, in three layers, by dural flaps, Palacos® as well as a pedicled galeo-periosteal flap.

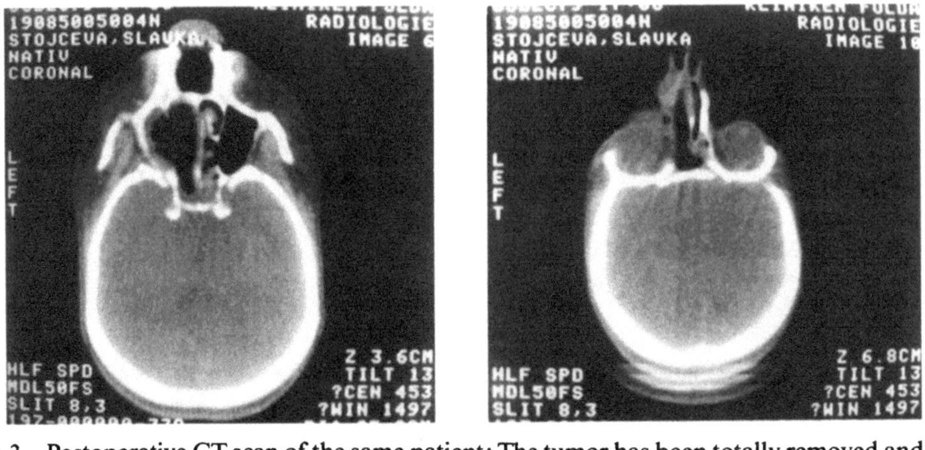

Fig. 3 Postoperative CT scan of the same patient: The tumor has been totally removed and the skull base defect is bridged by means of Palacos®.

slightly when touched. The CT scan (fig. 1) demonstrated that it also involved the adjacent paranasal sinuses; however there was no unequivocal proof of the skull base having been eroded. The tumor in the nose was biopsied and reported to be an olfactory neurocytoma.

A bifrontal craniotomy was done. Both olfactory tracts were exposed and transected just in front of the optic nerves. The cut ends were drawn up in the direction of the bulb and the tiny nerves traversing the cribriform plate were transected. The olfactory nerves were thus excised. The dura covering the anterior base of skull was stripped off, laying bare the lamina cribrosa, the ethmoidal roof and anterior part of the planum sphenoidale all of which were removed. The crista galli was also exposed and cut away, allowing the bony skull base to be shifted caudally. The defect in skull base was repaired in 3 layers. The initial layer was repair of the dura; then a sheet of sterile acrylic (incorporated with Refobacin, Trade name Palacos® by E. Merck) was laid over it. Finally a flap of galea and periosteum was dissected off the reflected scalp flap to which it remained attached by a pedicle, and its free edge was sutured to the frontal dura, thus offering further coverage to the base of the skull (fig. 2). The craniotomy was closed.

The ENT surgeon now took over, and by a nasal approach excised the tumor en bloc, which included removal of the underlying mucous membrane and the adjacent bone. The operation and the post-operative phase were uncomplicated. The postoperative CT scan (fig. 3) demonstrates both the total tumor removal and the skull base repair, evidenced by the radio-opaque Palacos.

Pathology

During the last few years we have seen and studied 7 cases of esthesioneuroblastoma. Three of the patients suffered a recurrence after varying intervals; of these, one case also had metastases in the lung and the skin (tab. 1).

On account of many important histological features of the tumor necessary for its identification, an exact diagnosis can only be made after electron microscopic examination; however, detection of Catecholamines by histochemical tests can be helpful. Besides identification of the tumor, the histological findings of pseudorosettes (rather than true rosettes), and neurofibrils, are important points to be considered when diagnosing esthesioneuroblastoma (fig. 4). The finding of desmosomes, neurofilaments, microtubules and secreting granules on electron microscopical examination confirms the diagnosis (fig. 5).

As far as histological examination is concerned there is considerable literature to suggest a primary tumor of the neural crest; this, we believe, is not the case. Instead, it is a regeneration of cells from the olfactory islands. It is still unclear as to whether the parent cells of the tumor are olfactory or interstitial. It is our opinion that there exist noticeable parallels between esthesioneuroblastomas and carcinoids, although the latter are not tumors of the neural crest. Contrary to the opinion of Pearse [4], we feel they develop much more from indifferent totipotent stem cells, which can also develop into a single functional endocrine cell. The neurogenic structures develop, like the APUD-system. In the histogenetical classification of the tumor, it should therefore be placed under the category of the large group of tumors of the APUD-system.

Table 1 Special observations

Age Sex	Case history	Local findings	Op.-specimens	Growth	Relapse (R) Metastasis (M)
49 f	unilateral respiration obstructed	left lower concha	biopsy bulbus and tractus olf.	local, aggressive	R: after half a year
29 f	unilateral respiration obstructed	left nasal cavity and paranasal sinus	tumor biopsy	local, aggressive	
59 f	unilateral respiration obstructed	right nasal cavity	biopsy	local, aggressive	R: after 2 years
40 f	unilateral respiration obstructed	right middle meatus and nasal septum	biopsy	local, pedunculated	
81 f	nose bleeding, unpleasant	right ethmoid bone	pedunculated tumor		
57 f	nose bleeding, unpleasant	middle and lower concha	pedunculated tumor		
71 f	nose bleeding, unpleasant	ethmoid bone	pedunculated tumor		R: local after 1 year M: lungs and skin after 3 years

This table depicts relevant details of all 7 cases of esthesioneuroblastoma.

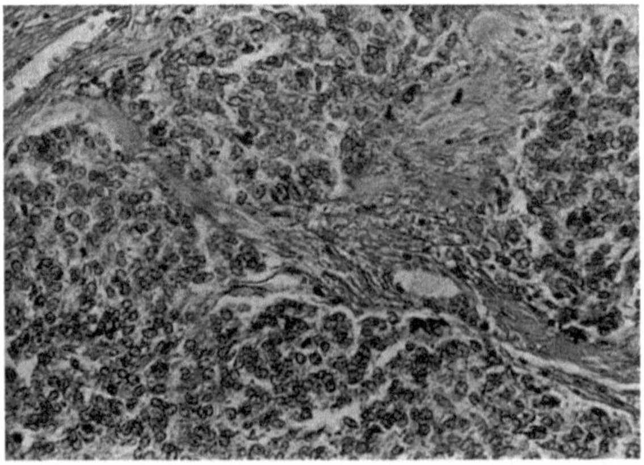

Fig. 4 Histological findings of a case of esthesioneuroblastoma: pseudo-rosettes and neurofibrils.

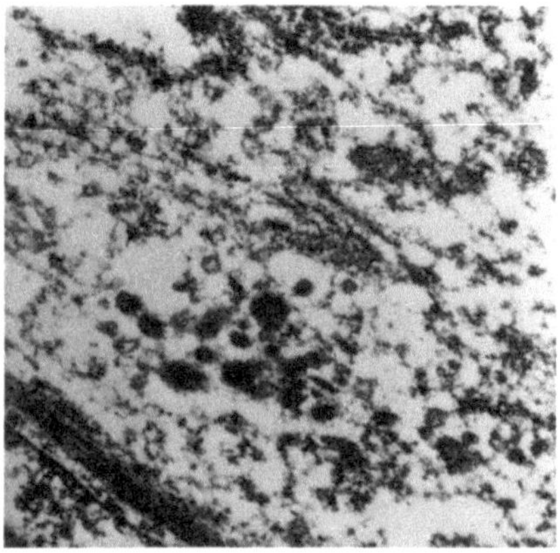

Fig. 5 Electron-microscopic features: Desmosomes, neurofilaments, microtubules and secreting granules.

Metastasis of esthesioneuroblastoma is uncommon and even when it occurs the prognosis is better than that of carcinomas. The surgical management is to be viewed in the light of the fact that the tumor does not arise basically from the olfactory tract or bulb, both of which are regarded as structures of the brain; thus they may be spared whilst planning an operation on a tumor which does not infiltrate the base of skull.

Brain metastases are very rare and occur only after the tumor breaks through the skull base anteriorly or alternatively embolises through vascular channels.

References

[1] Blockmanis, A.: Esthesioneuroepithelioma: A report of two cases and discussions of the management. Can. J. Otolaryng. **1** (1972) 43.
[2] Caballes, R. L.: Psammoma bodies in olfactory neuroblastoma. Laryngoscope **75** (1965) 1749.
[3] Huet, P. C. et al.: Un cas d'andiohistiocytome des fosses nasales. Ann. Otolaryngol (Paris) **70** (1953) 785-789.
[4] Pearse, A. G. E.: The cytochemistry and ultrastructure of polypeptide hormone-producing cells of the APUD series and the embryologic, physiologic and pathologic implications of the concept. J. Histochem. Cytochem. **17** (1969) 303-313.
[5] Skolnik, E. M. et al.: Olfactory neuroepithelioma. Arch. Otolaryngol. (1966) 61-67.
[6] Tringwald, F. R.: Olfactory placode tumors. Laryngoscope **76** (1966) 267.

Juvenile angiofibroma

M. Weidenbecher

Juvenile angiofibroma is a rare, histologically benign tumor in the nasopharynx whose etiology, pathogenesis and site of origin are still unknown. The tumor has a tendency for local invasion and destruction of surrounding structures.

Classification

Fisch has classified juvenile angiofibroma according to size:

Type I: Tumor limited to the nasopharynx and nasal cavity, no bone destruction.

Type II: Tumor invading the pterygopalatine fossa, maxillary sinus, ethmoid or sphenoid.

Type III: Tumor involves the infratemporal fossa, the orbit and the parasellar region.

Type IV: Infiltration of the cavernous sinus, the chiasma and the sella.

Diagnosis

Diagnosis is usually straightforward and is based on the patient's age and sex, the typical nasal symptoms of epistaxis, nasal airway obstruction and rhinorrhoea, and the typical location of the tumor.

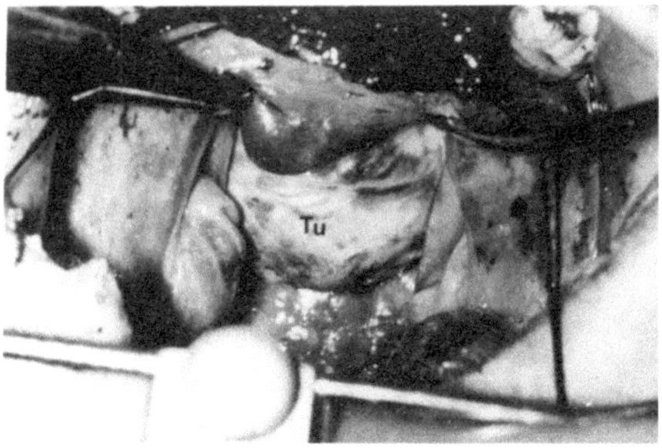

Fig. 1 The endoscopic picture shows the angioma in the mesopharynx.

Additional diagnostic information is obtained by
1. Endoscopy (fig. 1);
2. Computerized tomography (CT);
3. Superselective angiography;
4. Biopsy.

Preoperative procedures

The extremely rich blood supply of these tumors is one of the main problems in their surgical resection. A knowledge of the feeding vessels (external carotid, ascending pharyngeal, vertebral and internal carotid arteries) and how safely to occlude them is important in obtaining maximal access and visibility [4].

Many diverse methods have been used to decrease the vascularity and to minimize blood loss. These include:
1. Pre-operative radiotherapy [1];
2. Pre-operative therapy with oestrogen and androgen [7, 9];
3. Cryosurgery;
4. Ligation of the external carotid artery;
5. Embolization of the feeding vessels by superselective angiography and use of lyophilized dura [8] (figs. 2 and 3).

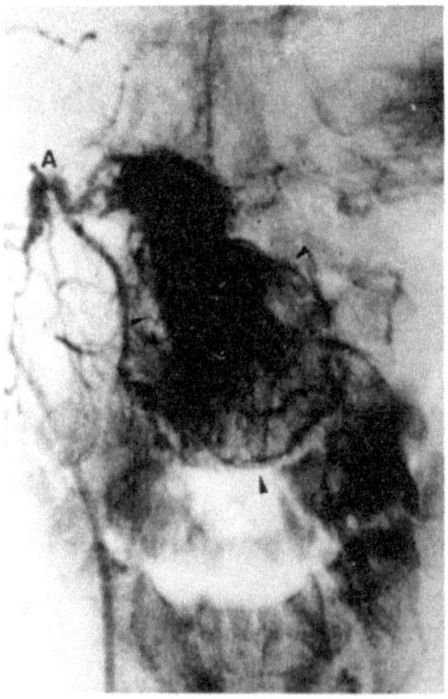

Fig. 2 Selective angiography of the maxillary artery shows the massive blood flow into the tumor. Arrows: Size of the tumor; A = Maxillary artery.

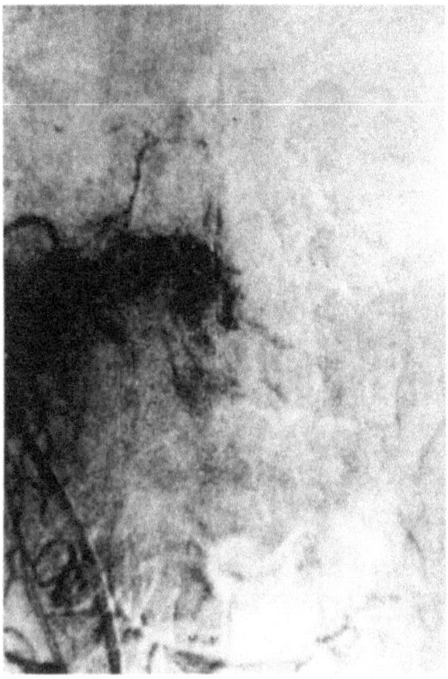

Fig. 3 The same patient after embolization with pieces of lyophilized dura.

Treatment of juvenile angiofibroma

Surgical treatment

Total exstirpation is the safest method, most commonly used for the treatment of these tumors. Total removal may be difficult if the tumor arises in the area of the sphenopalatine foramen and grows into the pterygopalatine and infratemporal fossae or through the infraorbital fissure, or through the foramen lacerum to involve the clivus and cavernous sinus.

The approach selected, depends on the extent and site of the tumor and its extensions, and may include any of the following
1. transpalatal;
2. transpalatal in combination with a transmaxillary approach;
3. lateral rhinotomy;
4. transcervical-transmandibular [6];
5. infratemporal [2];
6. transmandibular-transfrontal route: this approach has been shown to be necessary since the detection by CT of intracranial extensions. Tumors with intracranial extension require the cooperation of neurosurgeon and rhinosurgeon [5].

Radiotherapy [3]

The recurrence rate after radiotherapy on its own is higher than that after surgical treatment. Good results, however, have been reported with 4000 rads on small intracranial remnants of tumor, which had to be left in order to preserve important intracranial structures.

Results

From 1972-1981 fourteen patients with an angiofibroma of the nasopharynx were treated surgically. All patients were male, the ages ranging from 10-19 years. Twelve patients had tumors of size type I and II, two patients type III and IV. Twelve patients had a transpalatal, transmaxillary or a lateral rhinotomy approach. Two patients were treated by a transcervical-transmandibular approach and were given 4000 rads to the non-resected intracranial tumor remnant. No recurrence or tumor growth has been seen in any case up to the present time.

References

[1] Christiansen, T. A., A. J. Duvall, R. B. Carley: Juvenile nasopharyngeal angiofibroma. Trans. Am. Acad. Ophthalmol. **78** (1974) 140.
[2] Fisch, U.: The infratemporal fossa approach for nasopharyngeal tumours. Laryngoscope **93** (1983) 36.
[3] Fitzpatrick, P. J.: The nasopharyngeal angiofibroma. Arch. Otolaryngol. **106** (1980) 234.
[4] Jaffek, B. W., et al.: Juvenile nasopharyngeal angiofibroma: Management of intracranial extension. Head and Neck Surg. **2** (1979) 119.
[5] Krekorian, E. A., L. G. Kempe: The combined otolaryngology, neurosurgery approach to extensive benign tumors. Laryngoscope **79** (1969) 2086.
[6] Kremen, A. J.: Surgical management of angiofibroma of the nasopharynx. Ann. Surg. **138** (1953) 672.
[7] Martin, H., W. E. Ehrlich, J. C. Abels: Juvenile nasopharyngeal angiofibroma. Ann. Surg. **127** (1940) 513.
[8] Roberson, G. H., H. Biller, D. G. Sessions et al.: Presurgical internal maxillary artery embolization of juvenile angiofibroma. Laryngoscope **81** (1972) 1524.
[9] Schiff, M.: Juvenile nasopharyngeal angiofibroma. Laryngoscope **69** (1959) 981.

Malignant tumors of the paranasal sinuses*

W. Draf, M. Samii

It is now almost 14 years since we have been working as a close ENT-Neurosurgical team, when it comes to management of skull base problems [2–8, 10, 11]. During this time we have operated on about 60 cases with tumors of the *anterior* skull base.

There is a fundamental difference in the *surgical concept.* Whereas the *benign growths* are removed making sure the important functional structures are preserved, one has to resect *malignant neoplasms* as much as possible *en bloc,* including a sufficient margin of normal tissue.

In cases of malignant growths operation is *indicated* only when a radical removal is expected. This is not justified if the neoplasm has grown into the cavernous sinus or if for instance both eyes have to be included in the specimen.

Surgical treatment

For the *surgical treatment* of malignant tumors of the paranasal sinuses some *basic considerations* are necessary:

1. An *anatomical one:* Approaching the skull base from below, which means extracranially, or intracranially from above, the surgeon is confronted with three different vascular levels which from without inwards are the ethmoidal vessels, located on or inside of the osseous skull base, the intradural meningeal vessels and the subarachnoid branches of the anterior cerebral artery.
2. In patients with small malignant lesions it is justifiable to preserve the eye. The *tear drainage* can then be *preserved* if the area is free of tumor infiltration. For that we have developed the following technique [4]: The nasolacrimal duct is dissected with a drill out of its osseous channel as far as the nasal mucosa. The orifice in the inferior nasal meatus is peritomized, so that the nasolacrimal duct and the lacrimal sac can be moved away from the operating field. At the end of the operation the orifice is sutured back into the cheek flap. With this technique we have achieved good functional results.

---

* Herrn Prof. Dr. med. W. Kley zum 65. Geburtstag

3. *Hemostasis of the vessels in the skull base* and the bony walls of the paranasal sinuses has proved to be adequate with the use of chisel according to Passow, the bone wax, the diamond burr without irrigation and the bone punch.

The *surgical strategy* depends on the location and size of the malignant growth. An important factor is "whether it has infiltrated the skull base or not".

The *partial or radical resection of maxilla and ethmoid with or without orbital exenteration* is the method of choice provided there is at least one cm distance between the skull base and the neoplasm.

When there are signs of *skull base infiltration* several approaches can be consider:
1. Extracranial *partial resection of the anterior skull base* with partial or total removal of paranasal sinuses, and *preservation of orbital contents.*
2. Extracranial *radical resection* of maxilla, ethmoid and anterior skull base *with orbital exenteration.*
3. *Combined intracranial-extracranial approach.*

There are *different incisions* linked to the various techniques. Most of them carry the names of famous surgeons of the 19th and 20th century: The paranasal incision of Moure, the enlarged incision to create a cheek flap according to Dieffenbach, Weber and Fergusson and subciliary modification of Zange, the upper lid incision for orbital exenteration, Barbosas incision for the additional approach to the infratemporal fossa, the Siebenmann-eye-glass incision and the coronal incision according to Souttar, Mygind and Unterberger.

The *extracranial resection of ethmoid roof and cribriform plate with partial or total resection of paranasal sinuses and preservation of orbital contents* is indicated, if the bony orbital walls are intact. In addition the tumorous infiltration of the skull base must be slight.

Moures paranasal incision is sufficient in most of those circumstances. In cases where the maxillary sinus is involved, the enlarged incision gives a better exposure.

The resection of the skull base is done after the major part of the tumor has been removed. It is cut around with a drill at a place sufficiently distant from the tumor often using the microscope. The orbital contents are retracted laterally. The dura mater is exposed and the olfactory nerve filaments may be cut. After excision of the basal mass the dura graft for repair is positioned laterally between the skull base and the dura, medially between the nasal septum and the septal mucoperiosteal layer. It is fixed with fibrin glue.

The *extracranial approach to the anterior skull base with orbital exenteration* is indicated, if the tumor has infiltrated the orbit and the skull base. The growth is usually rather extensive. This demands a wide exposure of the midface and the skull base.

After resection of the tumor including the maxilla, ethmoid and orbital contents a wide excision of the anterior skull base on one side, if necessary, also of cribriform plate and ethmoid roof on the contralateral side is possible from caudally. For mobilisation of the dura the angled flap knife is useful. The dura specimen is examined as frozen section in order to see if the margins are free of tumor.

The repair of the dura follows in a similar way as already described. Larger grafts should be sutured additionally to the fibrin seal. The graft is covered with gelfoam. At the end the whole area of operation is protected with a large piece of silastic sheath, which is kept in place with a pack for about three weeks. It facilitates the re-epithelization of the dura with the mucoperiostal layer from the margins of resection. This way free split thickness skin grafts which often cause crusting, can be avoided.

The *combined intracranial-extracranial approach* to the anterior skull base was first published by Ketcham and co-workers in 1963 [9] and later on by other authors, for example Derome [1], the Bordeaux-group, and ourselves [2]. The combined approach in one session is indicated in malignant neoplasms with a wider intracranial spread. This method, especially when using the microsurgical technique, facilitates preservation of function and reconstruction. It contributes to improving the prognosis.

The sequence of the surgical steps may vary depending on the individual situation. In malignant neoplasms of the cranial paranasal sinuses and the orbit one can first expose the tumor caudally and mark how much of the skull base is to be excised. This way the length of time when the cranial cavity is open is shorter and the danger of infection reduced. In the second stage there follows the intracranial-intradural resection of the skull base and if necessary of the involved brain. The third step is the reconstruction of the skull base. The coronal scalp incision and an enlarged paranasal sinus incision are combined. A bifrontal osteoplastic or osteoclastic craniotomy provides a good exposure from intracranially. The extracranial part with or without orbital exenteration has been discussed already.

The *intracranial stage of the operation* begins with a bifrontal craniotomy which has to be osteoclastic if the tumor has invaded the cranium. The dura is opened after double purse-string ligature of the superior sagittal sinus. After retraction of the frontal lobes, the whole anterior skull base is exposed and the area to be resected is cut around. The dura is left in contact with the bone of the specimen and shifted downwards. Then follows the *reconstruction of the skull base in three layers.*

The *first,* caudal *layer* is achieved with two lateral pedicled dural flaps, which are rotated and sutured together in the midline. The *second layer* is an individually shaped implant of methylmethacrylate, which we perforate, to obtain an appropriate stabilizing scar. The *third layer* is a caudally pedicled galea-periostal flap which covers the implant. It is fixed in place with sutures and fibrin glue. In cases of

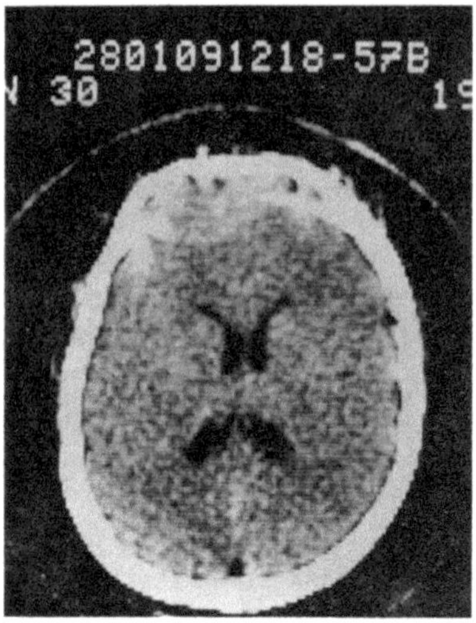

Fig. 1 Combined intracranial-extracranial approach in a case of extensive adenocarcinoma of the ethmoid and frontal sinuses. The CT shows the tumor invading the anterior fossa (Prof. Dr. S. Wende, Neuroradiological Department University of Mainz).

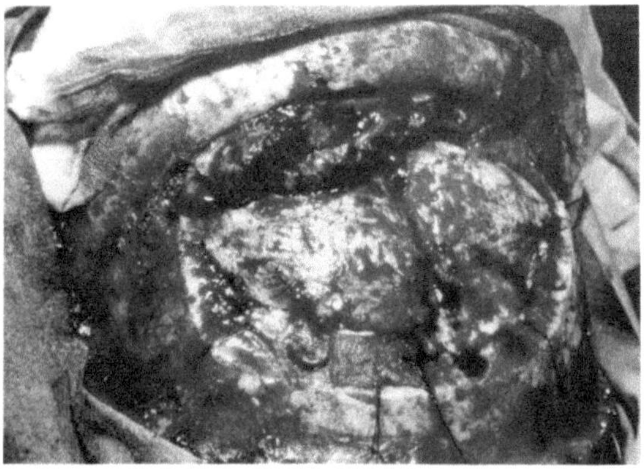

Fig. 2 After osteoclastic craniotomy the marked extent of the tumor and the infiltration of the dura are visible.

widely extensive resection of the dura, the outer aponeurosis of the temporalis muscle on one or both sides may be used, to build the caudal soft tissue layer. In any case the important thing is that the artificial implant is covered on both sides by adequate pedicled soft tissue. The cranial cavity is closed with the osteoplastic bone or with another implant and the scalp incision is sutured. After that we remove the block of skull base from below. The reconstructed area is checked from the facial cavity and the silastic sheath with pack is placed into the cavity before the facial incision is closed.

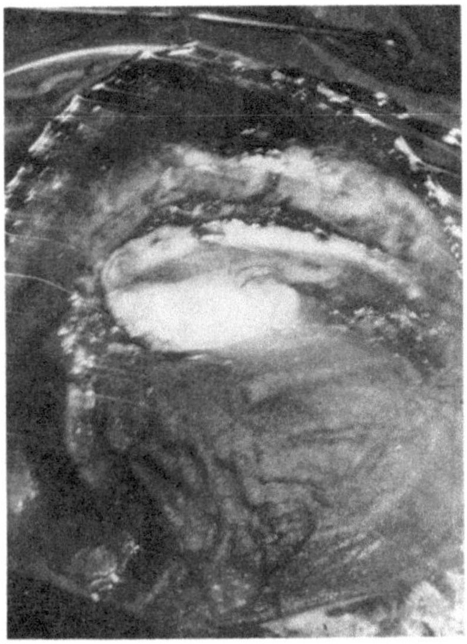

Fig. 3 Reconstruction of the forehead and skull base using methylmethacrylate as the middle of three layers.

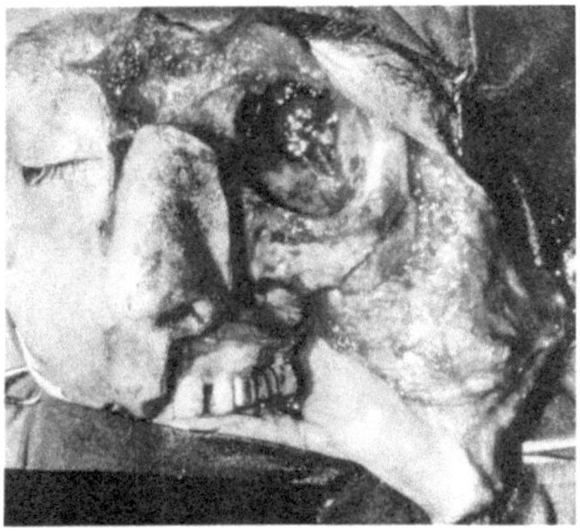

Fig. 4 Facial resection including the orbit.

A 55-year-old patient (figs. 1-6) suffered from an extensive, predominantly left-sided ethmoid frontal sinus adenocarcinoma which was invading the anterior fossa. A bifrontal osteoclastic craniotomy including the left supraorbital margin, was performed as the tumor invaded the posterior wall of the frontal sinus. As a large intracranial tumor mass had infiltrated the dura to a larger extent the anterior fossa was exposed after a relatively high incision. The brain did not seem to be involved. The intracranial resection included the posterior wall of the left frontal sinus, the ethmoid roof, the whole cribriform plate and the anterior part of the

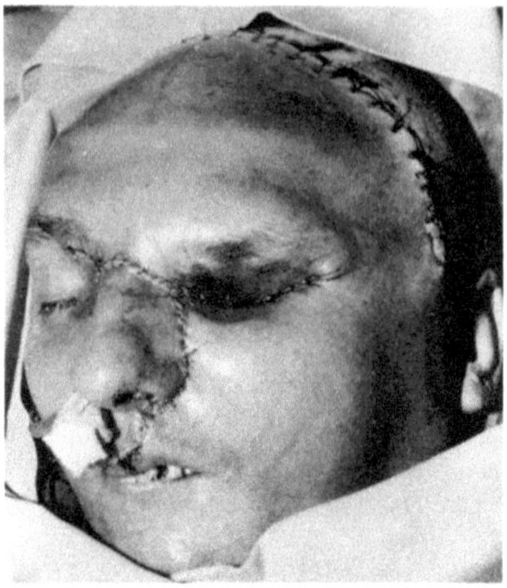

Fig. 5 End of operation. The methylmethacrylate is protected from below with lid skin.

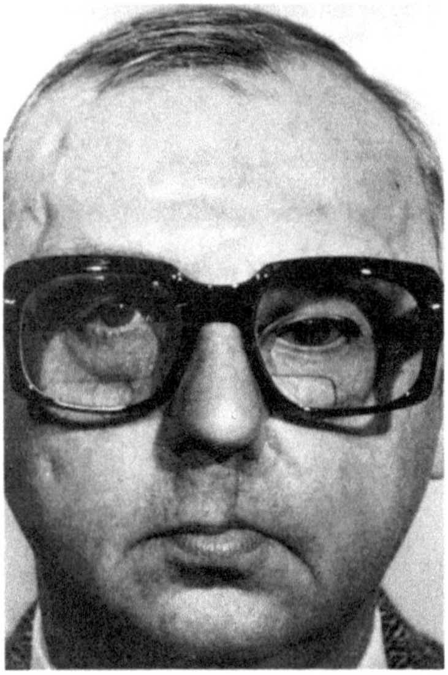

Fig. 6 The patient 18 month after operation.

planum sphenoidale. The cranium and the skull base were reconstructed with methylmethacrylate, a galea-periostal flap and from caudally with skin from the upper lid because of the extensive resection of dura.

Figure 5 shows how it looked at the end of the operation and figure 6 the patient 18 months later.

Summary

Many problems in tumor surgery of the skull base involving different specialities can be solved by cooperating during the procedure. The mortality and morbidity rate after such an intervention has decreased remarkably. This justifies the indication for a more radical intervention. Interdisciplinary team work and combined macro- and microsurgery bring better results regarding survival, function and esthetics.

References

[1] Derome, P.: Les tumeurs spheno-ethmoidales. Neurochirurgie **18** (1972) 1.

[2] Draf, W., M. Samii: Otorhinolaryngo-neurochirurgische Probleme an der Schädelbasis. Laryng. Rhinol. Otol. **56** (1977) 1007.

[3] Draf, W., M. Samii: Microsurgery of the lateral skull base. Proceedings of the 5th International Congress of International Microsurgical Society 4.-7.10. 78 Bonn. International Congress No 465. Excerpta Medica, Amsterdam-Oxford (1979).

[4] Draf, W.: In: M. Samii, W. Draf: Surgical treatment of tumors in the anterior skull base. Course on the surgery of the anterior skull base, Hannover 26.-29. March 1980.

[5] Draf, W., M. Samii: Intracranial-intratemporal anastomosis of the facial nerve after cerebello-pontine angle tumor surgery. In: Disorders of the facial nerve (M. D. Graham, W. F. House, eds.), pp. 441-449. Raven Press, New York 1982.

[6] Draf, W., M. Samii: Diagnostik und operative Strategie bei großen Glomustumoren der lateralen Schädelbasis. In: Aktuelles in der Otorhinolaryngologie (E. H. Mayer, C. H. Rieder, eds.), pp. 61-70. Österr. HNO-Kongreß Linz 1981. Thieme, Stuttgart-New York 1983.

[7] Draf, W., M. Samii: Frontobasal Injuries - Principles in Diagnosis and treatment. In: Traumatology of the skull base (M. Samii, J. Brihaye, eds.), pp. 61-69. Springer, Berlin-Heidelberg-New York 1983.

[8] Draf, W., M. Samii: Reconstruction of frontobasal fractures. In: Fractures of the frontobasis (V. Vecsei, ed.), p. 105. Proceeding of the I. Vienna Workshop International College of Surgeons. Vienna October 3.-6. 1982.

[9] Ketcham, A. S., R. H. Wilkins, J. M. Van Buren et al.: A combined intracranial-facial approach to the paranasal sinuses. Amer. J. Surg. **106** (1963) 699.

[10] Samii, M., W. Draf: Indikation und Versorgung der frontobasalen Liquorfistel aus HNO-chirurgischer und neurochirurgischer Sicht. Laryng. Rhinol. Otol. **57** (1978) 689-697.

[11] Samii, M., W. Draf: Neurosurgical-ENT-Treatment of lesions of the skull base. Advances in Neurosurgery 5. Springer, Berlin-Heidelberg-New York 1978.

Malignant maxillofacial tumors and the skull base – operative procedures and prosthetic management

N. Schwenzer

Introduction

The topographic situation of tumors growing in the oro-maxillofacial region is the reason why their malignant infiltration frequently involves the skull base. Less frequently than by direct invasion the skull base is affected by metastases from more distant primary tumors. The damage to the skull base depends on the tumor type, its primary location and its size. On surgical grounds the skull base may well be involved by radical operating techniques even in the absence of any malignant invasion.

Tumor types and their spread

Carcinomas of the oral cavity are the most common ones in our specialty; those situated in the cranial parts, i.e. hard and soft palate, tuber and sulcus palatinus area, demonstrate very early involvement of the skull base – for very obvious anatomical reasons [6]. Carcinomas developing from the mucosa of the maxillary cavity reach the skull base after having penetrated the orbit and the ethmoidal cells. The same principle applies to cystoadenoid type carcinomas and mucoepidermoidal type tumors starting in the maxilla.

Primary osteocarcinomas occur extremely rarely. However the maxilla and the area adiacent to the temporomandibular joint is quite often the site of metastatic involvement by tumors in different organs such as the prostate or thyroid gland. Tumor activity in the head of the mandible will spread into the glenoid fossa and may easily reach the skull base from there.

Osteogenic tumors including osteo-, chondro- and fibrosarcomas and tumors originating from soft tissue such as myosarcomas and the so-called malignant Schwannoma show also an ascending type of growth. Sometimes large nasopharyngeal fibromas may degenerate and then show malignant infiltrating features.

Another type of tumor with invasive characteristics is represented by the ameloblastoma, an odontogenic tumor, which requires to be managed like a malignant lesion. Its tendency to relapse is well known and may lead to the invasion of the surrounding soft tissue and end up by involving the cranial cavity. If located in the maxilla the tumor may spread alongside its ascending ramus and gain access to the skull base via the infratemporal region.

Basaliomas (basal cell carcinomas) and squamous cell carcinomas infiltrate different structures including the bony tissue. Basal cell carcinomas predominantly located in the periorbital area tend to invade the orbit as well as the ethmoidal cells and may eventually reach the anterior skull base [1, 5]. Many of them appear to be small and innocuous but then, as a consequence of incompetent treatment they may go a head and cause a fatal outcome.

Operative procedures in different locations

For efficient treatment of all these tumors an interdisciplinary cooperation by the maxillofacial surgeon, the ear, nose and throat specialist and, sometimes, the neurosurgeon is required. Each of the specialties can contribute their specific knowledge and skill as well as materials and methods, and such a fruitful combination is mostly mutually appreciated. In my view the maxillofacial surgeon's task is as follows:
1. to choose the anatomical approach optimal for exposure of the tumor and its removal, as well as for the handling of the skull base,
2. to confirm his experience in facial bone handling,
3. to substitute any tissue defect caused by the surgical procedure and to re-establish form and function of the organ by surgical as well as prosthetic means.

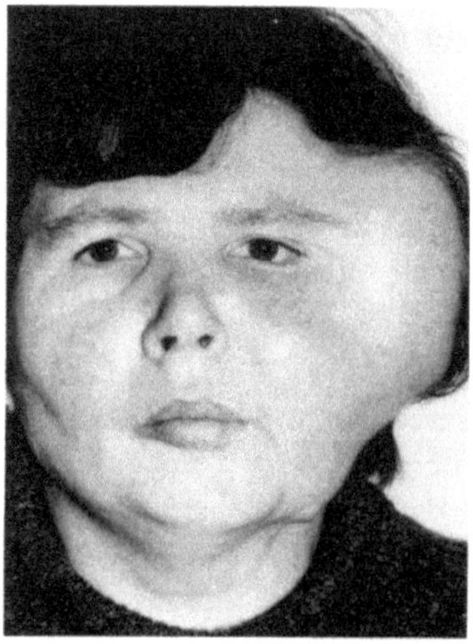

Fig. 1 Recurrence of an ameloblastoma of the mandible growing alongside the ascending ramus and involving the skull base.

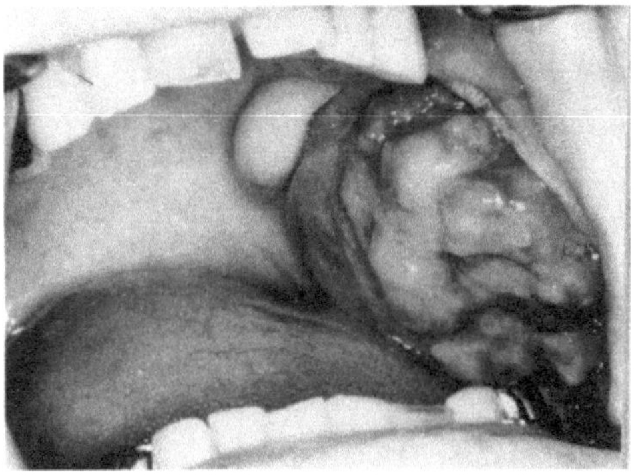

Fig. 2 Intra-oral findings.

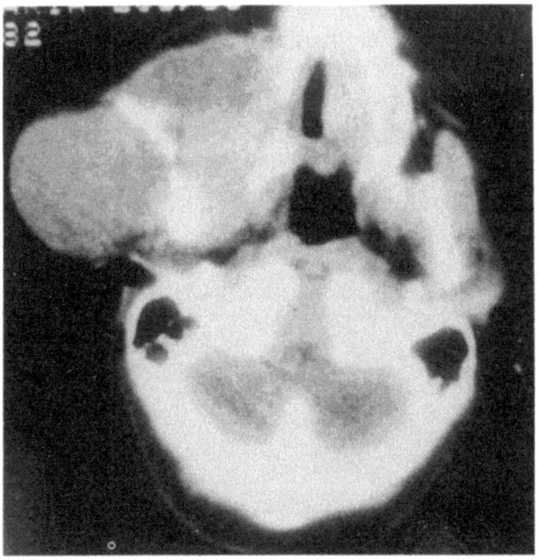

Fig. 3 The computer tomogramm shows that the tumor involves the infratemporal and temporal region.

The aim of treatment is, of course, to remove the tumor from within the healthy area, to correct any tissue defect and to keep the degree of inevitable mutilation as low as possible. The relation of the tumor to the skull base has to be investigated during the surgical procedure so that the extent of the resection can be graded accordingly. If affected the skull base has to be carefully revised and reconstructed or restored with dura and/or corresponding materials.

The different routes for surgical approach depend on the site of the tumor. In cases of maxilla carcinomas affecting the orbit a transmaxillary approach will be the first choice, and it can be combined with an incision useful for exenteration of the

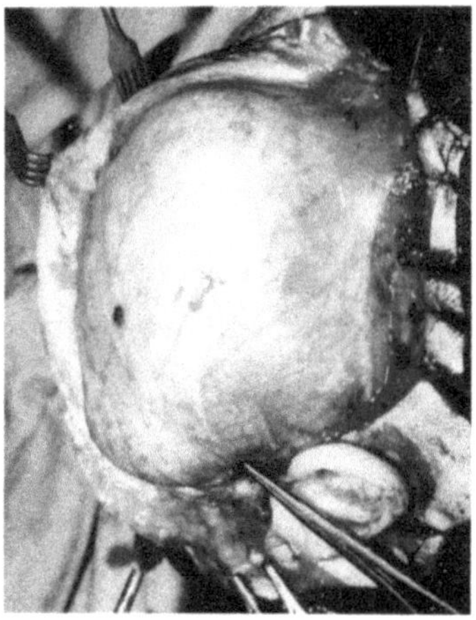

Fig. 4 Intraoperative view. The upper portion of the tumor could be removed from the skull base by a temporal and preauricular incision.

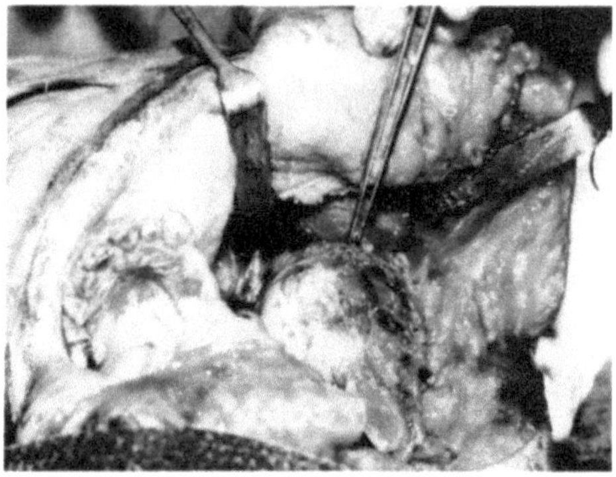

Fig. 5 The lower part was resected 6 weeks later together with the mandibular bone by a submandibular incision.

orbit. If the skin of the lid can be partially or totally spared from the procedure it can be used to cover the bone in the cranial orbit. This technique favors the epithelializing process of the wound and allows an early prosthetic management. Alternatively, in the case of bony defect the cranial parts of the orbit may be lined and padded with a flap, mobilised from the forehead, in a second session.

A transpalatine approach allows one to reach tumors situated between the skull base and the palate. Tumors of the lid invading the orbit can be dealt with by transorbital access, which also allows the revision of the ethmoidal cells. Skin tumors in the frontal and temporal area of the face may be approached from the forehead, and any defects can be reconstituted with flaps, only. Tumors growing alongside the ascending ramus of the mandible tend to reach the temporal and infratemporal

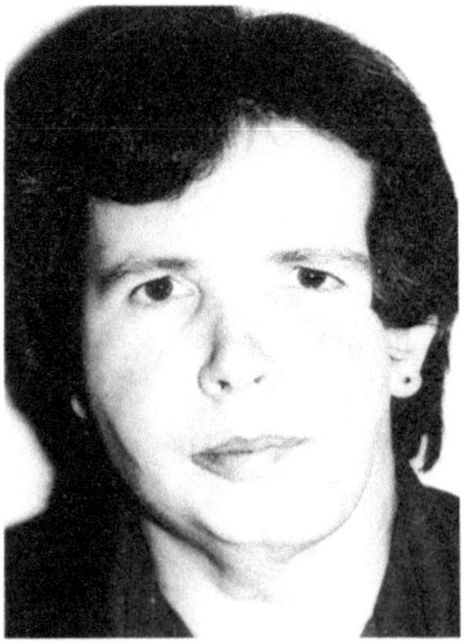

Fig. 6 Postoperative finding one year later.

region and sometimes may even be found above the zygomatic arch; they can be dissected from their temporal aspect. The incision is made from the preauricular to the temporal region and may be prolonged caudally to give a good view of the zygomatic arch and temporomandibular joint. In very extensive non-malignant tumors we prefer to proceed in two sessions, from the temporal area first and later from the submandibular area (figs. 1-6). The commonly practiced submandibular incision allows a transmandibular access for dissecting the mandible at its angle, and a consecutive plate osteosynthesis, or the resection of the diseased part. This is also the classical way to a carcinoma of the oral cavity.

Reconstructive measures

Tissue defects involving the anterior and lateral parts of the skull base require immediate restitution. According to the size and nature of the defect additional reconstructive steps may be necessary during the first surgical intervention. Pedicle flaps moved from intact neighbouring tissue of the forehead and/or the parietal area of the skull may lend themselves for this purpose. The skin, muscle, and periosteum can also be handled independently, if this is more convenient.

Excessive scar tissue shrinking following resection of the maxilla is prevented by the integration of a plastic resection plate, which may be coated with a free skin graft. This procedure usually shows satisfactory results.

A further possibility consists in pedicle flaps [7] and free musculocutaneous flaps including their microvascular bonding. Branching with the facial and temporal artery and vein is here the common practice. If it is desirable to keep the facial resection cavity patent for easy follow up of any potential tumor activity, there is only some prosthetic management to be considered. For secondary reconstruction, however, tubed pedicle flaps can be used.

Prosthetic management

An essential auxiliary measure in maxillofacial surgery is provided by prosthesis such as splints, resection plates and maxillofacial prostheses.

1. Splints and plate osteosyntheses are indicated after hemimandibulectomy to secure occlusion and to prevent any mechanical deviation of the mandibular remnant, due to scar tissue growing. Every dental splinting known in traumatology will serve the purpose.

2. Bone defects left from partial or total maxillary resection have to be replaced by dental plates or other alloplastic substitutes, so that a substantial reconstruction of the oral cavity and the skull base can be fixed [2]. We use plastic plates, which are usually made before the operation and tailored to the individual size and shape during the operation. The plates are then wired to the teeth or screwed into the neighbouring bone and give hold to tamponades, support soft tissue and last but not least facilitate normal speaking and feeding for the patient. Later, after the healing process has come to an end, we remove those provisional plates and replace them with surgical prostheses. The total prosthetic replacement of the maxilla is, of course, extremely difficult.

3. In principle, resection defects can be repaired by maxillofacial prosthetic management either as a temporary measure or as a definitive solution [3]. The latter

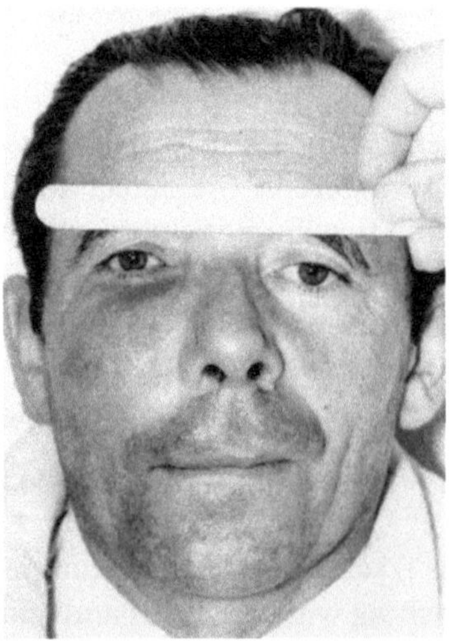

Fig. 7 50-year-old man with a carcinoma of the upper jaw involving the orbit.

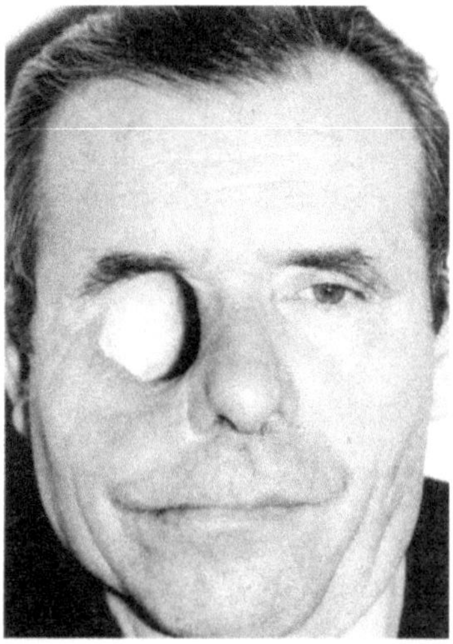

Fig. 8 Postoperative finding ten years later. After resection of the maxilla and exenteration of the orbit. The resection cavity had been covered by a free skin graft.

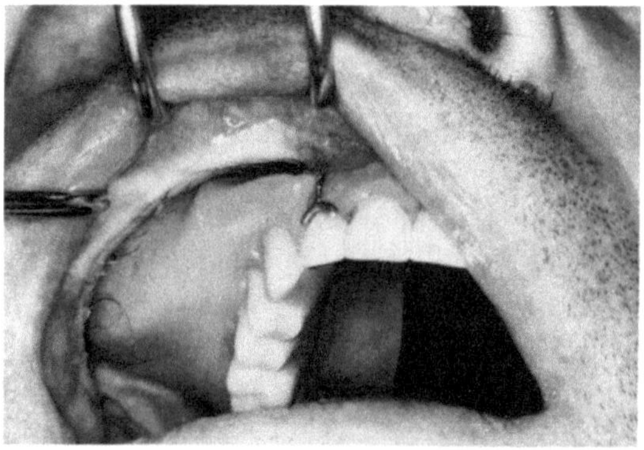

Fig. 9 The intraoral defect is covered by a surgical prosthesis.

may include further surgical stages [5]. Prosthetic substitution is required for orbital defects following exenteration or extensive resection in the nasomaxillary area. In the majority of cases one has to deal with orbital defects. Prosthetic devices can be fixed either externally to spectacles or internally to the walls of the resection cavity. Acrylic and silicon based materials are now in general use and give good results from the aesthetic point of view, particularly for little or non-mobile areas of the face. If the resection cavity communicates with the oral cavity an additional prosthetic device has to be provided (figs. 7–10).

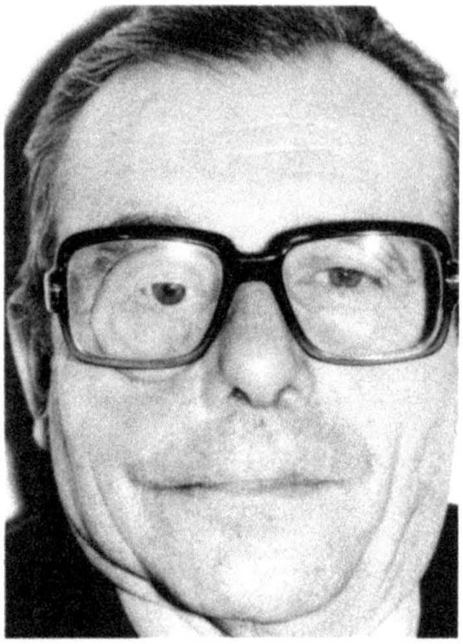

Fig. 10 The maxillofacial prosthesis (epithesis) of the orbit is fixed to the walls of the resection cavity. It consists of cured polymer.

Summary

Malignant maxillofacial tumors invading the vicinity of the skull base require interdisciplinary cooperation. The surgical approach has to guarantee an optimal view of the tumor as well as easy access to the skull base. Therapeutic considerations have to include the necessity or possibility of surgical and/or prosthetic management of all kinds of resections involving the orbit, the maxilla and the cranial parts of the oral cavity.

References

[1] Ehmann, G., W. Schmidt-Hoberg, G. Kessler: Zur unterschiedlichen Prognose von vorbehandelten und nicht vorbehandelten Basaliomen der Periorbita. Fortschr. Kiefer- u. Gesichtschir. **22** (1977) 147–149.
[2] Grimm, G. In: Zahn-Mund-Kieferheilkunde (N. Schwenzer, G. Grimm, eds.), vol. 2. Thieme, Stuttgart-New York 1981.
[3] Schwenzer, N.: Technik und Ergebnisse der epithetischen Versorgung von Gesichtsdefekten. Fortschr. Kiefer- u. Gesichtschir. **10** (1965) 115.
[4] Schwenzer, N.: Indikation zur chirurgischen und epithetischen Deckung von Gesichtsdefekten. Fortschr. Kiefer- u. Gesichtschir. **23** (1978) 21–23.
[5] Sooss, G., F. Schmetzer, N. Schwenzer: Klinik und chirurgische Therapie des Gesichtshautbasalioms. Fortschr. Kiefer- u. Gesichtschir. **27** (1982) 35–39.
[6] Spiessl, B.: Plattenepithelkarzinom der Mundhöhle. Thieme, Stuttgart 1966.
[7] Spiessl, B., J. Prein: Vorteile des myokutanen Pektoralislappens gegenüber dem autonomisierten Brustlappen bei der operativen Therapie des extrem ausgedehnten Basalioma terebrans. Fortschr. Kiefer- u. Gesichtschir. **27** (1982) 112–115.

Radiotherapy of the skull base

M. Wannenmacher, W. Hinkelbein, H. Knüfermann

Introduction

Tumors located in the base of the skull represent a special challenge for radiotherapy. There are great differences in the radiosensitivity of the tumors in this region as well as of the surrounding normal tissues. Therefore, exact treatment planning and careful performance is essential. The different tumors of the skull base show different radiocurability and should, whenever possible be treated in combination with surgery. A survey on radiosensitivity and radiocurability of primary skull base tumors t ogether with the required tumor doses is given with table 1.

Tumors of the skull base

The esthesioneuroblastoma is an uncommon tumor. Elkon et al. [2] analysed 97 cases from the world literature. The patients were treated in different ways. At stage A and B it makes no difference whether the patient is treated with radiotherapy or operation alone or a combination of both. Only at stage C a combination of radiotherapy and operation seems to bring better results. A total dose of at least 50 Gy should be reached (see tab. 2).

Chondromas can be said to be radioresistant and, therefore radiotherapy is not indicated.

Table 1 Tumors of the skull base

	Treatment		Radio-sensitivity	Radio-curability	Dose (Gy)
	Operation	Rad.			
Esthesioneuroblastoma	+	+	+	+	50
Chondroma	+	–	–	–	-
Chordoma	+	+	–/+	–/+	60–70
Juvenile angiofibroma (for multiple recurrences)	+	+	+	+	35–40
Plasmocytoma	–	+	+	+	50
Ewing-sarcoma	+	+	+	–/+	50–60
Hemangioma	+	+	+	+	30–40
Paraganglioma	+	+	+	–/+	45–50

Table 2 Esthesioneuroblastoma: Results of treatment by method and stage (78 patients; 6 mo-32 yr follow-up) [2]

Technique	Stage A			Stage B			Stage C		
	Initial Treatment	For Recurrence	Total Control Rate	Initial Treatment	For Recurrence	Total Control Rate	Initial Treatment	For Recurrence	Total Control Rate
Radiotherapy alone	2/5	5/5	70%	4/7	3/4	64%	1/5	1/1	33%
Operation alone	5/9	4/4	69%	3/6	1/2	50%	1/1	0/0	-
Radiotherapy *and* operation	7/10	0/0	70%	12/20	0/1	57%	7/15	0/0	47%

There is no doubt that the chordoma has a low radiosensitivity. Nevertheless, it was found out that chordomas of the skull base have a longer recurrence-free period with postoperative radiotherapy, but doses of at least 60-70 Gy are required. Suit [18] recommends a dose of 60 Gy with an additional proton beam of 10 Gy. Pearlman and Friedmann [14] were able to prove that the 5-year survival rate improved considerably with an irradiation dose exceeding 60 Gy.

In cases of juvenile angiofibroma the treatment of choice is preoperative vascular embolization followed by surgical removal. Results have been satisfactory. For a few patients without complete surgical resection or with multiple recurrences after repeated operation, a course of radiation therapy has been found to be effective in tumor control. The required doses range between 35-40 Gy [7]. It has to be emphasized that with radiotherapy of benign lesions there is always a risk of malignant transformation. Such risks must be carefully weighed against the benefits, before radiation therapy is considered.

Only solitary plasmocytomas are usually treated by radiotherapy alone. Primary radical operation is not justified because of the good radiosensitivity and radiocurability of this tumor. Operation may be used in the management of recurrences after irradiation, however. For solitary plasmocytomas a dose of 50 Gy in 5 weeks is effective [15].

Apart from the plasmocytoma the Ewing-sarcoma is the only radiosensitive bone tumor. Up to now, only 2 Ewing-sarcomas of the skull base have been described in the literature. The required dose would be 50-60 Gy.

Operation should be the main form of treatment for osseous hemangiomas. In case of inoperability or incompletely resected tumors radiotherapy can induce tumor regression.

Most of the paragangliomas occur in the temporal bone and should be treated by temporal bone resection if the lesions are operable. Postoperative radiation therapy is effective in reducing the incidence of local recurrences. Therefore, radiation therapy should be considered as part of an integrated program with a dose of 45-50 Gy in 5 weeks. Irradiation alone is the preferred form of treatment for the nonresectable lesions, with satisfactory local control [17, 6].

Table 3 Tumors invading the skull base site

	Therapy	
	Operation	Rad. therapy
Orbital tumors	+	+
Maxillo-ethmoidal tumors	+	+
Nasopharyngeal tumors	(+)	+
Tumors of the middle ear	+	(+)
Pterygo-palatine tumors	+	+
Basal meningiomas	+	(+)
Craniopharyngiomas	+	+
Tumors of the pituitary gland	+	(+)
Tumors of the cranial nerves	+	(+)

Table 4 Tumors invading the skull base histological type

	Radiosensitivity	Radiocurability	Dose (Gy)
Retinoblastoma	+	+	40-50
Lymphomas	++	++	40-50
Gliomas	(+)	(+)	50-60
Neurinomas	(+)	(+)	60
Soft tissue tumors	(+)	(+)	60
Squamous sell carcinoma	+	+	60
Adenocarcinoma	(+)	(+)	60
Adenoid cystic carcinoma	(+)	(+)	60
Lympho-epithelioma	++	++	60-65
Anaplastic carcinoma	+	+	65-75

Tumors invading the skull base

More frequent are those tumors invading the skull base from the upper or lower level (see tabs. 3 and 4).

Postoperative irradiation should be given to all tumors of the orbital and paranasal regions, at higher stages. Undifferentiated meningiomas have low radiosensitivity, but with a sufficient dose of e.g. 70 Gy retardation of tumor growth can be obtained [4]. For craniopharyngiomas postoperative irradiation is indicated in cases of incomplete resection [13].

With tumors of the pituitary gland irradiation depends on the histologic grading [12]. From all tumors possibly involving the skull base, lymphomas and lympho-epitheliomas have the highest radiosensitivity and curability. Radiosensitivity of squamous cell and anaplastic carcinomas is commonly lower but still with a satisfactory chance of curability.

Table 5 Nasopharyngeal carcinoma 5-year survival rate with radiotherapy only [9]

	Stage			
	I	II	III	IV
Study I (until 1965) (437 patients)	67.9%	62.2%	32.9%	11.0%
Study II (1969-71) (616 patients)	83.9%	67.9%	40.3%	-

Table 6 Nasopharyngeal carcinoma survival rate with radiotherapy only [11]

	Stage			Total
	I	II	III	
Study I (1958-1973) 1605 patients 70 Gy in 7-8 wk				
5-year survival rate	75.2%	56.9%	32.2%	43.5%
10-year survival rate	64.3%	48.5%	22.1%	33.6%
Study II (1974-1978) 1032 patients 70 Gy split course				
5-year survival rate	79.0%	63.2%	43.6%	56.0%

Table 7 Nasopharyngeal carcinoma 5-year survival rate

Institution/author	Year of report	Number of patients	5-year survival
Albrecht [1] (collected statistics)	1959	397	13.8%
Scanlon [16]	1967	142	30.0%
M. D. Anderson (Fletcher) [3]	1981	251	52.0%
Stanford (Hoppe)	1976	74	59.0%
Frommhold [5]	1984	63	46.5%
Wannenmacher [21]	1984	94	45.0%

Nasopharyngeal carcinomas can be cured by radiotherapy alone, and therefore, operation is not indicated. Analysing the published results, the outstanding number of patients from Asia becomes evident together with a high rate of cure, whereas the European and American results do not come up to the same level. In this connection the results of Ho [9] and Huang [11] are especially interesting, with cure rates of 80% at stage II, and 40% at stage III (see tabs. 5 and 6). Lately a distinct improvement in the results could be observed. In 1959, Albrecht [1] published collect-

Table 8 Total dose in nasopharyngeal carcinoma (Gy)

	Primary site		Related lymph nodes (without involvement postop.)		Related lymph nodes (with involvement without operation)	
Lympho-epithelioma	60-70	6-8 wk	45-55	5-6 wk	60-65	7-8 wk
Squamous cell carcinoma (unclassified carcinoma)	65-75	8-9 wk	50-60	6-7 wk	65-75	8-9 wk

ed statistics with a recurrence-free 5-year survival rate of 13.8%; 1980 the rate was 50% for the large material of the M. D. Anderson Hospital [3] and 59% for the Stanford group [10]. In Germany a rate of 46.5% to 45% was found comprising all stages (The 5-year survival rates are shown in table 7).

The difference results from the fact that in America there are a higher number of lymphoepitheliomas, whereas in Europe the squamous cell carcinomas and undifferentiated carcinomas predominate. Prognosis depends on destruction of skull base and involvement of the facial nerve. The squamous cell carcinomas have a recurrence rate of 30% and the lymphoepitheliomas of 10%.

The protection of the radiosensitive structures surrounding the nasopharynx calls for careful, well-planned techniques of treatment. The skull base is included in the irradiation field. Optimal dose distribution is reached with opposing fields or by a 3-field technique. Even in the early stages therapy should include the regional lymph nodes. The total dose depends on histology (see tab. 8).

Skull base metastases

Apart from the primary skull base tumors and the tumors involving the skull base, the metastases affecting the skull base can also be treated with radiotherapy. Megavoltage irradiation has a good palliative effect, which implies symptomatic relief for the patients. A study of Vikram [19] shows that most skull base metastases originate from breast cancer (see tab. 9). With radiotherapy living conditions can be improved in 78% of the cases. In particular cranial nerve affections cause great discomfort for the patient (see tab. 10).

If any involvement of the brain can clearly be excluded, the irradiation field will be confined to the skull base. In the more frequent cases - with additional brain metastases - the whole brain is irradiated with 40 Gy followed by a local boost of 10 Gy on the skull base. Only patients with a Karnofsky index exceeding 70% obtain a distinct benefit from therapy; it is the same with brain metastases.

Table 9 Primary sites with intervals from diagnosis of primary malignancy to diagnosis of metastases at the base of the skull [19]

Primary site	Number of patients	Interval from diagnosis of primary		
		Median	Range	
Breast	18	5.5 yrs.	1 mo.	– 20 yrs.
Lymphoma	9	1.5 yrs.	3 mos.	– 4 yrs.
Lung	7	1.0 mo.	1 mo.	– 3 yrs.
Head and neck	7	1.0 yr.	6 mos.	– 6 yrs.
Miscellaneous	5	3.0 yrs.	1 yr.	– 11 yrs.
Total	46	2.0 yrs.	1 mo.	– 20 yrs.

Table 10 Results of radiation therapy in 46 patients [19]

Improved	36 (78%)
complete relief of all symptoms	14 (30%)
partial relief	22 (48%)
Not improved	10 (22%)
No relapse following improvement (until death or last follow-up)	29 (81%)
Relapse of disease at bos	4 (11%)
Lost to follow-up	3 (8%)

Future prospects for treatment

Late clinical results require a combination of chemotherapy and radiotherapy improving the results with additional application of radiosensitizing agents, like misonidazole. During the last few years, fast neutrons, proton beams or pions first came into clinical use. The therapeutic results may be improved by a better response of hypoxic tumor fraction with fast neutrons and the application of higher tumor doses because of a more favourable depth-dose distribution in the case of protons and pions. The combination of radiotherapy and local hyperthermia, as well, could enhance the destruction of tumor cells, and thus improve the results.

From our opinion a significant progress can be achieved with interstitial therapy, using new radionuclides. Because of its favourable physical properties iodine-125 seeds can be used at operation without any exposure of the clinical personnel involved. At the skull base this allows the application of high doses in small volumes.

In case of head and neck tumors the interstitial implant is used like a local boost preceeding percutaneous irradiation. Goffinet [8] observed in a limited number of cases better results with a combination of operation + interstitial implantation + percutaneous irradiation. But, if the tumor is not encompassed by the necessary tu-

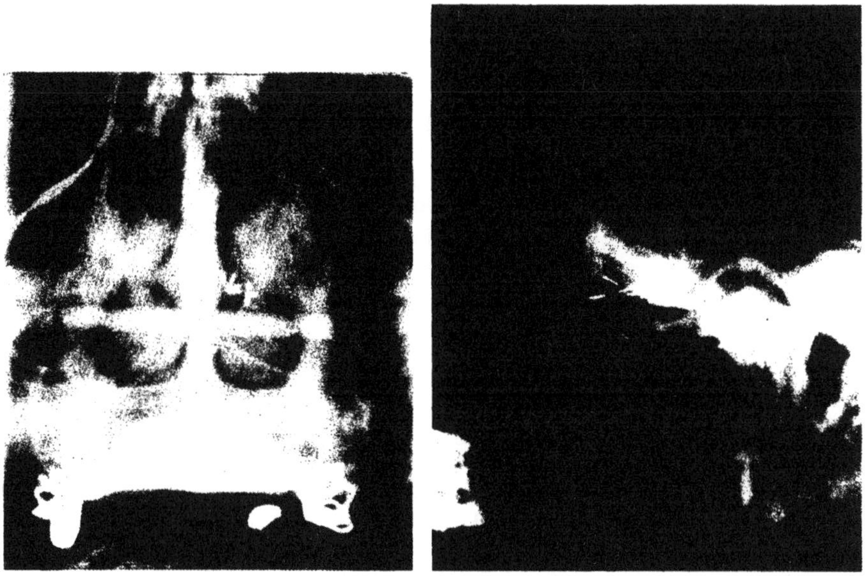

Fig. 1 Interstitial implant in a local recurrence of nasopharyngeal carcinoma in AP (a) and lateral view (b)

mor dose, recurrences may occur. Vikram and Hilaris [20] described a technique for transnasal interstitial iodine-125 implantation for carcinoma of the nasopharynx. We, also, have some experiences with the skull base area, such as implantations in nasopharyngeal and paranasal tumors (see fig. 1).

We would like to emphasize that with interstitial radiation therapy the local tumor dose can be increased to a level which can never be reached with external radiotherapy alone. Thus, local tumor control is improved implying the increase of the overall survival time.

References

[1] Albrecht, R.: Die Nasenrachentumoren und ihre Behandlung. Arch. Ohren-Nasen-Kehlkopf-Heilk. **175** (1959) 217-221.

[2] Elkon, I., S. L. Hightower, M. L. Lim et al.: Esthesioneuroblastoma, Cancer **44** (1979) 1087-1094.

[3] Fletcher, G. H., J. B. Mesic, H. Goepfert: Megavoltage Irradiation of the nasopharynx Int. J. Rad. Oncol. Biol. Phys. **7** (1981) 447-453.

[4] Friedmann, M.: Irradiation of meningioma: A prototype circumscribed tumor for planning high-dose irradiation of the brain. Int. J. Radiation Oncology Biol. Phys. **2** (1977) 949-958.

[5] Frommhold, H.: Strahlentherapie der Nasopharynxmalignome. In: Nasopharynxtumoren (M. Wannenmacher, ed.), pp. 36-48. Urban & Schwarzenberg, München-Wien-Baltimore 1984.

[6] Gibbin, K. P., J. M. Henk: Glomus jugulare tumours in South Wales - a twenty year review. Clin. Radiol. **29** (1978) 607-609.
[7] Gill, G., D. H. Rice, F. N. Ritter et al.: Intracranial and extracranial nasopharyngeal angiofibroma, Arch. Otolaryngol. **102** (1976) 371-373.
[8] Goffinet, D. R., A. Martinez, D. Pooler et al.: Intraoperative pterygo-palatine interstitial 125-I-seed implants. Int. J. Rad. Oncol. Biol. Phys. **9** (1983) 103-106.
[9] Ho, J. H. C.: An epidemiologic and clinical study of nasophapharyngeal carcinoma. Int. J. Radiat. Oncol. Biol. Phys. **4** (1978) 183-198.
[10] Hoppe, R. H., D. R. Goffinet, H. A. Bagshaw: Carcinoma of the nasopharynx. Eighteen years experience with megavoltage radiation therapy. Cancer **37** (1976) 2605-2612.
[11] Huang, S. C., G. L. Chu: Nasopharyngeal Cancer: study II, Int. J. Radiat. Oncol. Biol. Phys. **7** (1981) 713-716.
[12] Kramer, S.: The value of radiation therapy for pituitary and parapituitary tumours. Canad. Med. An. J. **99** (1968) 1120-1127.
[13] Lichter, H. A., W. M. Wara, G. E. Sheline et al.: The treatment of craniopharyngiomas. Int. J. Radiation Oncology Biol. Phys. **2** (1977) 675-683.
[14] Pearlmann, A. W., M. Friedmann: Radical radiation therapy of chordoma. Am. J. Roentgend. Radium Ther. Nucl. Med. **108** (1970) 331-341.
[15] Petrovich, Z., B. Fishkin, R. E. Hittle et al.: Extramedullary plasmocytoma of the upper respiratory passages, Int. J. Radiol. Oncol. Biol. phys. **2** (1977) 723-730.
[16] Scanlon, P. W.: Cancer of the Nasopharynx, Amer. J. Roentgenol. **99** (1967) 313-325.
[17] Simko, T. G., T. W. Griffin, A. J. Cerdes et al.: The role of radiation therapy in the treatment of glomus jugulare tumors, Cancer **42** (1978) 104-106.
[18] Suit, H.: Neoplasms of the Central Nervous System (by P. L. Kornblith, M. D. Walker, I. R. Cassady). In: V. T. De Vita, S. Hellmann, S. Rosenberg: Cancer (1982) 1242.
[19] Vikram, B., F. C. H. Chu: Radiation therapy for metastases to the base of the skull. Radiology **130** (1979) 465-468.
[20] Vikram, B., B. Hilaris: Transnasal permanent implantation for carcinoma of the nasopharynx. Int. J. Radiat. Oncol. Biol. Phys. **10** (1984) 153-155.
[21] Wannenmacher, M. (ed.): Nasopharynxtumoren. Urban & Schwarzenberg, München-Wien-Baltimore 1984.

Present role of chemotherapy in the treatment of head and neck cancer

G. B. Snow, J. B. Vermorken, H. M. Pinedo

Introduction

The experiences with chemotherapy in malignant tumors of the head and neck other than squamous cell carcinoma are very restricted. This review therefore is limited to a discussion of the role of chemotherapy in the management of squamous cell carcinoma of the head and neck. When chemotherapy is used in patients with end-stage locally or regionally recurrent or metastatic disease, palliation has not been associated with a significant prolongation of life, despite the fact that chemotherapy in this setting can induce objective tumor regression in 20–50% of patients, depending on the drug(s) regimens applied. During the last decade there has been an increasing interest in the use of chemotherapy as an adjuvant to operation and/or radiotherapy in the primary treatment of advanced head and neck cancer. The objective of this paper is to report on these recent developments.

Response of chemotherapy

Definition of response

For meaningful reporting of data objective standards of response must be defined. By convention, there are four response grades: complete response (CR), partial response (PR), no change (NC) and progressive disease (PD). A complete response (CR) refers to the disappearance of all measurable tumor. Partial response (PR) is defined to be at least a 50% decrease in tumor area (multiplication of the greatest diameter by its perpendicular diameter) or a 50% decrease in the sum of the products of the perpendicular diameters of multiple lesions for at least 4 weeks. Response rate is expressed as a percentage and could be expressed for patients having CR or PR alone or CR and PR together for total response rate. Response with less than 50% regression of measurable disease is considered no change (NC) or stable disease. Progressive disease (PD) is defined as more than 25% increase in measurable disease and/or appearance of new lesions during therapy.

In many instances tumor masses in the head and neck do not lend themselves to convenient or precise measurements. Assessments of response therefore should preferably be carried out by the regional expert who is familiar with the techniques of examination and investigation of the head and neck area and the medical oncologist together, so as to minimize measuring errors [1]. When operation is carried out after chemotherapy the response to chemotherapy can also be assessed histopathologically and this appears to enhance the validity of the data. Micheau et al. [2] have proposed a histopathological assessment scale for the response to chemotherapy.

Factors affecting response

Factors affecting response can be divided into patient-factors, tumor- and treatment-factors and these will be reviewed in this order.

Patient factors

The performance status of patients affects the response to chemotherapy. Patients who are ambulatory respond significantly better to chemotherapeutic agents than those who are bedridden [3]. patients with head and neck cancer often abuse alcohol and tobacco and may be malnourished. Patients with poor nutritional status do not tolerate chemotherapy well. A variety of scales is used to record the physical state of the patients. In table 1 the WHO Performance Status Scale is listed. This is preferred because of simplicity. This scale corresponds well with the Eastern Cooperative Oncology Group Scale (ECOG) that is frequently used in the USA. The Karnofski scale [4] is more detailed.

In general higher response rates to chemotherapy are reported in previously untreated patients than in those with disease recurred after prior treatment with radi-

Table 1 WHO performance status scale

Status	Scales
Fully active, able to carry out all predisease activities without restriction	0
Restricted in strenuous activity but ambulatory and be able to carry out light work or pursue sedentary occupation	1
Ambulatory and capable of all self care but unable to carry out any light work. Up and about more than 50% waking hours	2
Capable of only limited self care; confined to bed or chair more than 50% waking hours	3
Completely disabled. Unable to carry out any self care and confined totally to bed or chair	4

ation or operation [5]. Previous chemotherapy also affects response rates to subsequent second line chemotherapy.

Tumor factors

Several studies demonstrate that T and N (UICC, 1978) tumor staging standards are directly related to response rates to chemotherapy with smaller tumors responding more frequently [6, 7]. Furthermore it has been shown that regional metastases respond less frequently than primary tumors [8]. It is generally reported that local regional disease responds better to chemotherapy than distant metastases. Williams et al. [9], however, found that distant metastases are significantly more likely to respond than local regional disease.

The influence of site of origin within the head and neck on response rate to chemotherapy remains unclear. In 1975 Bertino et al. [10] reported that the highest response rates with methotrexate were seen with primary tumors in the oral cavity and oropharynx and the lowest response rates were found in tumors of the nasopharynx and hypopharynx. A recent review of the literature on the subject by Pitman and Bertino [5], however, fails to confirm a response advantage of oral cavity cancer over other sites. Despite suggestions of higher response rates to combinations of drugs for particular sites, no head and neck site clearly benefits more from chemotherapy than another [11].

Degree of histological differentiation may be another prognostic variable. Bleomycin for instance has been reported to be more effective against well differentiated squamous cell carcinomas as compared to poorly differentiated carcinomas [12]. However, Hong and Shapsay [13] found no difference in overall response rates among well differentiated and poorly differentiated lesions, using a combination of cisplatin and bleomycin. Also, no relationship between histological grading of head and neck carcinoma and response to chemotherapy was found by Jorgensen [14]. The influence of histological differentiation, therefore, remains to be defined.

Treatment factors

Single agents

To date, the best single agents for squamous cell carcinomas of the head and neck are methotrexate, cisplatin and bleomycin. Methotrexate is the single drug for which most experience has been accumulated. Response rates for this drug have varied from 75% to 24% in various series. Reported response rates for bleomycin varied from 93% to 6% and for cisplatin from 71% to 23% [15]. The optimal way to administer these drugs has been a matter of debate for a long time. The weekly administration of methotrexate seems to be the most optimal one, and high-dose methotrexate with leucovorin rescue does not seem to be superior to the standard dose of 40-60 mg/m^2/week [16]. It has been suggested that response to bleomycin is dose-dependent rather than schedule-dependent [17]. Different schedules of administration of cisplatin have been investigated in patients with advanced head and neck cancer. The response rates were quite comparable between series [15]. In a randomized trial Sako found no difference in response after 120 mg/m^2 of cisplatin as compared with 20 mg/m^2/day × 5 [18].

Although methotrexate is considered standard palliative treatment for patients with advanced head and neck cancer, a recently performed randomized study indicated that cisplatin and methotrexate are equally effective in the treatment of recurrent head and neck squamous cell carcinoma [19]. In this trial cisplatin was given at a dose of 50 mg/m^2 i.v. on days 1 and 8 every four weeks, while methotrexate was given at what is considered the optimal dose of 40-60 mg/m^2/week i.v.

Multiple drug regimens

In many trials it has been attempted to improve the response rate by combining antineoplastic agents. However, few of these studies have been performed in a randomized fashion, comparing one single agent with a combination. In table 2 randomized studies comparing single agent chemotherapy versus multiple drug regi-

Table 2 Comparison of combination and single-agent chemotherapy for recurrent head and neck cancer in randomized studies

Investigator	Drugs used	No. of patients	Response rate (%)	
Williams [9]	methotrexate	68	16	n. s.
	cisplatin, vinblastine, bleomycin	66	20	
Kaplan [45]	methotrexate	61	26	s. s.
	methotrexate, bleomycin, cisplatin	61	46	
Deconti [16]	methotrexate	81	26	n. s.
	methotrexate + leucovorin rescue	80	24	
	methotrexate + LR, cyclophosphamide and cytarabine	76	18	
Drelichman [46]	methotrexate	24	33.3	n. s.
	cisplatin, vincristine, bleomycin	27	40.7	
Jacobs [47]	cisplatin	40	18	n. s.
	cisplatin, methotrexate	39	33	
David [48]	cisplatin	30	13	n. s.
	cisplatin, methotrexate, bleomycin	27	11	

mens have been summarized. Only one of these studies showed superiority of combination over single agent chemotherapy.

Non-randomized trials suggest that cisplatin-containing regimens reveal higher response rates than non-platinum-containing regimens [20, 21]. The majority of the 2-drug combinations reported in 1982 have a 30-40% response rate in advanced recurrent head and neck cancer when cisplatin is included in the combination compared with 25-30% when it is not. An exception is the combination of cisplatin and 5-Fu which showed a response rate of 70% [22]. This is not quite unexpected since this combination was found extremely effective also when used as initial therapy before operation and/or radiotherapy, showing response rates of 88.5% to 94% [23, 24]. 5-Fluoro-uracil has only limited activity, when used as a single agent [25]. Reported response rates are in the order of 15% (range 0-33%). The reported clinical efficacy of the combination is in accordance with experimental data and suggest a synergistic effect of the two drugs [26, 27]. No data are available comparing this interesting combination with cisplatin alone. Recently a prospective randomized trial has been activated within the European Organization for the Research on Treatment of Cancer (EORTC) comparing cisplatin and 5-fluoro-uracil versus cisplatin alone versus cisplatin, methotrexate, bleomycin and vincristin in patients with advanced squamous carcinoma of the head and neck.

Adjuvant chemotherapy

The concept of integration of chemotherapy into combined modality treatment for the primary management of advanced head and neck cancer is increasingly being applied. The rationale of this approach is the recognition that operation and radiotherapy have reached a plateau in their ability to cure head and neck cancer and that even combinations of radiotherapy and operation have not so far significantly improved survival figures for patients with advanced stages of disease. There are three theoretical mechanisms whereby chemotherapy may be effective as an adjuvant to operation and/or radiotherapy: initial tumour shrinkage, sensitization of radiotherapy and the destruction of micrometastases. The use of adjuvant chemotherapy in its various settings will be discussed.

Induction chemotherapy

Induction chemotherapy aims at initial tumor shrinkage. Chemotherapy ranks first in the order of treatment based on the experiences that chemotherapy is more effective when the blood supply to the tumor has not been seriously interfered with by operation or radiotherapy.

Induction chemotherapy has been reported in many studies regarding patients with advanced head and neck cancer to have a favorable influence both in terms of tumor volume reduction and survival [20, 24, 28, 29]. Improved survival has been demonstrated for patients achieving a complete response to chemotherapy prior to local therapy, compared to patients with a partial response or no response to chemotherapy [30, 31, 32]. The design of induction chemotherapy regimens therefore, should allow for a high percentage of complete responders. Weaver et al. [33] have shown that the number of cycles of initial chemotherapy is of importance in this regard: three cycles of initial 5-fluoro-uracil and cisplatin result in a much higher complete response rate than one or two cycles [33]. In most of the studies carried out to date delay of standard treatment has been considered a potential disadvantage of induction chemotherapy, but thus far this has not been shown to be detrimental to patients' survival.

Induction chemotherapy did not appear to affect wound healing or limit surgical reconstructive techniques. It is essential that the margins of excision after chemotherapy are determined on the basis of the original extent of the tumor before chemotherapy. It has been a general experience that in patients demonstrating complete response to chemotherapy subsequent determination of adequate margins for surgical resection constitutes a difficult problem. The extent of the tumor, therefore, should be recorded on diagrams before the start of chemotherapy as accurately as possible. The evidence on the value of plotting out the extent of the tumor with submucosal injected deposits of Indian ink is conflicting. Radiation therapy following initial chemotherapy and operation also does not result in increased adverse effects of radiation.

Almost all of the studies in which induction chemotherapy has been used, however, are of a retrospective nature. The few prospective randomized studies on the value of induction chemotherapy so far carried out have not shown that this type of adjuvant chemotherapy significantly alters overall survival, disease-free survival or patterns of relapse [34, 35, 36]. The chemotherapy regimens used in these prospective studies, however, certainly do not meet todays standards of effective chemotherapy. The value of induction chemotherapy therefore has yet to be proven through well designed prospective randomized trials.

Chemotherapy and simultaneous radiotherapy

The object of combining chemotherapy with radiotherapy is to improve local complete responses to radiotherapy and decrease local recurrences. To take advantage of any enhanced effects resulting from direct interaction between drug and radiation, it is necessary that the two modalities be administered simultaneously or in close temporal proximity.

Bleomycin has been most frequently used in this setting. Two recent reports on randomized trials of simultaneous bleomycin and radiation therapy showed improved response rates, but no differences in survival [37, 38]. Cachin et al. [39] in an older study also could not demonstrate any difference between radiotherapy alone and combined radiation and bleomycin. In a randomized study Lo et al. [40] have found improved local control as well as survival from combining 5-fluoro-uracil and irradiation only in patients with oral cancer. Various multiple drug regimens have been used concurrently with radiotherapy without resulting in any significant increase in survival. In the majority of the above mentioned studies enhanced normal tissue reactions have been seen from the simultaneous use of these two treatment modalities.

Recently there is much interest in the use of cisplatin as a radio-enhancer. In several studies with combined cisplatin and radiotherapy higher complete response rates were observed than expected from radiation alone [41-43]. Pinedo et al. [44] demonstrated the feasibility of daily administration of cisplatin as a radio-enhancer. Within the EORTC a phase II study combining radiation and cisplatin has recently been started.

Maintenance chemotherapy (after local/regional treatment)

Adjuvant chemotherapy following surgery and/or radiotherapy - i.e. adjuvant chemotherapy in its strict sense - aims at destruction of micrometastases or microresidual tumor. Chemotherapy is started shortly after operation or radiotherapy when the total number of tumor cells, if any are still present, is in the chemotherapeutically curable range. This type of adjuvant chemotherapy has been shown to be effective in several tumors in other areas. However, no data are available in head and neck cancer of studies comparing patients having adjuvant chemotherapy following operation and/or radiotherapy versus no further treatment. In the few studies in which maintenance chemotherapy has been attempted, for a variety of reasons only a small percentage of patients were able to complete the chemotherapie programs. Lack of patient compliance was an important factor*. Another more basic problem associated with the design of studies of this type is the present lack of accurate knowledge of the prognostic factors that put patients with head and neck cancer at high risk for distant metastases.

---

* Wolf, G. T., Personal communication.

Summary

Active drugs and combinations of drugs against head and neck cancer are available today. A combination of cisplatin and 5-fluoro-uracil appears to be the most effective one. Palliation with chemotherapy for recurrent or metastatic disease has not been associated with a significant prolongation of life. The main emphasis on the use of chemotherapy in head and neck cancer should be on its integration into combined modality primary treatment. Such adjuvant chemotherapy at present, however, is still to be considered in the investigational stage. It is of paramount importance that adjuvant chemotherapy studies are well designed and carried out in a prospective randomized way to ensure that meaningful data will be obtained.

References

[1] Warr, D., S. McKinney, I. Tannock: Influence of measurement error on assessment of tumor response. Proc. Am. Soc. Clin. Oncol. **2** (1983) 226.
[2] Micheau, C., J. M. Richard, P. Marandas et al.: La régression tumorale après chemothérapie locale dans les carcinomes des voies aéro-digestives supérieures. Ann. Oto-Laryng. (Paris) **100** (1983) 577.
[3] Amer, M. H., M. Al-Sarraf, V. K. Vaitkevicius: Factors that affect response to chemotherapy and survival of patients with head and neck cancer. Cancer **43** (1979) 2203.
[4] Manual for staging of cancer. American Joint Committee on Cancer, second edition. J. B. Lippincott Company, Philadelphia 1983.
[5] Pitman, S. W., J. R. Bertino: Chemotherapy of squamous head and neck cancer. In: Oral oncology (I. van der Waal, G. B. Snow, eds.), pp. 217–249. Martinus Nijhoff Publishing, The Hague 1984.
[6] Decker, D. A., A. Drelichman, J. Jacobs et al.: Adjuvant chemotherapy with cis-diamino-dichloroplatinum II and 120-hour infusion 5-Fluorouracil in Stage III and IV squamous cell carcinoma of the head and neck. Cancer **51** (1983) 1353.
[7] Baker, S. R., R. W. Makuch, G. T. Wolff: Preoperative cisplatin and bleomycin therapy in head and neck squamous carcinoma. Arch. Otolaryngol. **107** (1981) 683.
[8] Kraut, M., M. Kies, L. Gordon et al.: Primary head and neck cancers are more responsive than metastatic nodal disease to combination chemotherapy. Proc. ASCO **24** (1983) 166.
[9] Williams, S. D., L. H. Einhorn, E. Velez-Garcia et al.: Chemotherapy of head and neck cancer: comparison of cisplatin and vinblastine and bleomycin (PVB) versus methotrexate (MTX). Proc. Am. Soc. Clin. Onc. **1** (1982) 202.
[10] Bertino, J. R., B. Boston, R. L. Capizzi: The role of chemotherapy in the management of cancer of the head and neck. A review. Cancer **36** (1975) 752.
[11] Mead, G. M., C. Jacobs: Changing role of chemotherapy in treatment of head and neck cancer. Amer. J. of Med. **73** (1982) 582.
[12] Ichikawa, T.: Bleomycin a new antitumor antibiotic (as a specific agent against squamous cell carcinoma). J. Jap. Med. Assoc. **61** (1969) 487.
[13] Hong, W. K., S. M. Shapsay: Treatment of previously untreated stage III and IV squamous cell carcinoma of the head and neck. Otolaryng. Clin. N. Am. **13** (1980) 521.
[14] Jorgensen, K., J. Schlichting: Relationship between histologic grading of head and neck tumours and regression after chemotherapy. Acta Radiol. Oncol. **19** (1980) 357.

[15] Taylor, S. G.: Head and neck cancer. In: Cancer chemotherapy 1979. The EORTC Cancer Chemotherapy Annual I (H. M. Pinedo, ed.), pp. 237-256. Excerpta Medica, Amsterdam 1979.
[16] DeConti, R. C., D. Schoenfeld: A randomized prospective comparism of intermittent methotrexate, methotrexate with leucovorin, and a methotrexate combination in head and neck cancer. Cancer **48** (1981) 1061.
[17] Issell, B. F., G. Borsis, J. C. D'Aoust et al.: Dibromodulcitol plus bleomycin compared with bleomycin alone in head and neck cancer. Cancer Chemother. Pharmacol. **8** (1982) 171.
[18] Sako, K., M. S. Razack, J. Kalnius: Chemotherapy for advanced and recurrent squamous cell carcinoma of the head and neck with high and low dose cis-diamminedichloroplatinum. Amer. J. Surg. **136** (1978) 529.
[19] Hong, W. K., S. Schaeffer, B. Issel et al.: A prospective randomized trial of methotrexate versus cisplatin in the treatment of recurrent squamous cell carcinoma of the head and neck. Cancer **52** (1983) 206.
[20] Taylor, S. G.: Head and neck cancer. In: Cancer Chemotherapy 1983. The EORTC Cancer Chemotherapy Annual V (H. M. Pineda, ed.), pp. 291-306. Excerpta Medica, Amsterdam 1983.
[21] Mika, H.: Studie zur intraarteriellen mono- und polychemotherapie von Mundhöhlen- und Oropharynxkarzinomen: Methotrexat (MTX) im Vergleich zur Kombination Vincristin-Methotrexat-Bleomycin-Cisplatin (VMBP). Arch. Oto-rhino-laryngol. **237** (1982) 59.
[22] Kish, J., A. Drelichman, A. Weaver et al.: Cis-platinum and 5-fluoro-uracil infusion in patients with recurrent and dissiminated epidermoid cancer of the head and neck. Proc. Am. Soc. Clin. Oncol. **1** (1982) 193.
[23] Kish, J., A. Drelichman, J. Jacobs et al.: Clinical trials of cisplatin and 5-FU infusions as initial treatment for advanced squamous cell carcinoma of the head and neck. Cancer Treat. Rep. **66** (1982) 471.
[24] Weaver, A., S. Fleming, H. Vandenberg et al.: Cis-platinum and 5-fluoro-uracil on initial therapy in advanced epidermoid cancers of the head and neck. Head & Neck Surg. **4** (1982) 370.
[25] Carter, S. K.: The chemotherapy of head and neck cancer. Seminars in Oncology **4** (1977) 413.
[26] Vierri, T., D. Coulter, F. Valeriore: Interval and sequence dependent lethal effects of cis-diamminedichloroplatinum (Cis-Pl) in combination with other agents. Proc. Am. Soc. Clin. Oncol. **20** (1979) 202.
[27] Schabel, Jr. F. M., M. W. Trader, W. R. Laster Jr., et al.: Cis-dichlorodiammineplatinum (II): combination chemotherapy and cross-resistance studies with tumors of mice. Cancer Treat. Rep. **63** (1979) 1459.
[28] Schuller, D. E., H. E. Wilson: Preoperative reductive chemotherapy for locally advanced carcinoma of the oral cavity, oropharynx and hypopharynx. Cancer **51** (1983) 15.
[29] Al-Sarraf, M., A. Drelichman, S. Peppard, et al.: Adjuvant cisplatinum and 5 Fu 96 hour infusion in previously untreated epidermoid cancers of the head and neck. Proc. Amer. Soc. Clin. Oncol. **22** (1981) 428.
[30] Perry, D. L., R. K. Davis, R. B. Weiss: Combined modality treatment with combination chemotherapy for advanced squamous cell carcinomas of the head and neck. Proc. Amer. Soc. Clin. Oncol. **1** (1982) 93.
[31] Schwert, R., J. R. Jacobs, J. Crissman, et al.: Improved survival in patients with advanced head and neck cancer achieving complete clinical response to induction chemotherapy. Prof. Amer. Soc. Clin. Oncol. **1** (1982) 193.
[32] Kies, M., M. Kraut, L. Gorden, et al.: Improved survival and pretreatment characteris-

tics of complete responders to combination chemotherapy in advanced head and neck cancer. Proc. Amer. Soc. Clin. Oncol. **2** (1983) 159.
[33] Weaver, A., J. A. Kish, J. Ensly, et al.: Superior clinical complete response rate and survival with initial cisplatinum and 120 hours 5 FU infusion before definitive therapy in patients with locally advanced head and neck cancer. Book of Abstracts Joint Meeting of the Society of Surg. Oncol. and the Society of Head and Neck Surgeons, New York, NY. (May 1984) 168.
[34] Wolf, G. T., C. Jacobs, R. W. Makucj, et al.: Cisplatin (DDP) and bleomycin (BLM) adjuvant chemotherapy in head and neck cancer. Results of the head and neck contracts program. Proceedings Intern. Conf. on head and neck cancer, Baltimore. **130** (1984) 43.
[35] Taylor, S., E. Applebaum, D. Caldarelli, et al.: A randomized trial of methotrexate with leucovorin as adjuvant treatment of patients with head and neck squamous cancer. Proceedings Intern. Conf. on head and neck cancer, Baltimore. **44** (1984) 43.
[36] Kun, L. E., R. U. Toohill, P. S. Ritch, et al.: Effect of induction chemotherapy in advanced cancers of the upper aerodigestive tract (UAD): a prospective, randomized trial. Proceedings Intern. Conf. on head and neck cancer, Baltimore. **199** (1984) 43.
[37] Shanta, V., S. Krishnamurthi, M. Sharma: Irradiation, bleomycin and hyperbaric oxygen in the treatment of oral carcinoma. Acta Radiol. Oncol. **22** (1983) 13.
[38] Fu, K. K., T. L. Phillips, I. J. Silverberg, et al.: Combined radiotherapy and chemotherapy with bleomycin and methotrexate for advanced head and neck cancer: interim rapport of an NCOG randomized trial. Proc. Amer. Soc. Clin. Oncol. **2** (1983) 160.
[39] Cachin, Y., A. Jortay, H. Sancho, et al.: Preliminary results of a randomized EORTC study comparing radiotherapy and concomittant bleomycin to radiotherapy alone in epidermoid carcinomas of the oropharynx. Eur. J. Cancer **13** (1977) 1389.
[40] Lo, T. C., A. L. Wiley, F. J. Ansfield, et al.: Combined radiation therapy and 5-fluorouracil for advanced squamous cell carcinoma of the oral cavity and oropharynx. A randomized study. Am. J. Roentgenol. **126** (1976) 229.
[41] Haselow, L. E., G. S. Adams, M. M. Oken, et al.: Cisplatinum with radiation therapy for locally advanced unresectable head and neck cancer. Proc. Em. Soc. Clin. Oncol. **2** (1983) 159.
[42] High, M., L. Heuser, C. H. Schmidt, et al.: Simultane Cisplatin- und Bestrahlungstherapie lokal fortgeschrittener Plattenepithelkarzonome der Kopf-Hals-Region. Dtsch. Med. Wochenschr. **46** (1983) 1743.
[43] Leipzig, B.: Cisplatin sensitization to radiotherapy of squamous cell carcinomas of the head and neck. Am. J. Surg. **146** (1983) 462.
[44] Pinedo, H. M., A. B. M. F. Karim, W. H. van Vliet, et al.: Daily cis-dichlorodiammine platinum (II) as a radioenhancer: a preliminary toxicity report. J. of Cancer Res. Clin. Oncol. **105** (1983) 79.
[45] Kaplan, B. K., S. E. Vogl: Methotrexate, bleomycin and diamminedichloroplatinum in squamous cancers of the head and neck, cervix and other sites. Proc. Am. Soc. Clin. Oncol. **19** (1978) 312.
[46] Drelichman, A., G. Cummings, M. Al-Sarraf: A randomized trial of the combination of cisplatinum, oncovin and bleomycin (COB) versus methotrexate in patients with advanced squamous cell carcinoma of the head and neck. Cancer **52** (1983) 399.
[47] Jacobs, C., F. Meyers, C. Hendrickson, et al.: A randomized phase III study of cisplatin with or without methotrexate for recurrent squamous cell carcinoma of the head and neck. Cancer **52** (1983) 1563.
[48] David, S., W. Kessler: Randomized comparison of Cis-diamminechloroplatinum versus Cis-diamminedichloroplatinum, Methotrexate and Bleomycin in recurrent squamous cell carcinoma of the had and neck. Cancer Chemother. Pharmacol. **3** (1979) 57.

Transmaxillary and transoral approach to invasive tumors of the skull base

E. Halves, J. Reuther, W. Richter

We will report some of the special problems in the treatment of invasive tumors of the skull base. An analysis of the last 100 benign skull base tumors from the last 2 years revealed about 34% of problematic cases. Those are tumors, that probably could not be removed with one single operation. We had 8 recurrent and 16 invasive adenomas of the pituitary gland, 6 craniopharyngiomas, 1 invasive meningioma and 1 chordoma. Two of these cases will now be presented.

The first patient was 33 years old when he came to our department in January 1983 with a recurrent inactive pituitary adenoma. He had already been operated on by the ethmoidal and sphenoidal route, but now had a suprasellar mass proved by an air study. The surgeon could only remove the tumor subtotally with partial filling of the tumor cavity by a muscle graft. On admission in 1983 the patient now had a

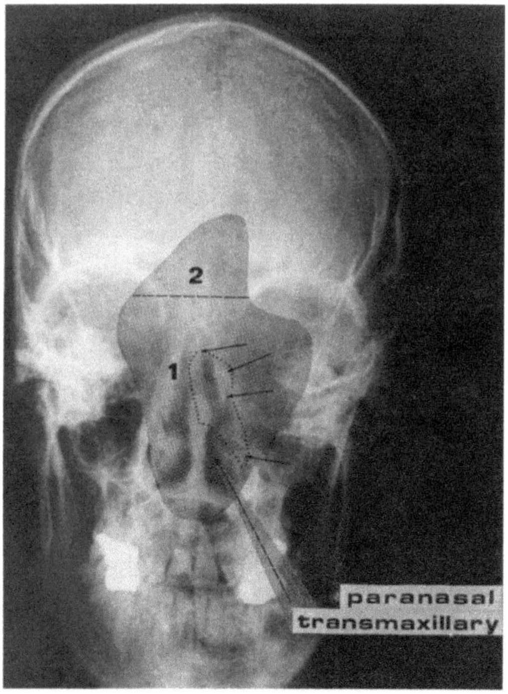

Fig. 1 P.H., 33 years. Invasive pituitary adenoma. Bone reconstruction after paranasal transmaxillary approach (dotted line, wire marked by arrows).

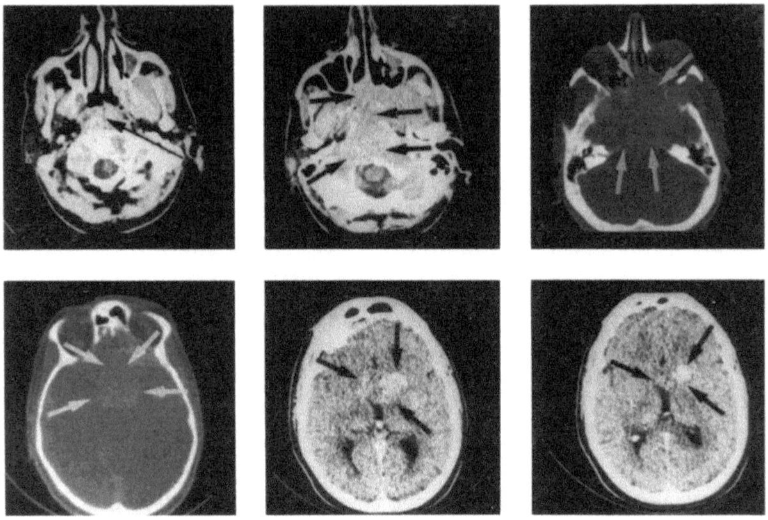

Fig. 2a H. P., 33 years. Hormonal inactive pituitary adenoma invading the skull base and the brain from the lower clivus to the paraventricular region.

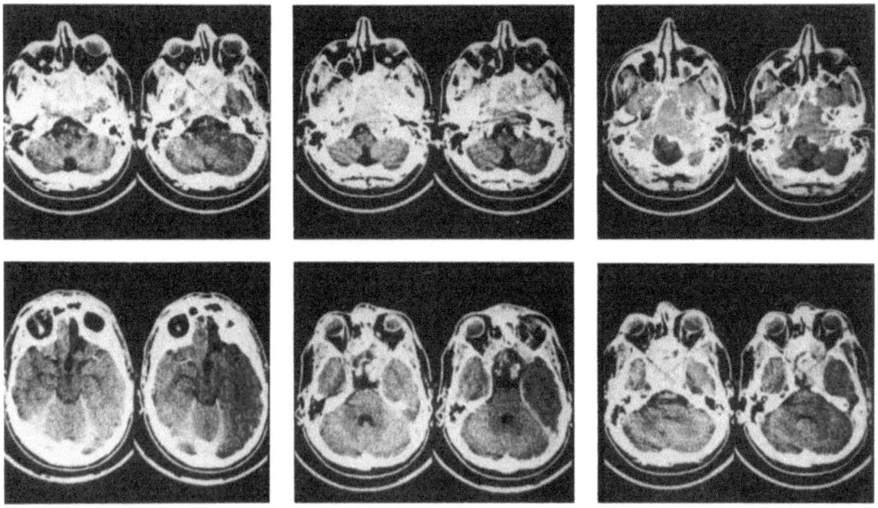

Fig. 2b CT scan 1 year after the two stage operation.

6 years history of blindness in the left eye with visual deterioration on the right and the CT scan revealed a giant recurrent adenoma with a large suprasellar mass and a huge ethmoidal and sphenoidal cavity filled by an inhomogenous mass (fig. 2a).

The huge mass of intrasphenoidal and suprasellar tumor made it impossible to reach all, or even most, of the tumor by one single approach. Although over the last ten years we have had very good experience with the transnasal approach even

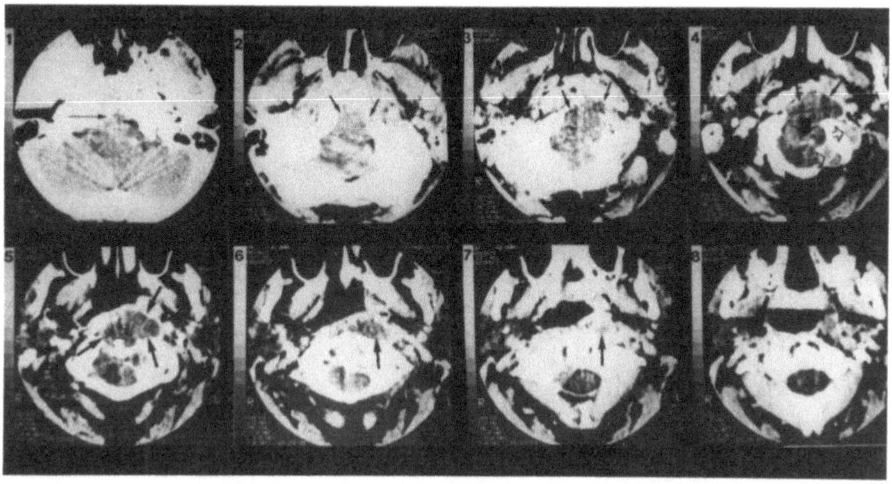

Fig. 3 F. M., 26 years. Chordoma of the lower clivus (1) and the intra- (4) and para-atlantal region (6–8).

in giant pituitary adenomas, in this individual case the bilateral ethmoidal and caudo-clival extension required a wider opening than the narrow rhinoseptal approach. That is why we chose a left paranasal incision after Moure, with partial resection of the nasal and maxillary bone and subsequent reconstruction (fig. 1). The disadvantage of all oblique approaches to the sella turcica was mainly abolished by an extensive resection of the ethmoid bone on the left. Nevertheless there were many problems within the huge tumor cavity including profused bleeding from the tumor and the granular tissue and strings of connective tissue surrounded by the soft tumor, so that an anatomical separation was nearly impossible and consequently topographical orientation was very difficult. The goal of this approach should be a tumor resection below the sellar entrance line (fig. 1) in order to leave the suprasellar portion of the tumor (fig. 1) for the second operation of the two stage procedure by the subfrontal route. This was achieved sufficiently on both sides within the ethmoid and the sphenoid bone down to the medial borders of the cavernous sinus.

The profused bleeding and the extensive destruction of the clivus made complete dissection at the basal part of the tumor too dangerous. To achieve sufficient haemostasis nearly the whole tumor cavity had to be refilled with haemostyptics. The further progress of the patient was uneventful and the reconstructed bone (fig. 1) led to a good cosmetic result. Three months later the suprasellar part of the tumor was nearly completely removed, by using a right frontal craniotomy and a subfrontal approach. Only in the left cavernous sinus some adenomas tissue might have been left. At the end of this operation we reconstructed the diaphragm of the sella by a periostal flap in order to separate the subarachnoidal space from the ethmoidal and sphenoidal tumor cavity.

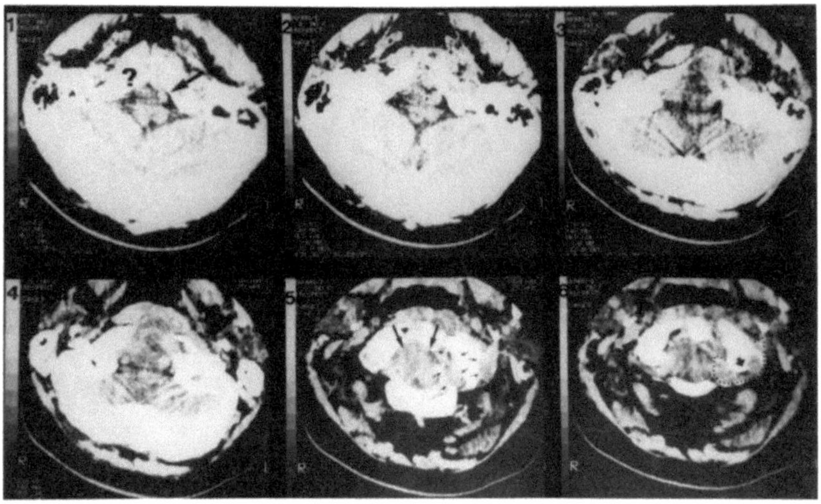

Fig. 4a F. M., 26 years. Cranio-cervical CT scan 1 month after transoral operation. Remnants of the tumor around the left condyle.

Postoperative ophthalmological controls revealed a slight improvement, the patient did well and he was soon able to work. The CT-control one year later (fig. 2b) demonstrated the residual tumor tissue around the lower clivus but no more tumor in the suprasellar area, whereas the tissue in the large cavity of the ethmoidal and sphenoidal bone could not clearly be differentiated by CT.

The question still at issue is how to deal with the remaining tumor whether we should wait, irradiate or operate a fourth time, possibly by a transoral route.

The second patient was 26 years of age when he came to our department with a chordoma of the lower clivus, proved by epipharyngeal biopsy. The tissue material did not show any indication of malignancy, so that we had to consider a similar therapeutic management as in the previous patient.

After a less characteristic history with headaches he developed pains and weakness in the right arm and shoulder and on admission he had acute dysarthria, dysphagia and other signs and symptoms of medullary compression. Craniocervical CT-scan (fig. 3) revealed destruction of the lower third of the clivus, the ventral margin of the foramen magnum and of the arch of the atlas. The spinal cord and medulla oblongata were displaced dorsally and to the right by a mostly isodense tumor without significant contrast enhancement. Angiography did not show pathological tumor vessels, but a nearly unilateral development of the left vertebral artery. The rapidly developing symptoms required an immediate decompressive operation, but the bilateral extension of the tumor around the medulla, the left vertebral artery, possibly surrounded by tumor and the unknown further invasion by the tumor made the decision for the most effective but less dangerous approach very difficult. We chose the transoral approach with the patient in a supine posi-

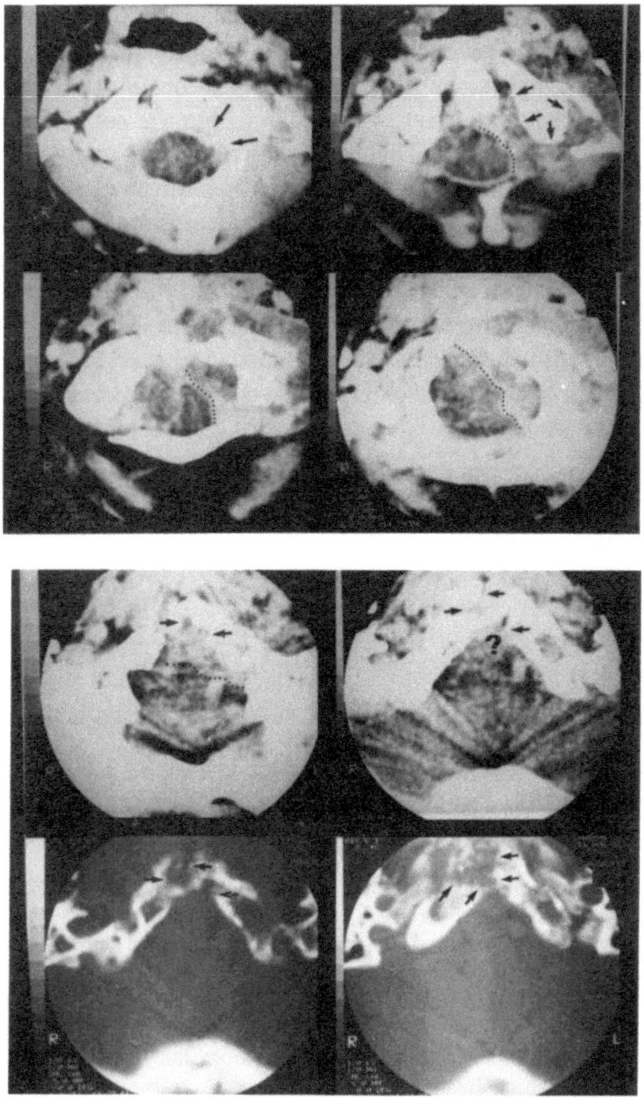

Fig. 4b, c Five months after the operation demonstrating tumor recurrence intraspinal (dotted line), around the condyle, and within the clivus (arrows).

tion, oral intubation and splitting of the soft palate. The posterior wall of the pharynx was incised in the midline from the lower third of the clivus down arch of the atlas, that had to be partially resected in order to remove the tumor from the ventral surface of the spinal dura. A separation of the purely extradural tumor from the body of the atlas, the medial circumference of the left condyle, and the clivus was achieved. Only the lateral parts around the left condyle could not be reached by this approach and had to be left behind. The pharyngeal wall and the soft palate were closed by a three layered suture and the postoperative course was uneventful. The patient improved very soon from his medullary and neural compression syndromes. The CT scan one month after the operation (fig. 4a) showed some tumor tissue round the left lateral mass of the atlas within the spinal canal and at the left lateral margin of the condyle. The good clinical results were the main reason, that we did no further intervention at this time, bus unfortunately the patient deteriorated rapidly four months later once more developing severe signs and symptoms of medullary and caudal nerves compression. The CT at this time (fig. 4b, c) revealed a large recurrence of the tumor around the ventral and left lateral part of the atlas narrowing the epipharynx as well as the spinal canal from the left. Further surgical or radio-therapeutical interventions seemed to be in vain considering the rapid growth and the extremely unfavourable location of the tumor and the patient died one month later from respiratory insufficiency.

This only temporary success in the removal of a histologically benign tumor raises the question whether a different therapeutical approach might have led to a more satisfactory result in the individual case.

References

Alonso, W. A., P. Black, G. H. Connor et al.: Transoral transpalatal approach for resection of clival chordoma. Laryngoscope **81** (1971) 1626.

Apuzzo, M. L. J., M. H. Weiss, J. S. Heiden: Transoral exposure of the atlantoaxial region. Neurosurgery **3** (1978) 201-207.

Arana-Iniguez, R., L. A. Castillo, P. Benedek, et al.: Transoral approach in clivus and high cervical chordomas. Acta Neurol. Latinoamer. **14** (1968) 65-73.

Bushe, K.-A., E. Halves: Modifizierte Technik bei transnasaler Operation der Hypophysengeschwülste. Acta Neurochir. (Wien) **41** (1978) 163-175.

Delgado, T. E., E. Garrido, R. D. Harwick: Labiomandibular, transoral approach to chordomas in the clivus and upper cervical spine. Neurosurgery **8** (1981) 675-679.

Gutkelch, A. N., R. G. Williams: Anterior approach to recurrent chordomas of the clivus. J. Neurosurg. **36** (1972) 670-672.

Halves, E., K. A. Bushe: Trans-sphenoidal operation on craniopharyngiomas with extrasellar extensions. The advantage of the operating endoscope. Acta Neurochir. (suppl.) **28, 2** (1979) 362.

Halves, E., N. Sörensen: Indications for the trans-sphenoidal approach to craniopharyngioma operations in youth and childhood. In: Tumours and the central Nervous System in Infancy and Childhood (D. Voth, P. Gutjahr, C. Langmaid, eds.), pp. 270-275. Springer Verlag, Berlin-Heidelberg-New York 1982.

Hamberger, C. A., G. Hammer, G. Norlen, et al.: Transantrosphenoidal hypophysectomy. Arch. Otolaryngol. **74** (1961) 2-8.

Hardy, J.: Trans-sphenoidal hypophysectomy. J. Neurosurg. **34** (1971) 582-594.

Harwick, R. D., A. S. Miller: Craniocervical chordomas. Am. J. Surg. **138** (1979) 512-516.

Krayenbühl, H., M. G. Yasargil: Cranial chordomas. Prog. Neurol. **6** (1975) 380-434.

Landolt, A. M., C. B. Wilson: Tumors of the sella and parasellar area in adults. In: Neurological Surgery, ed. 2 (J. R. Youmans, ed.), vol. 5, pp. 3107-3162. W. B. Saunders, Philadelphia 1982.

Laws, E. R., jr., M. J. Ebersold, D. G. Piepgras: The results of transsphenoidal surgery in specific clinical entities. In: Management of Pituitary Adenomas and Related Lesions with Emphasis on Transsphenoidal Microsurgery (E. R. Laws jr., R. V. Randall, E. B. Kern et al., eds.), pp. 277-306. Appleton-Century-Crofts, New York 1982.
Moure, E. J.: Des fibromes dits nasopharyngiens. Bull. et mém. soc. franc. d'ophthalm. Paris 1923.
Mullan, S., R. Naunton, J. Hekmat-Panah, et al.: The use of an anterior approach to ventrally placed tumors in the foramen magnum and vertebral column. J. Neurosurg. **24** (1966) 536-543.
Stevenson, G. C., R. J. Stoney, R. K. Perkins et al.: A transcervical, transclival approach to the ventral surface of the brain stem for removal of a clivus chordoma. J. Neurosurg. **24** (1966) 544-551.
Svien, H. J., T. J. Litzow: Removal of certain hypophyseal tumors by the transantral-sphenoid route. J. Neurosurg. **23** (1965) 603-611.
Windle-Taylor, P. C.: Cervical Chordoma: Report of a case and the technique of transoral removal. Br. J. Surg. **64** (1977) 438-441.
Windle-Taylor, P. C.: Cervical Chordoma: Report of a case and the technique of transoral removal. Br. J. Surg. **64** (1977) 438-441.
Wood, B., E. S. Sadar, H. L. Levine, et al.: Surgical problems of the base of the skull. Arch. Otolaryngol. **106** (1980) 1-5.

Transoral approaches for tumor operations on the skull base

R. Schmelzle, N. Schwenzer, K. Jahnke

Introduction

Transoral approaches through the hard and soft palate for the surgical treatment of skull-base tumors are used either alone or in combination with other approaches [1, 3, 5–10].

Besides a simple elevation of the velum and incision of the dorsal pharyngeal wall for exposure of the clivus, sagittal, transversal and curved incisions with partial or complete splitting of the hard and soft palate with or without preservation of blood vessels are performed. Additional approaches from the oral vestibulum to the pterygoid fossa, through the maxillary sinus and via the nose should also be mentioned (figs. 1 a and b).

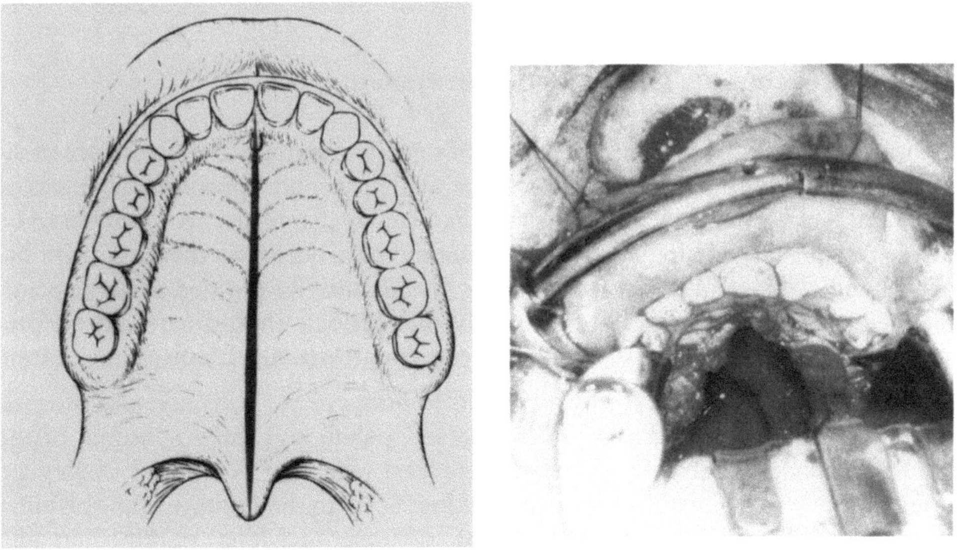

Fig. 1 a, b Midline incision of soft palate and dorsal part of hard palate for exposure of epipharynx and clivus.

Indications

The *indication* for the transoral approach to benign and malignant tumors of the skull-base exists for tumors situated in the nasopharynx, the retromaxillary area and the parapharyngeal space. The surgical techniques include diagnostic and curative procedures, such as exploratory excision, tumor resection and treatment of recurrent tumors. Depending on the size of the tumor, transpalatal, transmaxillary and transnasal approaches must be complemented by additional extraoral approaches.

Pathological data

Up to now, we have used the transoral approach in patients with benign and malignant tumors:

a) Benign tumors: odontogenic tumors such as ameloblastoma and cementoma, chondroma, chordoma, fibrous dysplasia (for biopsy), hemangioma, nasopharyngeal fibroma.
b) Malignant tumors: adenoid cystic carcinoma, carcinoma in pleomorphic adenoma, chondrosarcoma, fibrosarcoma, malignant melanoma, non-Hodgkin lymphoma, rhabdomyosarcoma, squamous cell carcinoma.

These lesions either originated at the skull-base or extended to it secondarily.

Oral approaches and stomatognathic system

Prior to transoral approaches, treatment of dental and gingival illnesses are obviously necessary. For prevention of postoperative infections, previous diagnosis of such illnesses - especially vitality testing and sulcus diagnosis - has proved to be indispensable. On one hand, the *incision* should clearly expose the tumor. On the other hand, damage of the stomatognathic system must be avoided as far as possible. Teeth, periodontal tissues and the alveolar process should carefully be preserved, and special care must be taken to prevent growth disturbances in children.

In edentulous patients, we try by all means to preserve the bony alveolar process, the hard palate, its borderline toward the soft palate and the vestibulum of the mouth. Scars on the alveolar ridge interfere least with later prostheses as they are often found in this place after tooth extraction. Scars in the midline of the alveolar process and the palate are unimportant. Oblique incisions, paramedian and curved scars of the hard palate interfere with the adherence of partial and complete prostheses (figs. 2a-c).

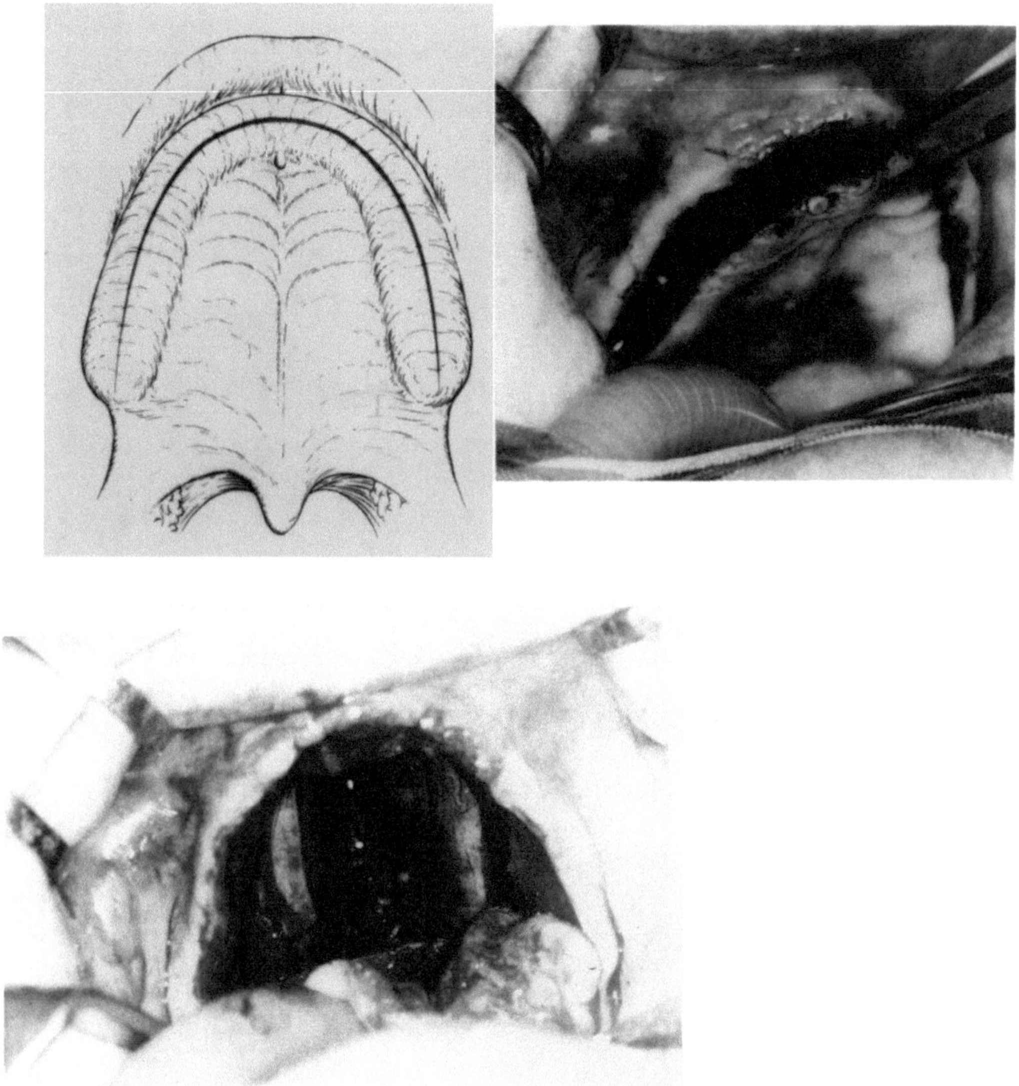

Fig. 2 a–c Transoral approach for removal of a melanoma in a 76-year-old female. After a palatal fenestration the anterior part of the alveolar process remains in its place.

While removing the palatal mucosa, the periosteum of the alveolar ridge should remain on the bone to prevent postoperative bone atrophy. This technique should also be applied with tumors that extend far anteriorly, thus affording an anterior extension of the approach.

In such cases we recommend a bimeatal approach with anterior fenestration and preservation of the bony alveolar process. The resulting bone-bridge does not enhance the viability but facilitates the exact positioning of prostheses in the follow-

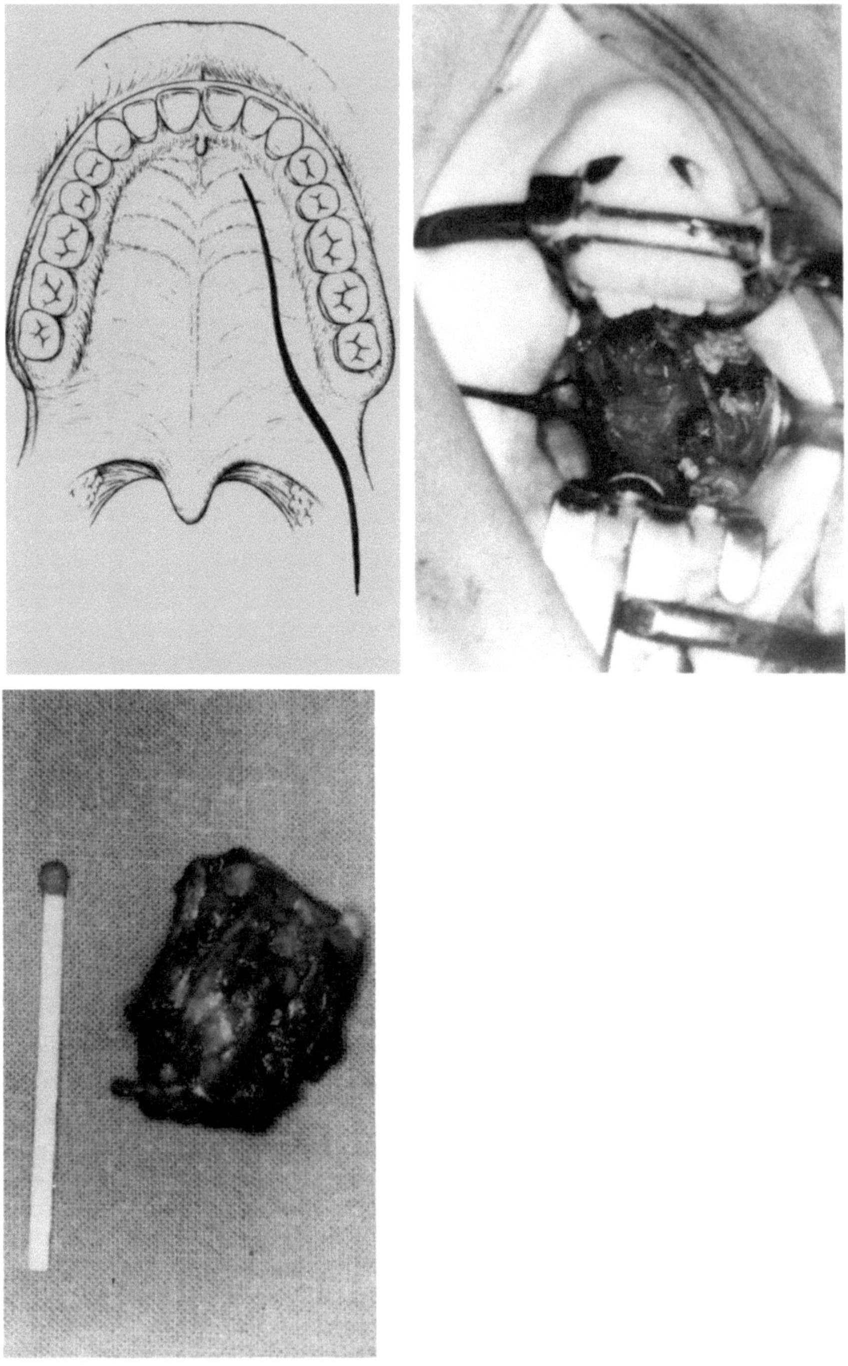

Fig. 3 a-c In a 14-year-old boy, excision of a rhabdomyosarcoma which has previously been irradiated and treated by chemotherapy. Transoral resection via intermaxillary plica and the lateral part of hard palate. The site of the tumor at the skull base is shown in figure 3 b.

up period. In special cases, preservation of the hard palate is also possible, especially by use of the approaches of Owens [5] and Steinzeug [9]. Palate bone and vomer are temporarily resected and are replaced at the end of the operation. For fixation wire osteosynthesis and cover plates are used.

As regards incisions of the soft palate, functional aspects should also be considered: if transverse incisions seem necessary, they should follow the method described by Nessel and Mündnich [4] as well as Denecke and Ey [2].

From our experiences in cleft-palate operations, we generally prefer sagittal midline and lateral incisions, which produce excellent functional results provided appropriate suturing technique of the different woundlayers is used. Elongation of a functionally inadequate velum can be achieved by a Z-plasty. Lateral approaches via the palate, the intermaxillary area and the oral vestibulum prove to be useful in the treatment of small benign lesions of limited size. By following the medial pterygoid muscle, we have even used a lateral oral approach in order to remove a recurrent rhabdomyosarcoma, 2.5 cm in diameter, in the upper parapharyngeal space (figs. 3 a–c).

By continuing the lateral incision of the soft palate to the retromolar region of the mandible the skull-base can be reached via the medial pterygoid muscle. This approach gives good access to the parapharyngeal space including the internal carotid artery and to the nasopharynx. In principle it is a combination of approaches which are usually used 1. in cleft palate operations and 2. in progenia surgery. This combined approach can be used instead of the trans-mandibular approach.

Postoperative treatment is always required to achieve correct and sufficient opening of the mouth. If defects in the hard palate are unavoidable, planning for sufficient retention areas is the prerequisite for defect-prosthetics and thus satisfactory functional results. In addition, the fixation of an artificial palate will prevent undesired cosmetic results and will facilitate later fitting of a permanent facial prosthesis.

Summary

Intraoral approaches play an important role in the treatment of skull-base tumors. Considering the different lesions, as well as the functional aspects of the stomatognathic system postoperatively, cooperation involving different medical specialities including maxillo-facial surgery is recommended. Our own surgical approach for exposing the nasopharynx and the upper parapharyngeal space is described. The approach is used instead of the transmandibular approach. It results in an excellent exposure and does not create any significant functional defect.

References

[1] Blair, V. P.: Congenital atresia or obstruction of air passage. Ann. Otol. **40** (1931) 1021.
[2] Denecke, H. J., W. Ey: Die Operationen der Nase und im Nasopharynx. In: Allg. und spez. Operationslehre, Band V, Teil 1, 3., völlig neubearb. Auflage. Springer Verlag, Berlin-Heidelberg-New York-Tokyo 1984.
[3] Loeb, H. W.: Operative surgery of the nose, throat and ear, pp 155-156. C.V. Mosby Co, St. Louis 1927.
[4] Nessel, E., K. Mündnich: Surgery of the nasopharynx. In: Head and Neck surgery, vol. 2, Face and Facial Skull (H. H. Naumann, ed.). Georg Thieme, Stuttgart 1980.
[5] Owens, H.: Observations in treating seven cases of choanal atresia by the transpalatine approach. Laryngoscope (St. Louis) **61** (1951) 304.
[6] Přecechtěl, L.: Transpalatine operation for choanal atresia. Ann. Oto-laryng. (Paris) **1014** (1938) 187.
[7] Ruddy, L. W.: A transpalatine operation for congenital atresia of the small child or in the infant. Arch. Otolaryng. **41** (1945) 432.
[8] Schweckendiek, H.: Transpalatinale Behandlung angeborener Choanal-Atresien. Z. Hals-, Nasen- u. Ohrenheilk. **42** (1937) 367.
[9] Steinzeug, A.: Ein neues Operationsverfahren zur Beseitigung der Choanenverwachsungen. Arch. Ohren-, Nasen-, Kehlkopfheilk. **137** (1933) 364.
[10] Wilson, C. P.: Observations on the surgery of the nasopharynx. Ann. Otol. (St. Louis) **66** (1957) 5.

Diagnosis - combined treatment of nasopharyngeal angiofibroma

A. S. Dimitriadis, L. Manolidis

Introduction

Essential for the diagnosis and the treatment of a nasopharyngeal angiofibroma is a thorough radiological examination. Juvenile angiofibromas are benign, vascular, locally agressive neoplasms that are preferably treated by surgical resection or irradiation.

In order to better define the tumor 11 patients with juvenile angiofibroma have been studied in a period of the last 5 years by plain films, thin section tomography, CT, angiography and two of them had pre-operative embolization.

The purpose of this paper is to present our experience in the pre-operative radiological examination, in the pre-operative embolization and in the surgical treatment of juvenile angiofibroma (J. A.). Juvenile nasopharyngeal angiofibroma, is a benign, highly vascular, non-infiltrative lesion, arising from the nasopharynx of pubescent males.

Material and methods

Radiological examination of the patients with juvenile angiofibroma begins with plain films of the nasopharynx and paranasal sinuses. Thin section tomography was a second step in AP and lateral projection (fig. 1).

Angiography, is the third step including selective internal and external carotid injections and CT is the fourth step using a fourth generation scanner (EMI 7070) with axial and coronal projections before and after intravenous injection (figs. 2 and 3).

Two of the patients had pre-operative embolization with silastic spheres and gelatin foam (gelfoam). The planning of the surgical treatment or the irradiation of the lesion based on Bryan's classification system.

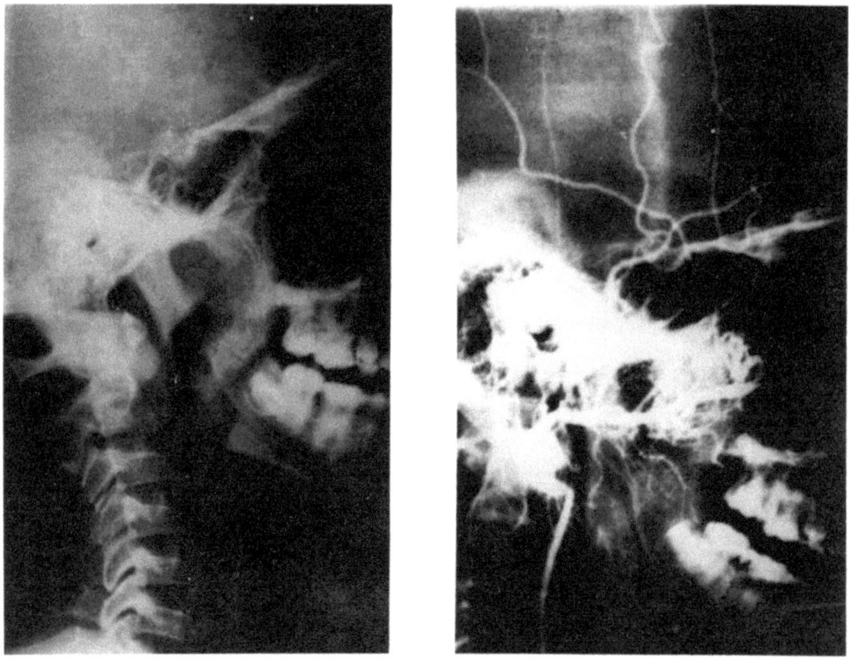

Fig. 1 Case I: a = lateral plain film reveals a nasopharyngeal mass with no erosion of the sphenoid bone or invasion of the surrounding structures, b = angiogram of the same patient.

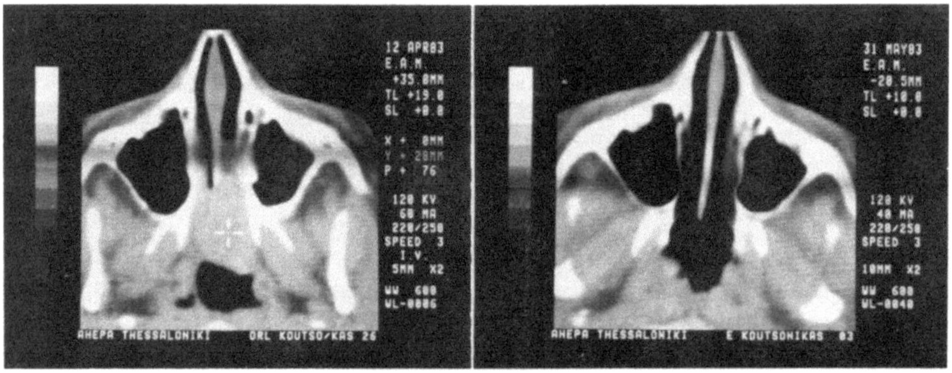

Fig. 2 Case I: a = pre-operative axial scan after contrast injection. Enhancing lesion within left posterior nasal cavity and nasopharynx (cross), b = postoperative axial scan of the same patient.

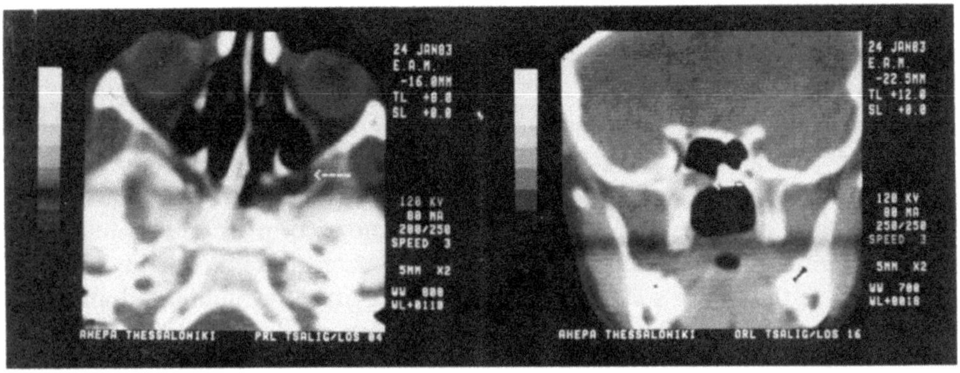

Fig. 3 Case II: Axial (a) and coronal (b) scan reveals a small tumor in the left pterygomaxillary fissure (arrow). Widening of the fissure is apparent.

Surgical technique

The transnasal surgical approach can be used in excising these tumors thus avoiding the various methods currently used in the past (transpalatal, endoral transmaxillary and transtemporal).

The operation is carried out under general anesthesia while the patient is in the classic tonsillectomy position.

After the tumor has been digitally palpated, the palate is retracted outwards and the tumor is removed, trying to avoid mechanical injuries to the adjacent soft tissues.

A strong snare is introduced into the nasopharynx through the nasal cavity and it is properly secured all around the base of the tumor. It is essential that the snare is tightly attached to the base of the neoplasm. As long as we are sure that the above requirement is met, the snare is pulled outwards and the tumor is completely eradicated. It should be kept in mind that the neoplasm is quite hard. It can only be removed completely by eradication as it cannot be expected to be excised sufficiently by using the snare. Postoperative bleeding is slight, therefore no nasopharyngeal packing is required.

Juvenile angiofibromas were treated in 11 patients according to the above-mentioned method. All of them have been followed up by CT scan.

Discussion

Angiofibromas are the most common benign tumors of the nasopharynx, representing 0.5% of all head and neck neoplasms. Common symptoms are nasal obstruction and spontaneous epistaxis. The treatment of the J.A cannot be considered as of a single entity, because of the occurrence in different anatomical compartments and it is the anatomic location that determines the method of treatment. We use the Bryan's classification for J.A. Clinical evaluation alone is not adequate for estimating the size and the extent of the tumor. Plain films and thin section tomography provides information as to tumor location by the indirect evidence of bone erosion and replacement of air-filled structures. However, this does not differentiate between tumorous and non-tumorous soft tissues. The antral bowing sign, the enlargement of the pterygomaxillary fissure (Hoffman sign) and the bony erosions are the radiological signs from the plain films and thin section tomography. The CT appearance of the juvenile angiofibroma has been well described. CT shows how far the tumor has extended and after contrast injection shows the vascular enhancing nature of the lesion. This is a crucial sign in the differential diagnosis. The axial projections show very easily the intracranial extent of the tumor. The intracranial extension to the cavernous sinus region is shown better by CT than other imaging techniques. Angiography may accurately demonstrate the tumor by its vascularity and thus confirm the histological diagnosis. However, angiography does not demonstrate the gross anatomical extent of the lesion because of its tendency to extend through fissures, foramina and sinus compartments. All angiofibromas enhanced more than adjacent muscle. Other nasopharyngeal lesions that may mimic angiofibromas (antral polyps, lymphoma, squamous carcinoma) enhance no more than adjacent muscle tissue. The midline extent of the tumor creates problems in the planning of the surgical treatment and in the planning of the pre-operative embolization or other hemostatic procedures. Our embolization technique, includes first angiography, and then selective catheterization of the appropriate feeding vessels. The embolization is performed by gelfoam. We perform the embolization before the operation (the first patient was operated on seven days after embolization, whereas the second, twenty days after the embolization) and have had no complications from embolization other than those expected.

Of the 11 patients that were operated on, the last two had pre-operative embolization. In these, the amount of blood needed during the operation, was 400 ml, in comparison to the 2000-2500 ml that were needed in the other cases. Two of our patients needed irradiation and were followed up by CT examination. In both of them, some residual tumor tissue was shown by the CT. Follow-up examination with CT is done in those patients who have had pre-operative embolization.

References

[1] Bryan, N. R.: Radiographic management of juvenile angiofibroma. AJRN **2** (1981) 157-166.

[2] Holman, C. B., W. E. Miller: Juvenile nasopharyngeal fibroma - roentgenologic characteristics. AJR **94** (1965) 292-298.

[3] Wilson, G. H., W. N. Hanafee: Angiographic findings in 16 patients with juvenile angiofibroma. Radiology **92** (1969) 279-284.

[4] Weinstein, M. A., et al.: Diagnosis of juvenile angiofibroma by CT. Radiology **126** (1978) 703-705.

[5] Roberson, G. H.: Therapeutic embolization of juvenile angiofibroma. AJR **133** (1979) 657-663.

[6] Lasjaunias, P.: Nasopharyngeal angiofibromas: hazards of embolization. Radiology **136** (1980) 119-123.

Extension of nasopharyngeal tumors to the posterior region of the skull base

J. Traserra, J. Romeu

Introduction

Tumors that arise from the posterior wall of the nasopharynx can follow anyone of these lines of growth:

1. Local growth, without deep infiltration of the mucosa and without bone destruction. Nevertheless, they can metastatize and also involve the related lymph nodes.
2. Sphenoidal invasion. This direction of growth usually implies intracranial spread.
3. Posterior invasion. This is the kind of spread referred to in this paper. The tumor invades the vertebral region from the posterior nasopharyngeol wall.

Anatomical region

The posterior wall of the nasopharynx is in direct relation of the skull base and the upper cervical vertebrae. The posterior wall does not present any clear limit from the superior wall; there exists a direct continuation between one and the other. However we may consider the sphenoid as forming the roof, and then, going back and downwards, we will find the basilar part of the occipital and the two first vertebrae, atlas and axis, which are not related to the superior wall, but to the posterior one and the nasopharynx. However, between the mucosa and the bone area, there is the pharingo-basilar fascia which is the one that makes possible the rigidness of the nasopharynx and, in addition, there are the prevertebral muscles, the longus capitis, rectur capitis, posterior major, rectus capitis anterior, and obliquus capitis superior. The relation between the nasopharynx and these muscles areas, explains the cervical symptoms caused by the posterior propagation of the tumors of this region, since we are talking about protractor, flexor, and rotatory muscles of the head: For this reason the infiltration and invasion by the cancer is the cause of the anomalous position of the head and of the immobility of the neck. The most decisive method of studying and obtaining exact knowledge of the relations existing between the posterior wall of nasopharynx and occipital and first two cervical vertebrae, seen both, from the normal and from the pathological point of view, consists in lateral radiography and tomography. Rizzuti [5] studies the efficiency of the radiological position of skull base in order to evaluate the relation between the posterior wall of the nasopharynx and anterior arch of the atlas.

Case Reports

Case 1: 28-year-old male. We want the emphasize the fact that at the age of eleven years this patient was operated on for a right nasofibroma. The symptoms started in November 1982 with occipital headache of moderate intensity and at the same time, the appearance of a right cervical adenopathy. Till January 1983, the intensity of his occipital headache and the size of the adenopathy increased and he developed dysphonia. From this moment we start the observation of this patient, showing the following ENT exploration. Posterior rhinoscopy: Tumor on posterior wall on the left side with cicatricial damage in the right choanal region. Laryngoscopy: Paralysis of right larynx (hemilarynx). We perform a CT, a complete X-ray examination and biopsy (fig. 1).

Tumor of nasopharynx was confirmed and the result of the biopsy is a lymphoepithelioma. The treatment comprises chemotherapy and cobalt therapy. He developed generalized bone metastasis, and died in December 1983.

Case 2: 41-year-old male. January 1983: Hemicranial headache on the left. One month after: torticollis, dysphonia, dysphagia and cervical adenopathy. On examination he showed torticollis, paralysis of larynx, paralysis of pharynx, paralysis of VII and paresis of left arm. X-ray: Luxation of lateral mass of the first cervical vertebra. Compression between first cervical vertebra. Compression between first cervical vertebra and occipital bone.

Scanner examination demonstrated bone destruction of the first cervical vertebra (fig. 2). Posterior rhinoscopy: A large pharyngeal lesion. Biopsy revealed undifferentiated carcinoma. The treatment was cobalt-therapy. One month after, he developed paralysis of the left half of the tongue and a mass of tumor appeared under the sternomastoid muscle in continuity with the tumor of the base of the skull. A new exploration with scanner shows osteolysis of the lateral mass of the atlas on the left and destruction of half of the posterior arch. Infiltration of the prevertebral muscular masses. Later general metastases appeared and in December 1983 the patient died.

Case 3: 55-year-old male. The clinical history starts in January 1980 with occipital headache of very slow progression and low intensity. After three month, there appear torticillis and difficulties in head movements. A rediological exploration showed destruction of the first cervical vertebra (fig. 3).

Owing to this symptoms and the radiological findings, a posterior rhinoscopy was performed and a large tumor of the nasopharynx was diagnosed. The treatment of

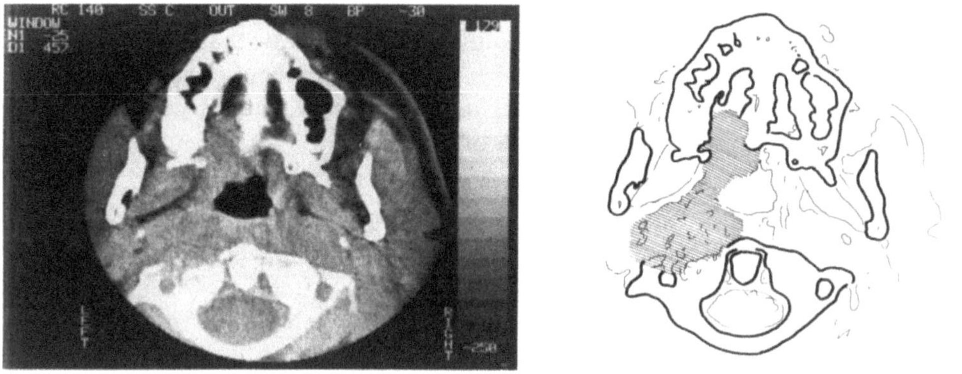

Fig. 1 Destruction of the atlas due to the posterior extension of the tumor, which is invading the lateral well and the choanal region.

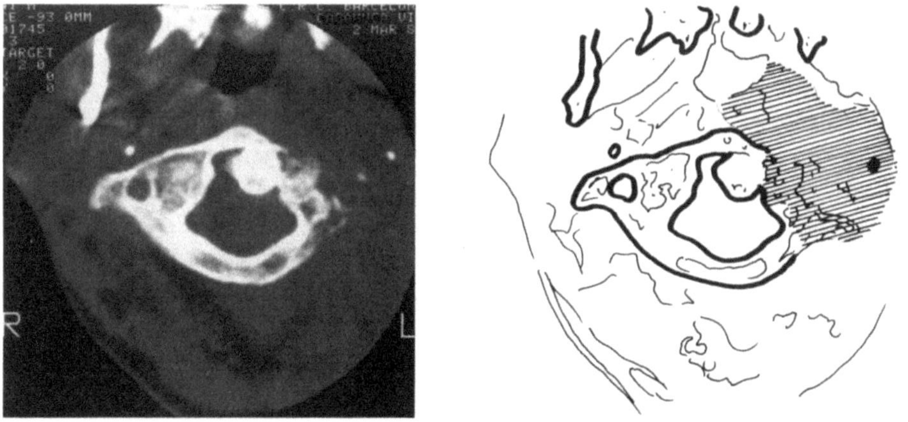

Fig. 2 Extensive nasopharyngeal tumor, involving the lateral mass of the atlas.

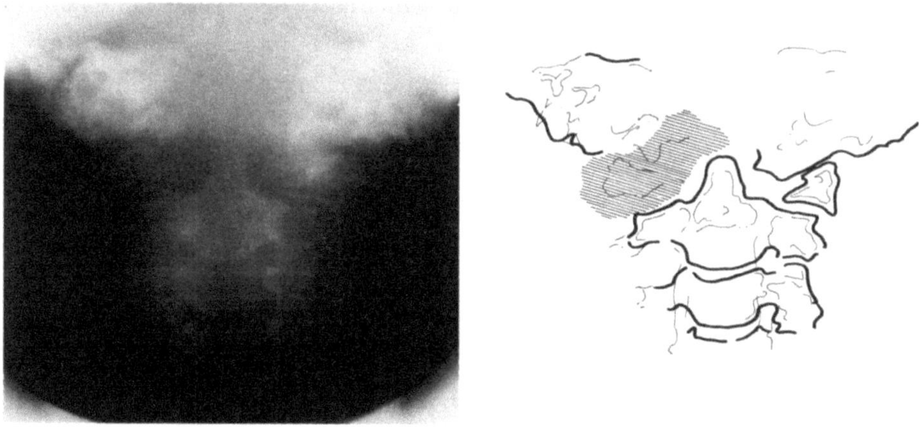

Fig. 3 Large tumor in the nasopharynx, destroying the lateral mass of the atlas and invading the prevertebral region.

the patient is by cobalt therapy. The progress of the patient was quite good, and from January 1981 on, the further radiological control show that the lesion in the nasopharynx has disappeared. In October 1982: development of scarring and destruction of first cervical vertebra posteriorly. At present: subject with favourable evolution, but has tetraplegia as a result of radiation.

Clinical manifestations

In our cases there has been prominent headache which showed several features: it was of an early presentation, posterior in location, mostly around the temporo-occipital or parieto-occipital areas with some irradiation towards the cervical region. On physical examination there was a limitation in the head movements and on testing them there was a marked increase in pain. The tumors of nasopharynx in which the extension was only posterior without otic or nasal symptoms, were diagnosed quite late because usually before going to an ENT specialist the patients used to seek the advice of a rheumatologist, orthopedic surgeon or even the psychiatrist (as one of our patients did). Due to this presentation a posterior rhinoscopy was never done initially. The posterior rhinoscopy should always be performed whenever we meet an association of posterior cervical pain and destructive lesions shown radiologicaly in the upper cervical spine or occipital region. At present, in addition to the classical posterior rhinoscopy, which can be done with retraction of the soft palate and even, if necesary, with general anesthesia, we can also practice an examination with a microscope or by means of the pharyngoscope, according the method popularized by Steiner [7]. In order to confirm the existence of a tumor it is necesary to perform a biopsy and this will practicaly always show the existence of a "lymphoepithelioma" or an undifferentiated carcinoma. However on other occasions, there are not only posterior vertebral symptoms but there are other associated clinical manifestations which make somewhat the diagnosis easier.

Posterior symptoms and otic symptoms: these are seen in cases of posterior tumors which present also a lateral evolution which give rise to tubal obstruction.

Posterior symptoms or neural symptoms: Posterior vertebral symptoms, associated with paralysis of the ninth, tenth, eleventh or twelfth cranial nerves certainly requires an examination of the nasopharynx.

Posterior symptoms/lymphadenopathy: Our cases showed enlarged nodes, a finding similar to the ones described by Guccione [3]. The presentation of a vertebral syndrome with enlarged lymph nodes specially if the biopsy of these nodes shows an undifferentiated carcinoma, will impose an examination of the nasopharynx.

Radiology

In order to study the nasopharynx there are several radiological projections, as described by K. Reiner [4]. The conventional lateral tomography of the nasopharynx is a very reliable method for studying the tumors with posterior extension because we can see in this study the primary tumor and its precise location. In the radiological examination we should also look for the possible existence of a sclerosis of the base of the skull. This sclerosis is the result of an inflammatory lesion produced by tumors of the nasopharynx and is not secondary to direct tumoral invasion. It is due to an osteoblastic reaction in the vicinity of the base of the skull. This sclerosis is quite characteristic in the posterior region (sphenoid, occipital bone, atlas, axis). Soo and Lim [6] described the sclerosis of the base of the skull observed in the radiological examination as an increase in the radiological shadows. Among 48 cases, four of them presented sclerosis of the anterior arch of atlas and one with sclerosis of the odontoid process. However all of them are very extensive, involving the sphenoid and with nasal symptoms but without vertebral symptoms. Teoh [9] found in 31 autopsies of patients with nasopharyngeal carcinoma, two cases with sclerosis of the base of the skull and both of them were squamous carcinoma. After the treatment, it is very important to perform a radiological examination of this area since this will be a very useful method to detect possible tumoral recurrence.

Method for radiologycal examination: Perform basic radiographs and tomographs. We consider quite basic and we aree with Fletchener [2] that we can observe the following signs: First a tumor shadow in the nasopharynx. Second tumoral spread to vertebral region. Xeroradiology in profile position is very important. Anterior-posterior tomographies. We can observe a destruction of the lateral masses of the atlas. Radiography of the base of the skull with the Hirtz position and tomography in the same position. Actually the examination with CT scanner is basic: This method of exploration means a significant progress in tumors previously diagnosed because it allows us see the deep extension into the mucosa, to the endocranium, the paranasal sinuses, the orbit and also the bone destruction of the base of the skull.

This method has the advantage of showing the submucosal soft tissue. Using this investigation when we suspect posterior invasion we will see:

1. Infiltration of soft tissue (muscles) located under the mucosa.
2. Destruction of anterior and posterior arch of the atlas.
3. Destruction of lateral masses.
4. Tumorous invasion of foramen lacerum and the condyloid foramen.
5. Extension outwards of the tumor that is growing from the nasopharynx involves the sternomastoid region.

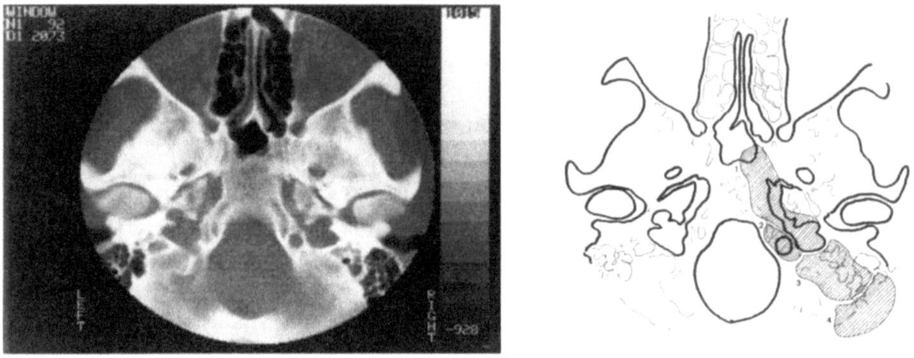

Fig. 4 Spread of tumor: On a normal TAC we can superimpose the diagram and see the extent of the tumor infiltration; 1 = Lateral mass of the atlas and the foramen laerum, 2 = Condyloid foramen, 3 = Mastoid and facial nerve, 4 = Extracranial extension.

Spread of Tumor

The posterior growth of these cancers, to the prevertebral muscles, atlas and axis, follows several predictable ways. As we have shown in previous papers, [10] the tumors of the nasopharynx extend along lines of least resistence, following a sort of preformed pathway. When the cancer arrives at the occipital bone, instead of infiltrating it, it goes downwards (fig. 4) extracranially to the atlas. It can then destroy the lateral mass on one side, the anterior arch, the posterior arch or the odontoid process, as described by Sundaresan et al. [8]. After that, the tumor can reach the foramen lacerum affecting the minth, tenth and eleventh cranial nerves extracranially but not intracranially a particularity which differentiates this pattern of growth from others in this region, but which does not change the clinical progression (fig. 4).

The tumorous spread can reach the foramen magnum and the twelfth cranial nerve, affecting movements of the tongue, and producing muscular atrophy. If the tumor continues its growth, it may reach the lateral part of the neck, where it is possible to biopsy it, as in our case report 2. The tumorous spread must be clearly diffentiated by means of radiology and CT scanner from a big metastatic mode. According to Guccione [3], the cancer can reach the intracranial cavity from the prevertebral area, penetrating into the posterior fossa through the foramen magnum.

Treatment

We will not discuss further the management of these patients, which is usually based on radiotherapy and sometimes on chemotherapy, but we must stress the accurrence sequelae to the radiation. Our only case of cure presents a tetraplegia, throught to be the result of radiation so close to the cerebrospinal axis. Bey et al. [1] who present 42 cases treated with radiation, report three neurologic complications: A hemiplegia, a transitory hemiparesis and a non-evolutive Brown-Séquard syndrome. In all three cases the dose of radiation that reached the medulla or brainstem was more than 5000 rads.

Prognosis

Prognosis is poor, because these patients are usually diagnosed when the disease is at an advanced stage, because of the failure to relate the symptoms with the nasopharynx and the difficulty of exploration of this part of the pharynx. The tumor can also infiltrate the submucosa and spread to the base of the skull and vertebral region, which also worsens the prognosis, as does the finding of metastatic lymph nodes.

Summary

We report three cases of undifferentiated carcinoma of the nasopharynx with posterior spread, destroying the atlas from the inferior part of the base of the skull. Diagnosis was late, and in two cases followed biopsy of a cervical lymph node metastasis. We stress the need for radiological exploration of the occipital bone and upper vertebrae when there is a complaint of posterior cervical pain, contractures or malposition of the head. If bone destruction or a tumorous mass is found, a careful exploration of the nasopharynx must be performed and the possibility of a submucosal tumor considered.

References

[1] Bey, P., B. Gueddari, L. Malissard et al.: Les Carcinomes du Naso-Pharynx. Ann. otolaryn. (Paris) **98** (1981) 43-46.

[2] Fletchner, G. H., R. R. Million: Malignant tumors of the nasopharynx. Amer. J. Roentgend. **93** (1965) 44.

[3] Guccione, G.: Atteggiamento viziato del Capo da Neoplasia della Rinofaringe. Archivio Italiano de Otologia, T. LXXIX, **1** (1968) 83-96.

[4] Reisner, K.: Radiologische Diagnostik der Nasopharynxtumoren. In: Nasopharynx-Tumoren (M. Wannenmacher, ed.), pp. 22-35. Urban & Schwarzenberg, München-Wien-Baltimore 1984.

[5] Rizzuti, R. J., J. P. Whalen: The Nasopharynx. Roentgen anatomy ans its alteration in the base view. N. Y. Radiology 104/**3** (1972) 537-540.

[6] Soo, Y. S., E. E. Lim: Nasopharyngeal carcinoma presenting with sclerosis in the base of skull. Med. J. Aust. 2/**22** (1971) 1126-1128.

[7] Steiner, W.: Endoskopische Diagnostik der Nasopharynxtumoren. In: Nasopharynx-Tumoren (M. Wannenmacher, ed.), pp. 1-7. Urban & Schwarzenberg, München-Wien-Baltimore 1984.

[8] Sundaresan, N., J. H. Galicich, J. M. Lane et al.: Treatment of odontoid fractures in cancer patients. J. Neurosurg. **54** (1981) 187-192.

[9] Teoh, T. B.: Epidemoid carcinoma of nasopharynx among chinese. J. Path. Bact. **73** (1957) 452.

[10] Traserra, J., R. Avellaneda: Modalités de l'extension tumorale des cancers du Thino-Pharynx. Bulletin du Cancer 62, **3** (1975) 307-318.

Sudden blindness by an esthesioneuroblastoma – case report

L. A. Rios-Nogales Garces, E. Heiss, E. Grote

Esthesioneuroblastomas belong to the rare tumors confronting the neurosurgeon. Case histories pointing to primary intracranial involvement are also rare. The following illustrative case is therefore presented.

A 25-year-old male patient complained 3 to 4 month prior to admission to our service of having intense headaches, especially at the back of the eye. In the preceding two months he had noticed a progressive bilateral visual loss followed by a right-sided exophthalmos. Three days before admission he developed a right-sided blindness and a left-sided loss of vision with merely light perception. Emergency admission followed because of massive papille. edema as well as a right-sided proptosis with normal eyelid closure, complete anosmia and a right-sided hypoacusis. Otherwise there were no significant neurological signs. In addition, the patient complained of having severe headaches, and his condition alternated between aggressiveness and severe apathy.

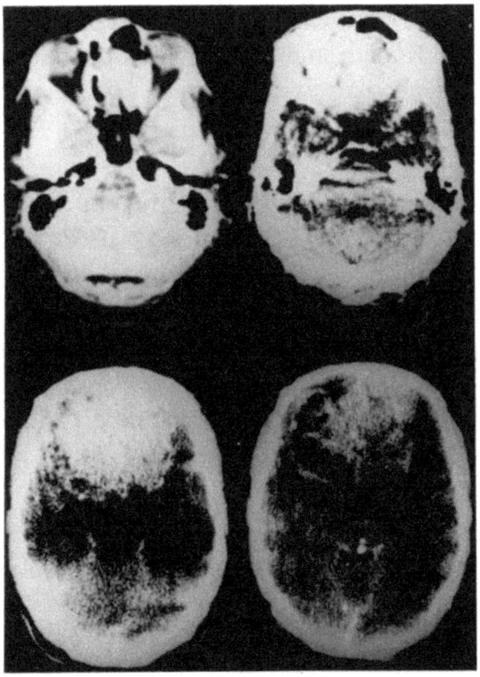

Fig. 1 The CT scan findings in a case of esthesioneuroblastoma. A large, round, midline, enhancing mass arising from the paranasal sinuses and filling the anterior fossa.

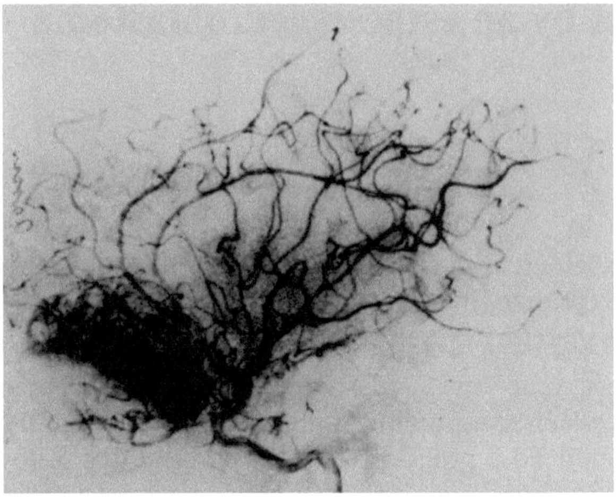

Fig. 2 The lateral angiogram shows a richly vascularized tumor with dorsal displacement of the anterior cerebral artery.

The CT scan (fig. 1) disclosed an extraordinarily large bifrontal tumor with marked enhancement after contrast medium injection, filling the base of the anterior fossa and invading the paranasal sinuses and both orbits, from the right side particularly, with compression of the optic nerves. Anti-edematous therapy was instituted and an biopsy was taken transnasaly. The histological diagnosis of the frozen sections was a non-hodgkin lymphoma. Radiation therapy was started and continued after the final diagnosis of esthesioneuroblastoma was made, since the radiosensitivity of these tumors is well known and the angiography (fig. 2) showed a richly vascularized tumor.

CT scan follow-ups showed a reduction of the tumor mass by one third after two weeks of radiation. Within two weeks after completion of radio-therapy a rapid regrowth of the tumor was demonstrated, so that a surgical removal was indicated.

During the operation a bifrontal tumor was found, which was solid and partly necrotic. It was so large that it had not only caused a compression of both frontal lobes but had also spread to the region of both optic nerves and orbits, as well as to the paranasal sinuses. After tumor extirpation the remaining defect of the anterior fossa and dura was closed with a fascia-muscle flap. The histological examination of all specimens confirmed the diagnosis of esthesioneuroblastoma.

The recovery from such an operation is even for a young patient very difficult. It must be underlined that postoperatively neither a frontal lobe syndrome nor other additional significant neurological deficits were present. The patient reported an improvement of vision on the left side as well as capability of finger counting. Two months later we obtained a final report from the attending clinic, and the patient was still in moderate condition; however, a tumor recurrence in the paranasal sinuses was already present. He returned to his home country for further care by his family. This rare tumor originates from the olfactory mucosa and was first reported in 1924 by Berger and Luc [1].

In 1973 Hamilton et al. [4] reviewed 128 cases and Djalilian [2] found a further 140 cases world wide. Histologically, esthesioneuroepithelioma (with rosettes), esthesioneuroblastoma (with pseudorosettes) and esthesiocytoma (with fibrin formation and without rosettes or pseudorosettes) can be differentiated.

The prognosis of the patients is less dependent upon the histological character then on the tendency toward local invasion and metastasisation. Since no relationship exists between histological maturity and tumor malignancy [8], the classification proposed by Kadish et al. [6] seems to be more practicable. In this clasification the stage A tumors are solely intranasal in location, stage B with additional invasion of the paranasal sinuses, and stage C with extension beyond the paranasal sinuses or with distant metastases.

Esthesioneuroblastomas are conditionally malignant tumors with a five year survival rate of 50% [5, 11]. Male and young patients are sightly predisposed. In 50% of the cases local recurrence occurred. In 14 to 20%, distant metastases are found not only in the cervical lymphatic nodes, but also in the lung, skeletal system, liver, spleen, kidney, ovaries and even in the face.

Initial symptoms are usually nonspecific and usually include a stuffed and runny nose, epistaxis, anosmia and headaches. Additional symptoms such as retrobulbar pain, diplopia, papilledema, increased lacrimation, trigeminal paresthesia and blurred vision occur in patients with tumor extension into the orbits, which is seen in 17% of the cases. In case of extension to the nasopharynx, hearing impairment can also be present.

In 12.5 to 20% of the patients an intracranial invasion is seen and followed by signs of intracranial hypertension; especially frontal lobe syndrome and even seizures are possible [3]. Obert et al. [9OZ reported two cases of patients with brain abscess as a further complication.

As previously mentioned, esthesioneuroblastomas rarely have the character of primary intracranial space occupation as the first sign. In 5 of the 10 cases reviewed in 1980 by Goldhammer et al. [3] a loss of visual acuity was present; in a further case reported by Wilson et al. [12] sudden blindness had ocurred. In 1979 Sanwar [10] presented a case of primary sellar-parasellar esthesioneuroblastoma.

Because of the mostly nonspecific symptoms in patients with esthesioneuroblastoma, despite CT and other additional diagnostic methods, the final diagnosis is only possible after biopsy. Differential- and mis-diagnoses are: anaplastic carcinoma, malignant lymphomas, rhabdomyosarcomas and even chordomas and meningiomas.

How difficult a realible diagnosis can be, was demonstrated in the case presented by Goldhammer et al. [3], which was subsequently diagnosed by Landolt et al. [7]

in 1981 as an osteoblastic metastasis. Our own case was primarily diagnosed as a non-hodgkin lymphoma.

The therapy of esthesioneuroblastomas is a combination of surgical removal and radiation. A review of the literature leads to the conclusion, however, that the tendency to regrowth of these tumors cannot be appreciably influenced.

References

[1] Berger, L., R. Luc: L'esthésioneuroépithéliome olfactif. Bull. Ass. Franç. Cancer **13** (1924) 410-421.

[2] Djalilian, M., R. D. Zujko, L. H. Weiland, et al.: Olfactory neuroblastoma. Surg. Clin. North America **57** (1977) 751-762.

[3] Goldhammer, Y., M. Sadeh, R. Tadmor, et al.: Intracranial esthesioneuroblastoma associated with unilateral visual loss. J. Neurosurg. **53** (1980) 836-840.

[4] Hamilton, A. E., L. J. Rubinstein, G. J. Poole: Primary intracranial esthesioneuroblastoma (olfactory neuroblastoma). J. Neurosurg. **38** (1973) 548-556.

[5] Hutter, R. V. P., J. S. Lewis, F. W. Foote jr., et al.: Esthesioneuroblastoma - a clinical and pathological study. Amer. J. Surg. **106** (1963) 748-753.

[6] Kadish, S., M. Goodman, C. C. Wang: Olfactory Neuroblastoma A clinical analysis of 17 cases. Cancer **37** (1976) 1571-1576.

[7] Landolt, A. M., U. Fisch, R. L. Friede: Esthesioneuroblastoma - letter to the editor. J. Neurosurg. **55** (1981) 154-155.

[8] Oberman, H. A., D. H. Rice: Olfactory neuroblastomas - a clinicopathologic study. Cancer **38** (1976) 2494-2502.

[9] Obert, G. J., K. D. Devine, J. R. McDonald: Olfactory neuroblastomas. Cancer **13** (1960) 205-215.

[10] Sarwar, M.: Primary sellar-parasellar esthesioneuroblastoma. AJR **133** (1979) 140-141.

[11] Skolnik, E. M., F. S. Massari, L. T. Tenta: Olfactory neuroepithelioma. Review of the world literature and presentation of two cases. Arch. Otolaryngol. **84** (1966) 644-653.

[12] Wilson, W. M. G., G. Cullen: Olfactory groove tumour causing sudden blindness. A case report. Can. J. Ophthalmol. **2** (1967) 133-138.

Bifrontal meningioma of the skull base

W. Köning, R. A. Frowein, O. Wilcke

A 50-year-old female with a 3 year history of an increasing frontal lobe syndrome and severe changes in social behaviour was admitted to our clinic 6 months ago and computerized tomography revealed a large frontal tumor.

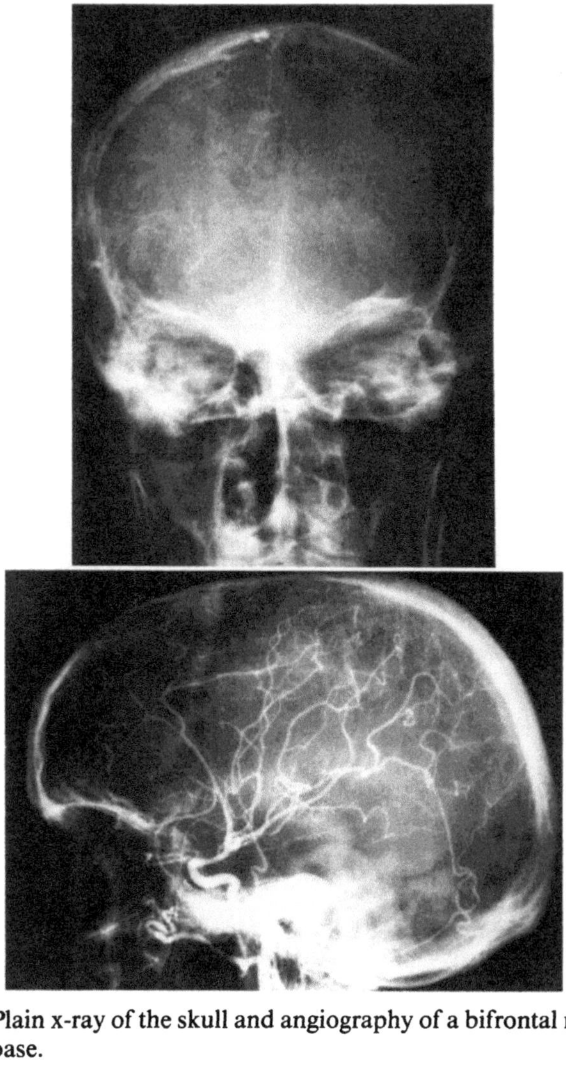

Fig. 1 Plain x-ray of the skull and angiography of a bifrontal meningioma of anterior skull base.

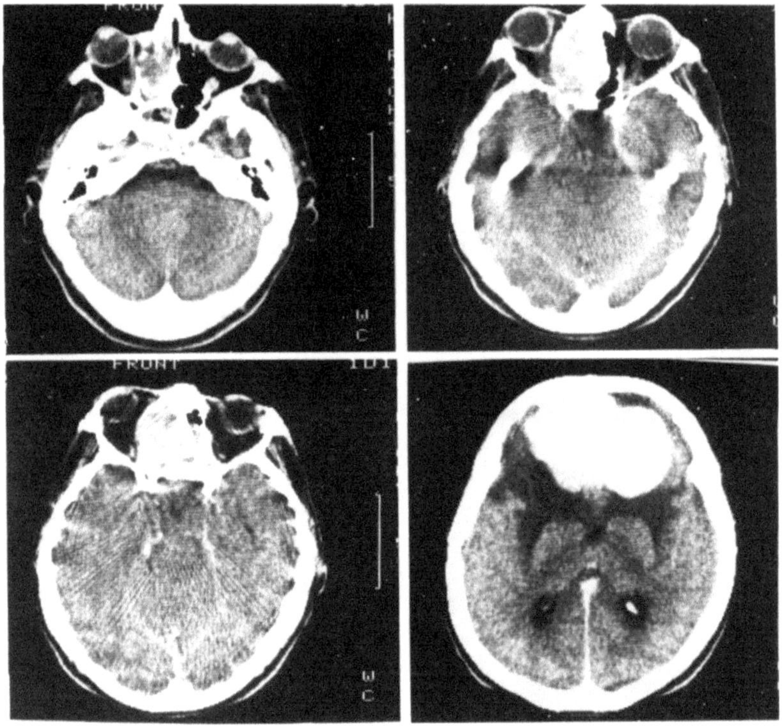

Fig. 2 Axial CT-sections of the meningioma extending into the ethmoidal cells, left orbit and nasal cavity.

At the first examination bilateral anosmia was found, visual acuity was 1.0 on the right and 0.5 on the left side with moderate exophthalmos on the left without visual field changes. Pupil reactions and eye movements were normal. Except for a mild dizziness walking with closed eyes no other neurological disturbances were present. General condition was poor.

Plain skull films (fig. 1) showed no transparency of the paranasal sinuses and upper nasal cavity. The anterior carotid arteries were displaced dorsally by a big space occupying lesion on the angiogramm and a marked vascularisation of the external vessels was seen in the fronto-basal area.

Axial CT-section (fig. 2) confirmed the enormous size of the intracranial tumor, extending into ethmoidal cells, medial wall of the left orbit and the nasal cavity. This was demonstrated very impressively by the coronal sections (fig. 3).

A typical advanced medial olfactory groove meningioma was diagnosed (as reported by Cushing [1]). Because of the very large intracranial extension and poor general condition a combined extra-intracranial approach was suggested in two stages.

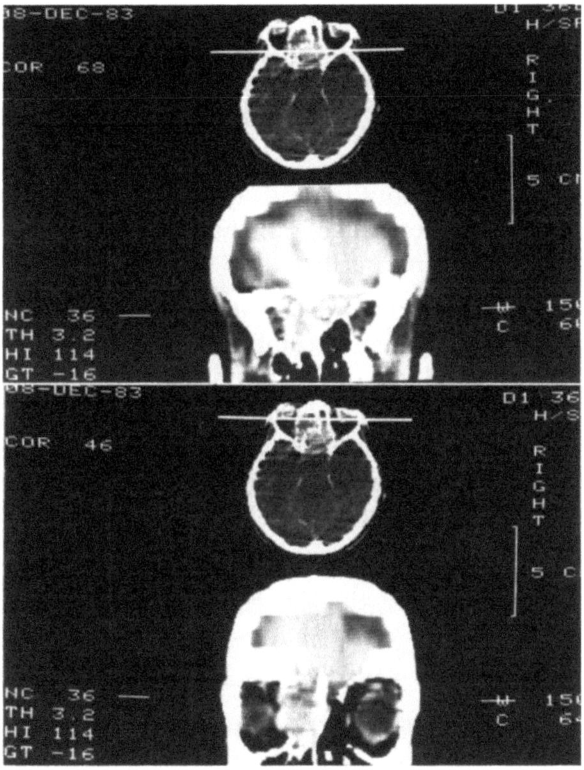

Fig. 3 Coronal CT-sections, revealing intracranial and basal tumor extension.

First the tumor was approached by a coronal incision and a bifrontal craniotomy. After ligating and dividing the anterior sagittal sinus the tumor was resected step by step together with the basal falx cerebri. The main vessels and the chiasm were identified and preserved.

The dura of the planum spenoidale, optic foramina, the clinoid processes and the dura of the dorsal portions of the lesser and greater wings of sphenoid bone were free of tumor.

The cribriform plate, ethmoidal cells, the frontal sinuses and the bony medial wall of the left orbit were invaded and destroyed.

By careful dissection a complete exision of the lesion was accomplished except for the deeper intranasal and ethmoidal portions of the tumor. The skull base defect was covered without osseous reconstruction only by a large graft of pericranial tissue, which was stitched to the normal dura to give a watertight closure. Four weeks later after an uneventful period the second operation was undertaken by the ENT surgeon, who removed the naso-ethmoidal portion of the tumor by a paranasal approach.

The patient made a good recovery, including the frontal lobe syndrome involved; visual acuity improved to 0.7 and motility of the ocular muscles was normal. There was no CSF leakage, no pulsating exophthalmos and the general condition continues to improve. Histologically the tumor was classified as a fibroblastic meningioma without malignancy.

Because of the clinical course, the operative findings and result in this case, the operative management and kind of cranioplasty of skull base defects communicating with the paranasal sinuses have to be reconsidered.

In this case with extensive intra- and extracranial extension of the tumor and because of the general condition of the patient a combined intracranial-extracranial operation in two stages was preferred to a one stage operation. In addition to the dural repair by a graft of pericranial tissue [5, 6] dermal graft [2] or fascia lata graft [4], bone reconstruction by bone grafts [2] or methylacrylate [3, 7] is not mandatory in all cases, but the suture of the basal grafts in a watertight fashion and the complete closure of the cranial cavity to avoid CSF leakage and ascending infection are essential in all cases.

References

[1] Cushing, H., L. Eisenhardt: Meningiomas. Hafner Pup. Comp., New York 1962 (Reprint of 1938).
[2] Derome, P., et al.: Les tumeurs spheno-ethmoidales. Neurochirurgie **18** (1972) Suppl.
[3] Harris, P., I. T. Jackson, et al.: Reconstructive Surgery of the Head. In: Advances and Technical Standards in Neurosurgery (H. Krayenbühl, ed.), vol. 8, p. 264. Springer Verlag, Wien-New York 1981.
[4] Malis, L. I.: Tumours of the parasellar Region. In: Advances in Neurology (R. A. Thompson, J. R. Green, eds.), vol. 15, p. 198. Raven Press, New York 1976.
[5] Offret, G., C. Haye: Tumeurs de l'Oeil et des Annexes oculaires. Masson, Paris 1971.
[6] Pertuiset, B.: Les tumeurs osseuses de la voute du crâne et les cranioplasties. Thèse Paris, 1949.
[7] Schürmann, K., D. Voth: Die Bedeutung der transfrontalen Orbitotomie für die Behandlung der intraorbitalen raumfordernden Prozesse. Advances Ophthal. **25** (1972) 188-239.

Surgical reconstruction of the Eustachian tube

C. Jansen

Tumors of the skull base cause problems with Eustachian tube function relatively frequently but one has to realize that especially in cases with malignant tumors the problem plays just a minor role for the patient. On the other hand there still remain cases who need treatment.

Patients who recover completely or almost completely are very interested to return to a normal existence which means having adequate hearing.

Our experience of about eight years with dysfunction of the Eustachian tube after skull base fractures or tumors shows that there are some typical findings. When the tube functioning is changing because of recurrent swelling of the mucosal lining the patient starts becoming nervous. The hearing varies and otitis media occurs frequently. The pressure of the tumor also reduces the caliber in its different portions. Complete closure mostly does not involve the whole length of the tube but partial obstruction is common.

When the Eustachian tube is closed a conductive hearing loss becomes evident. A severe drum head retraction follows immediately and the patient starts complaining of ear-ache or head-ache. Valsalva, Toynbee and other tests are negative. To get more information the surgeon needs special radiography. Conventional radiography can be sufficient when a contrast medium or a wire is used. For the diagnosis of an insufficient caliber of the bony part of the Eustachian tube we use Computer Tomography with a longitudinal plane of Stenvers [1, 2]. In our hands the combination of the conventional technique and the CT works very well. In case of a drum head perforation the wire can be introduced from the middle ear to find out where the obstruction is located. When the drum head is intact the wire is inserted using a tube catheter with a fiber optic. The straight optical system can ensure the catheter finding the right way [3]. On the other hand we also have the flexible fiber optic of 3.2 mm and 1.8 mm. The fiber optic system also allows direct inspection which is a great advantage. In cases where the bony part is obstructed it is possible to inject a contrast solution without the risk of filling the middle ear.

The solution can be sucked out immediately afterwards. So far we have not found many cases with hypersensitivity of the mucosal lining. On the other hand one has to realize that radiography is not able to help us with problems of the swollen mucosal lining of which we unfortunately have a lot of cases. We are looking forward to finding but what the NMR system might do. As far as the treatment is concerned there are not many possibilities available. When the middle ear is not yet infected a grommet can be inserted. Instead of the grommet a small hole is made in the posterior bony canal wall close to the annulus. The hole can be kept open by a teflon tube. A chronic middle ear infection does complicate the situation dramatically. Besides the bad hearing, mastoiditis and cholesteatoma can demand surgical intervention. The surgeon has to decide which kind of operation he should do, because he cannot expect any function of the Eustachian tube.

On one hand the removal of cholesteatoma is urgently needed, but on the other hand the reconstruction of any middle ear function seems to be worthless. Putting a silastic tube into the tympanic cavity as mentioned before was not found to be adequate. After removal of the skull base tumor and further recovery of the patient a special technique of Eustachian tube surgery can be used. The technical details of the procedure have been explained with articles and movies since 1976 but a short summary is given here. The procedure is based upon the technique of Posterior Tympanotomy [4] published in 1958 which allows the wide opening of the epitympanum without destroying the posterior bony canal wall. Detachment of the mucosal lining in the epitympanal area is one of the most important parts of the procedure. Keeping the mucosal lining intact, at least partially, is the key to a good result. In that way the mucosa can be folded forward and the enlargement of the bony part of the Eustachian tube can be started by drilling. The drilling is done in the posterior and posterior-superior part of the orifice. Our experience has shown that in about 82% of all cases the anatomical situation allows a wide opening without causing any problems. Critical points are the potential opening of the mandibular joint and producing a dural prolapse. At that stage of the procedure we try to use again the 1.8 mm straight or the flexible type of fiber optics. After enlargement of the tube orifice in its posterior portion it is interesting to find that the tube axis keeps going straight to the nasopharyngeal orifice. Sometimes we use the flexible system from the nasopharynx as well to find out what the cartilaginous part of the tube is like. Under microscopical view the osseus part is enlarged. Studies on quite a number of human temporal bones has shown that the cartilaginous part of the Eustachian tube does a turn from inferior to superior. That means the cartilage starts inferiorly close to the end of the osseus part. Thus the posterior-superior part is still bone which allows somewhat further opening.

Resection of the tensor tympani muscle has been performed in a number of cases to enable further enlargement. We found in about 12% of all cases the canal was dehiscent inferiorly and the pulsating carotid artery is visible. Widening of the cartilaginous part of the tube using the drill or using incisions has not so far been done.

Because of the widening of the bony part of the tube the mucosal lining has to be incised. In that way there does exist a dehiscence. Fibrin glue is used in order to keep the mucosa lining in place a conical silastic tube is inserted, also somewhat into the cartilaginous part. In our experience a sufficient aeration of the middle ear also plays a most important role for the healing of the mucosal lining in Eustachian tube surgery. Therefore the silastic tube is multiperforated and is turned daily circlewise. It remains *in situ* for about two or three weeks.

In most of the cases with cholesteatoma the above-mentioned procedure for surgical reconstruction was successful. The rate in tumor cases was much worse because the mucosal defect plays the most obvious role for adequate result. Small defects have an agreeable recover rate. Further details on statistics have been published before [5, 6].

In conclusion it should be stated that the adequate surgical reconstruction of the Eustachian tube in cases with tumors is still extremely difficult. Further experience will show whether the new technique is a really worthwhile procedure.

References

[1] Zonneveld, F. W., H. Damsma: Direct multiplanar CT of the petrous bone. Presented at 68th Annual meeting of the Radiological Society of North America 1982, paper 160.

[2] Stenvers, H. W.: Röntgenologie des Felsenbeines und des bitemporalen Schädelbildes. Springer, Berlin 1928.

[3] Jansen, C. W.: Endoscopy and Surgery of the Eustachian Tube. Politzer Society Proceedings of the Montreux Conference 1983. The American Journal of Otology, vol. 6 (1985) 3.

[4] Jansen, C. W.: Über Radikaloperation u. Tympanoplastik. Sitzungsber. Fortbild. Ärztek. Ob. **18** (1958) 2.

[5] Jansen, C. W.: Mikrochirurgie des Epitympanons. Arch. Ohren Nasen Kehlkopfheilkd. **231** (1981) 568.

[6] Jansen, C. W.: Topographisch-anatomische Details bei der Tubenchirurgie. Archives of Oto-Rhino-Laryngology *Supplement* **II** (1983) 311-312.

III Middle and posterior skull base tumors

Petroclival and medial tentorial meningiomas

L. N. Sekhar, M. Samii

Introduction

The operative treatment of petroclival and medial tentorial meningiomas continues to remain a great challenge to neurosurgeons and other physicians involved in the care of these patients [1]. The critical location in front of the brain stem, the close involvement of the cranial nerves, the vertebral basilar arteries and their branches, and the extensions of the tumor into multiple regions not amenable to a single operative approach, make their total removal often difficult and hazardous. Until recently, the surgical excision of these lesions was often accompanied by high operative mortality and morbidity [1, 8]. Even in the best neurosurgical clinics of today, the results are often suboptimal. This article will present the state of the art in the treatment of these lesions based on the experience at two neurosurgical institutions, the University of Pittsburgh Neurosurgical Clinic, and the Neurosurgical Clinic of the City Hospital of Hanover [2, 3]. A discussion of the optimal operative approaches, operative techniques, and of the current problems to be resolved will follow.

Clinical material

From the years 1973 through 1983, 22 petroclival and 13 medial tentorial meningiomas were operated at the University of Pittsburgh Neurosurgical Clinic. The operations were performed by P. J. Jannetta, L. N. Sekhar, or J. C. Maroon. During the years 1977 through 1983, 12 petroclival and 6 medial tentorial meningiomas were operated at the Neurosurgical Clinic of the City Hospital of Hanover by Professor Madjid Samii. Doctor Sekhar had the privilege of assisting some of the difficult operations during the time that he spent with Professor Madjid Samii.

The experience at the two clinics is combined to illustrate the similarities in the presentation of these patients, the common technical problems faced by the surgeon and certain different ways in which these lesions can be handled operatively.

Table 1 Symptoms and signs of petroclival and medial tentorial meningomas

	Petroclival		Medial Tentorial	
	Pittsburgh (n=22)	Hanover (n=12)	Pittsburgh (n=13)	Hanover (n=6)
Dementia	3	–	5	1
Psychomotor seizure	–	–	5	–
Coma: intermittent or persistent	–	–	4	–
Dysarthria	–	–	–	1
Cranial nerve problems				
II Postpapilledemic optic atrophy	1	–	1	2
III Paresis	–	–	2	2
IV Paresis	–	–	3	2
V Trigeminal neuralgia	11	2	2	1
sensory loss	14	5	6	4
IV Paresis or palsy	2	–	2	2
VII Hemifacial spasm	4	–	1	–
Paresis or palsy	8	4	4	4
VIII Vertigo, Dysequilibrium	4	5	3	2
Tinnitus	7	5	–	2
Hearing Loss	14	8	1	2
X Paresis	3	3	1	1
XI Paresis	–	1	–	–
XII Paresis	2	2	3	–
Hemiparesis	2	–	5	5
Hemisensory loss	1	2	1	1
Cerebellar deficit				
Gait ataxia	13	7	12	4
Extremity ataxia	6	3	8	3

Clinical signs and symptoms

The clinical signs and symptoms of the patients in both groups are summarized in table 1. Cerebellar signs and symptoms are equally common in both groups. Cranial nerve signs and symptoms were somewhat more frequent in the petroclival group. Dementia, hemiparesis and hemisensory loss were more frequent in the tentorial group. In addition, psychomotor seizures, and intermittent or persistent coma were also observed in some of the patients with medial tentorial tumors, the former presumably resulting from medial temporal lobe compression, and the later presumably due to severe compression of the mid brain, or to associated severe hydrocephalus.

Table 2 Petroclival meningiomas - CT findings

	Pittsburgh (n=22)	Hanover (n=12)
Size of lesion		
small < 1 cm	1	-
medium 1-2.5 cm	2	1
large > 2.5 cm	19	11
Tumor extension		
Tentorial notch	5	6
Clivus	8	8
Foramen magnum	-	3
Location on petrous ridge		
in front of IAC	19	8
behind IAC	3	4
Bony changes		
Erosion of petrous apex	2	2
Hyperostosis of petrous bone	5	1
No change	15	9

Preoperative studies

Cranial computed tomographic (CT) scans in the axial and coronal planes were the most useful preoperative studies. The coronal scans revealed the precise location of the tumor in relationship to the tentorium and this was useful in planning operative approaches. In general, the tumors were hyperdense in comparison with the brain in non-enhanced CT scans, and enhanced significantly in a homogenous fashion following the infusion of contrast material. The CT findings of petroclival meningiomas are summarized in table 2. The majority of the large lesions were more than 5 cm in diameter. On the basis of CAT scans, the lesions were classified as petroclival if its predominant location was in this area, or as medial tentorial if its predominant location was in the tentorial notch area. However, both tumors had a tendency to extend from one area into the other. Further extensions into the region of the cavernous sinus, Meckel's cave, foramen magnum, and extradural regions also occurred.

Cerebral angiography demonstrated the blood supply of the tumors in the majority of the cases, supply being most commonly derived from the meningohypophyseal branch of the internal carotid artery, and less commonly from the middle meningeal, the occipital, the ascending pharyngeal, and the vertebral meningeal arteries. In addition, the tumors were often supplied by branches of the vertebral basilar circulation. The most important value of cerebral angiography, however, was in demonstrating the relationship of the tumor to the arteries and branches of the vertebral basilar circulation. This information aided the surgeon intraoperatively.

Neurophysiological studies such as audiogram, brain stem evoked responses, and facial electromyography were of use in following the patients postoperatively, as well as for intraoperative monitoring, when this was used. Nuclear magnetic resonance scanning was not available when these patients were operated, and is therefore not commented upon.

Operative adjuvants

Preoperative embolization of vascular basal meningiomas has been suggested and practiced by other surgeons, but was not used in our cases. In every operation, excellent neuroanesthetic technique was essential. The majority of the operations were performed with the use of balanced neuroanesthetic technique, and with muscle paralysis. However, when intraoperative monitoring of muscle activity was essential, an inhalational technique using Halothane or Forane was practiced. With the use of hyperventilation and other adjuvants for relaxation, brain retraction problems were not experienced even with inhalational techniques.

In every patient, either Mannitol or Lasix were used to achieve excellent cerebral relaxation and to reduce the retraction pressure. In addition, cerebral spinal fluid drainage, either using a lumbar catheter or by opening of the cisterns, was used to relax the brain further. Hypotensive anesthesia was avoided since the combination of hypotension and brain retraction can increase the injury to the retracted brain.

In the recent years, neuroanesthetic monitoring techniques have been used in Pittsburgh with the help of Doctor Aage Moller, neurophysiologist. The techniques that have been most valuable have been the continuous monitoring of brain stem evoked responses by computer averaging techniques, and in selected cases, monitoring of facial EMG activity and intraoperative facial nerve stimulation. Most recently, Doctor Sekhar and Doctor Moller have developed and applied continuous monitoring of the electrical activity of the extra ocular muscles while operating on lesions involving the cavernous sinus, to minimize morbidity to the third and sixth cranial nerves [3]. In the future, continuous monitoring of the somatosensory evoked potential from the retracted brain may become commonplace to minimize retraction induced brain injury.

Table 3 Petroclival meningiomas, operative results and complications - Pittsburgh series (n=22)

Cranial nerve relationships					
IV	Rostral	21			
	Anterior	1			
V	Superior-anterior	18			
	Anterior	4			
	Invaded	3			
VI	Anterior	22			
VII, VIII	Posterior	16			
	Inferior	3			
	Superior	1			
	Anterior	3			
IX, X	Inferior	15			
	Not closely related	7			

Postoperative results					
Operative approach	*Total cases*	*Outcome*			
		Good	Fair	Poor	Dead
Retromastoid craniectomy					
Complete removal	12	11	1	0	0
Subtotal removal	7	4	3	0	0
Subtemporal craniotomy					
Complete removal	2	1	1	0	0
Subtotal removal	1	0	1	0	0

Follow up and recurrence rates		
Factor	*Complete excision*	*Subtotal excision*
Follow up (yrs)		
Mean	5	4
Range	1-10	1-7
Recurrence	1 (small)	1
Reoperation	0	1

Operation

Petroclival meningiomas

The operative approaches, cranial nerve relationships and follow-up data of petroclival meningiomas operated in Pittsburgh and Hanover are presented in tables 3 and 4. The different operative approaches available for treatment of these and medial tentorial tumors, as well as the selection of approaches, will be discussed subsequently. The *retromastoid approach* was a predominant technique

Table 4 Petroclival meningiomas operative findings and complications - Hanover series (n = 12)

Operative approach - retromastoid craniectomy		
Total Excision - with dura and bone drilling		11
Partial excision - with coagulation of dura		1 (cavernous sinus infiltration)
Cranial nerve relationships		
Tumor behind internal auditory canal - all nerves anterior		
Tumor in front of IAC:	V - cranial, often surrounded	12
	VII, VIII - dorsal, stretched	12
	IX, X, XI - posterior	9
	- surrounded	3

Complications		
IV	Permanent paralysis	1
VII	Temporary paralysis	5
VIII	Permanent total loss	2
	Partial loss	1
IX, X	Temporary paralysis	1
	Duodenal ulcer	1
	Operative mortality	none

used in the resection of the tumors both in Pittsburgh and Hanover. In terms of cranial nerve relationships, it was useful on preoperative CT to see if the tumor was located behind or in front of the internal auditory canal. When the tumor arose from the petrous ridge from behind the internal auditory canal, the seventh and eighth cranial nerves were consistently located in front of the tumor when approached from the retromastoid paracerebellar exposure. The trigeminal root was consistently displaced rostrally, either anterior or posterior to the tumor. It was often considerably stretched and sometimes invaded by the tumor, particularly near the Meckel's cave. The ninth, tenth, and eleventh nerves also had a relationship similar to the seventh and eighth nerves based on its location on the petrous ridge. However, in some instances, they were completely surrounded by the tumor on all sides and had to be dissected carefully.

There was no operative mortality either in Pittsburgh or Hanover. Meaningful follow-up data was available in the series operated in Pittsburgh. One tumor thought to be totally excised (with the coagulation of the basal dura), has recurred. However, since this tumor has been small on CAT scans, and the patient asymptomatic, a reoperation has not been necessary so far. Of the lesions excised subtotally, one patient has required reoperation, the others are being followed by repeated CT. In Hanover, of the tumors excised totally, none have recurred so far. Of the two tumors known to be excised partially on account of their invasive nature, both patients have undergone radiation therapy and are being followed.

Table 5 Operative treatment of medial tentorial meningiomas

	Pittsburgh (n=13)	Hanover (n=6)
Operations		
Cerebrospinal fluid shunt only	2	–
Retromastoid approach		
Total excision	1	–
Subtotal excision	3	1
Retromastoid subtemporal		
Total resection	2	–
Subtemporal		
Total excision	3	–
Subtotal excision	–	–
Frontotemporal Sylvian	1	1
Frontotemporal, drilling of petrous apex	–	3
Complications		
Death	–	0
Permanent hemiparesis	2	0
Cranial nerve deficits	5	3

Medial tentorial meningiomas

The operative approaches and complications of the medial tentorial group, both in Pittsburgh and Hanover, are summarized in table 5. A cerebral spinal fluid shunt only was used in Pittsburgh in two patients, in one patient on account of advanced age, and in the other patient, because of refusal to undergo operation. A variety of operative approaches were used in the treatment of these lesions. Of these, the combined retromastoid and subtemporal approach, and the frontotemporal approach with the drilling of the petrous apex were those that afforded the best view of the tumor and permitted the radical excision.

There were no deaths in the series, and permanent hemiparesis occurred in two patients in Pittsburgh. The quality of life has been excellent to fair in all the surviving patients.

Illustrative cases

Patient 1: Surgeon: P. J. Jannetta
This 41-year-old lady presented with a nine year history of right-sided facial numbness, initially intermittent and subsequently progressive, a six year history of right-sided hearing loss, and a several week history of headache, mild dementia and ataxia. She had been evaluated prior to referral and had undergone a ventriculoperitoneal shunt for treatment of hy-

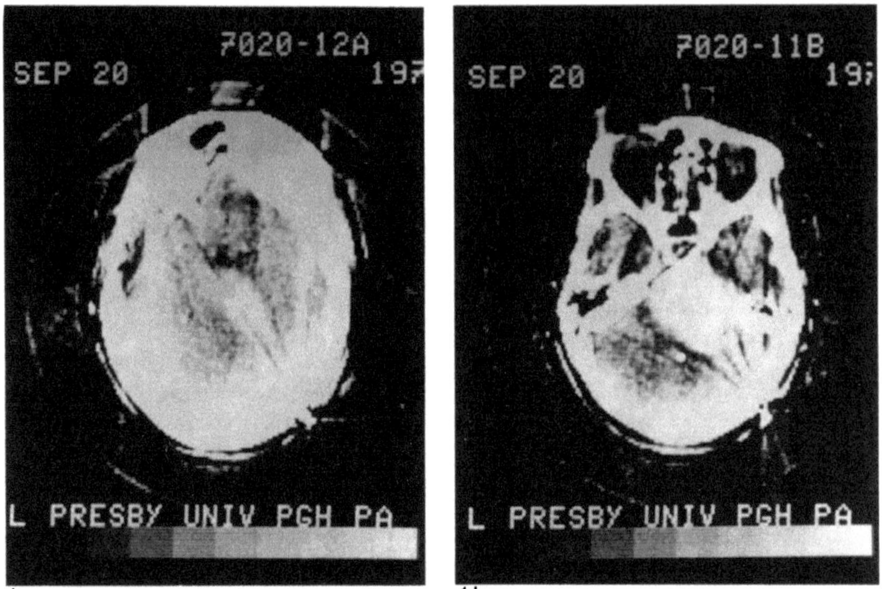

1a 1b

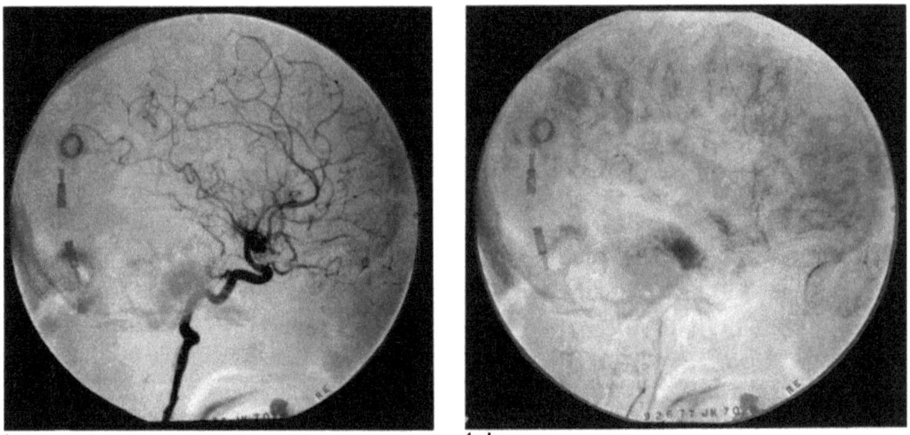

1c 1d

drocephalus. Examination revealed the involvement of all three divisions of the trigeminal nerve, partial paralysis of the facial nerve, almost total hearing loss, a mild gait ataxia, and a right arm dysmetria. CAT scan revealed a very large petroclival lesion extending from the right cerebellar pontine angle into the clivus on both sides, and up into the tentorial notch. Cerebral angiography revealed the blood supply to the tumor coming from the meningohypophyseal trunk of the internal carotid artery.

The lesion was approached by retromastoid craniectomy with a patient in the half sitting position. At operation, a very large vascular lesion was found and the tumor was difficult to resect on account of its tough and fibrous consistency and vascularity. The seventh and eighth nerves were pushed posteriorly and inferiorly, the ninth and tenth nerves were severly stretched caudally, the fifth nerve was pushed up cranially and was significantly thinned, the sixth nerve was stretched anteriorly and medially in a hairpin like fashion. The tumor

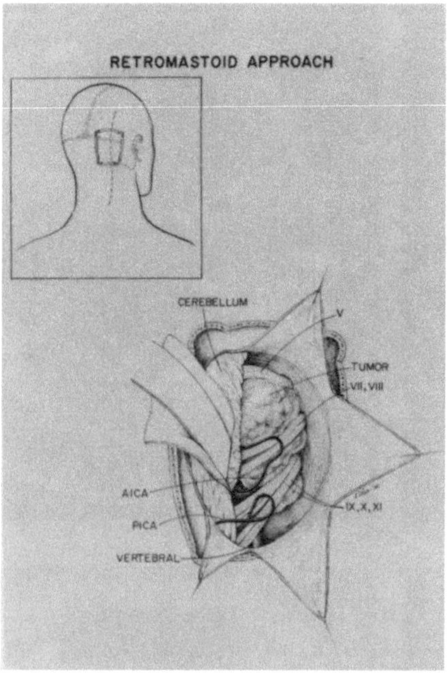

1e

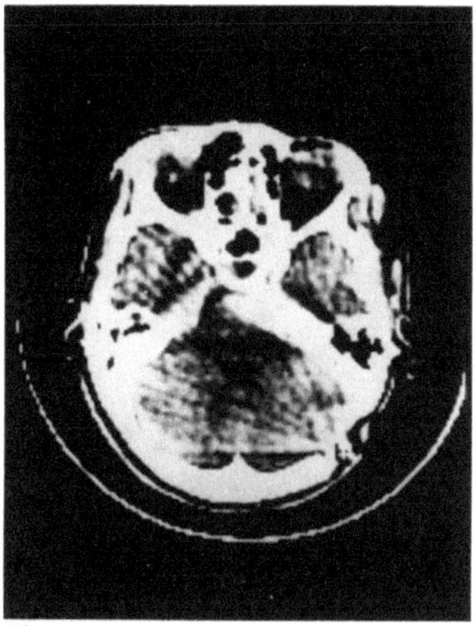

1f

Fig. 1 (Patient 1). Figs. 1 a and b are preoperative enhanced CT scans which reveal a large right petroclival meningioma starting in the right cerebellopontine angle, and extending across to involve the entire clival area, and up into the tentorial notch. Figs. 1 c and 1 d are right carotid arteriograms which show an enlarged meningohypophyseal artery supplying the tumor, and a tumor stain in the capillary phase. Fig. 1 e is an illustration of the retromastoid exposure for this kind of tumor. Follow-up CT scan 7 years later revealed a small tumor recurrence (Fig. 1 f), but the patient was asymptomatic.

surrounded the basilar artery and this area of tumor was coagulated. A small portion of the tumor was difficult to dissect off the brain stem and this was also coagulated. This lady made a good recovery postoperatively, her only deficit being a persistent trigeminal numbness. In follow-up, seven years later, CAT scan revealed a small recurrence, presumably from the portion left on the basilar artery. Since she is asymptomatic, she is being followed by repeated CT scans (figs. 1 a–f).

Patient 2: Surgeon: L. N. Sekhar
This 66-year-old man presented with progressive ataxia and dementia for six months. Axial and coronal CT scans revealed a very large medial tentorial meningioma extending into the region of the petrous ridge and the cavernous sinus. Cerebral angiography showed that the tumor was fed predominantly by the meningohypophyseal branch of the internal carotid artery. The posterior cerebral, the superior cerebellar, and the basilar arteries were displaced. Operation was performed by a combined right subtemporal and retromastoid approach. The tumor was completely resected, except for the portion within the cavernous sinus. The cavernous sinus was not entered because he had no extraocular muscle problems and because of his age. The trochlear nerve coursed through the tumor and was sectioned. The superior cerebellar artery entered the tumor and had to be dissected a fair amount in order to preserve it. The trigeminal nerve was pushed downwards below the level of the seventh and

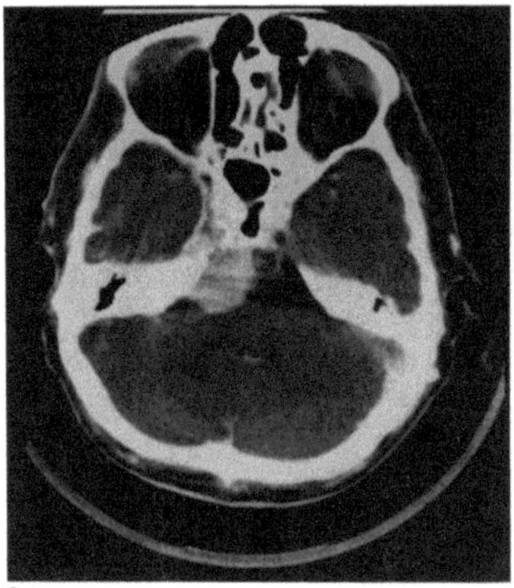
2a

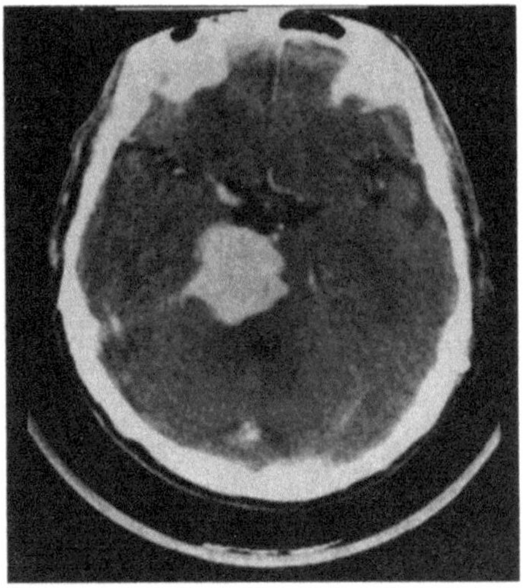
2b

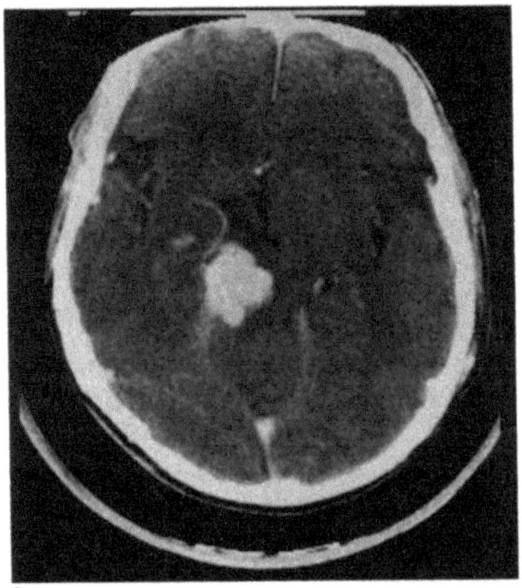
2c

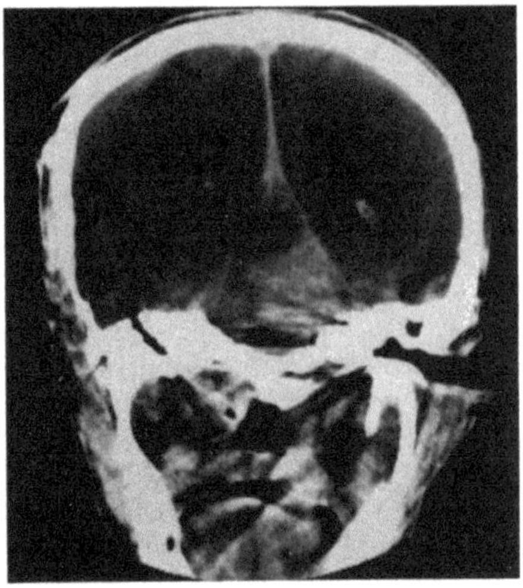
2d

eighth cranial nerves. The seventh and eighth nerves were pushed posteriorly and inferiorly. Postoperatively, the patient exhibited transient right facial palsy and left hemiparesis, both of which cleared subsequently. In follow-up, he was ambulatory and his dementia had cleared (figs. 2a-g).

Patient 3: Surgeon: M. Samii
This 56-year-old lady was referred with the history of progressive facial numbness, dementia, as well as ataxia. On examination, there was evidence of involvement of the trigeminal nerve with long tract signs. Computed tomography revealed a large meningioma occupying the medial tentorial notch area, and the petroclival region. Operation was performed by a left frontotemporal craniotomy without splitting of the sylvian fissure. After progressive debulking of the tumor, the trigeminal nerve was found to be significantly involved by infiltration of the tumor within its fascicles and was, therefore, divided. After division of the trigeminal nerve, the apex of the petrous bone was drilled using a diamond burr. This

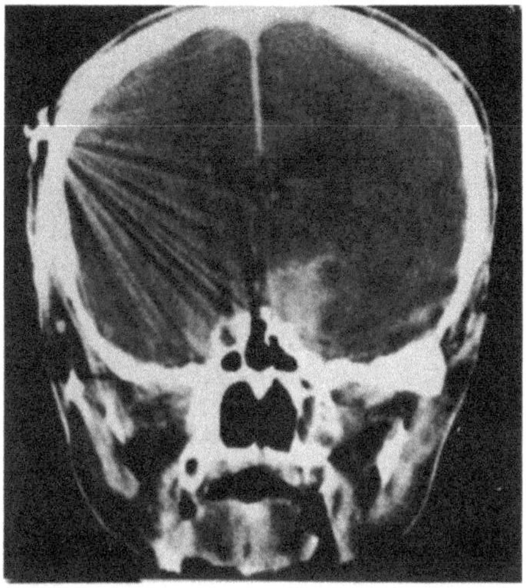

2e

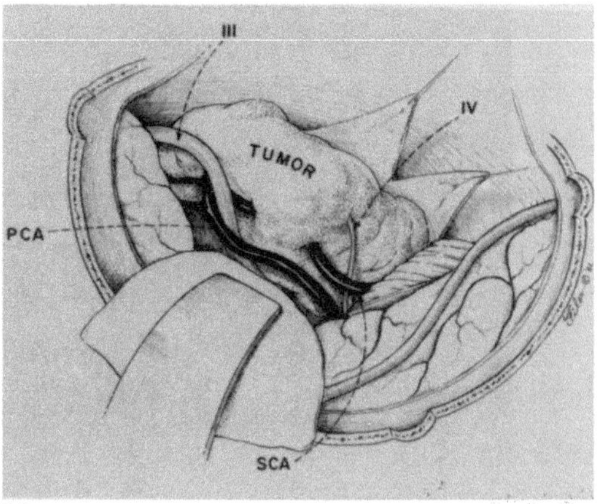

2f

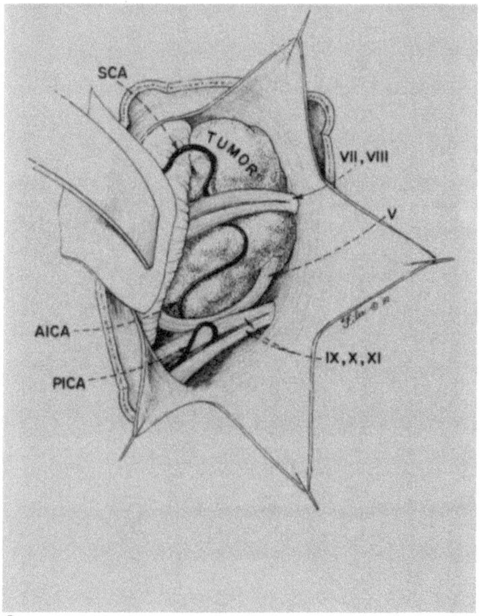

2g

Fig. 2 (Patient 2). Figs. 2a, 2b, and 2c are enhanced axial CT scans which illustrate a large tumor arising from the medial tentorial notch area, with extension onto the petrous ridge. The coronal CT scans (Figs. 2d and 2e) reveal that the tumor is both supra and infratentorial. This tumor was resected by a combined subtemporal-retromastoid approach. The exposure obtained by the subtemporal approach is illustrated in Fig. 2f. Note the superior cerebellar artery which runs through the tumor. Fig. 2g illustrates the exposure obtained by the retromastoid approach. Note that the trigeminal nerve is pushed down by the tumor, below the level of the facial and auditory nerves.

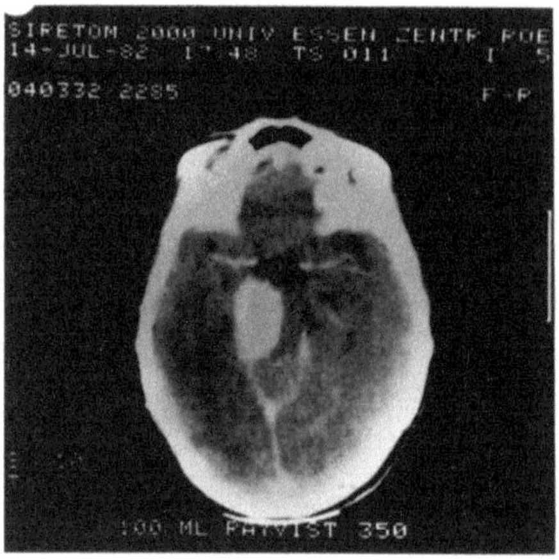

3a

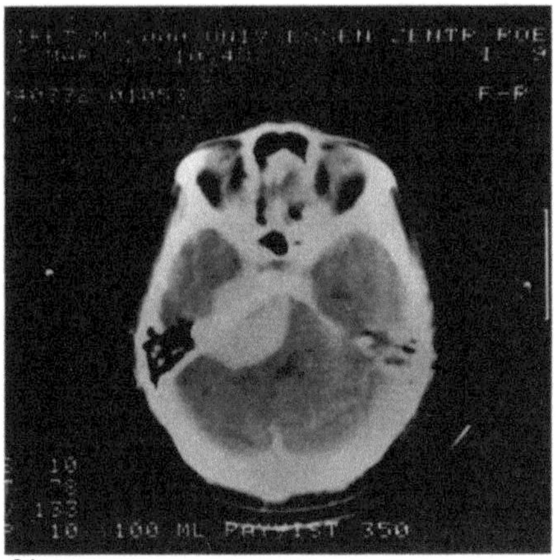

3b

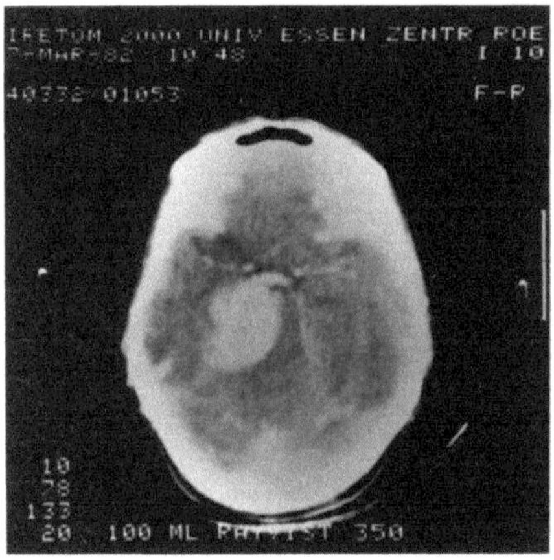

3c

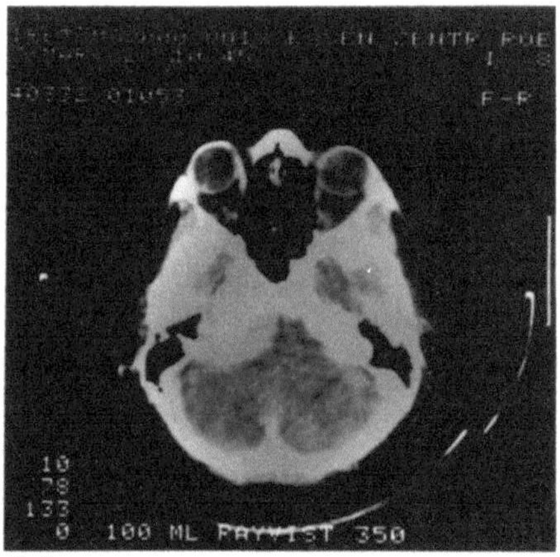

3d

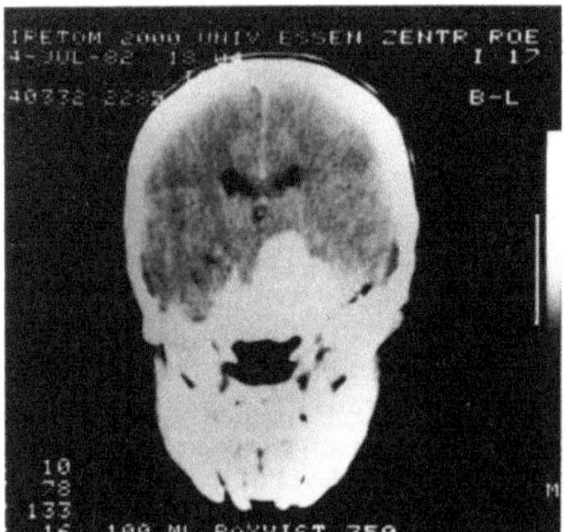

3e

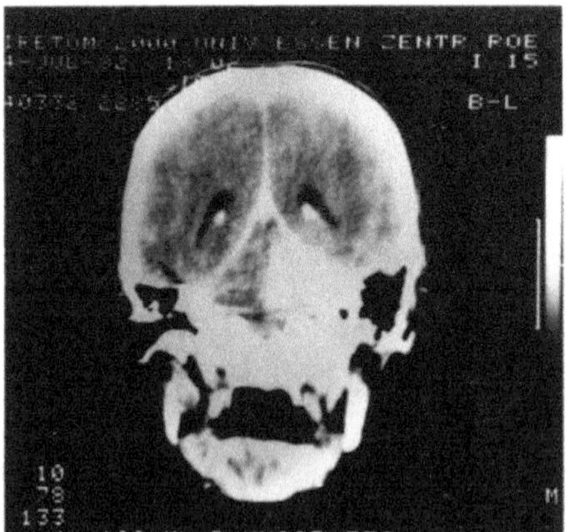

3f

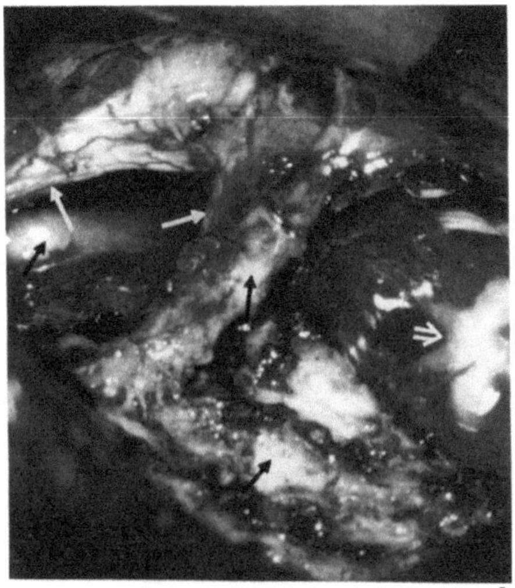

3g

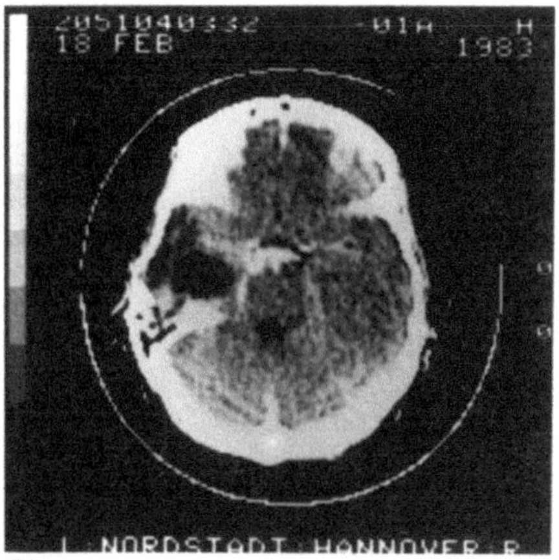

3h

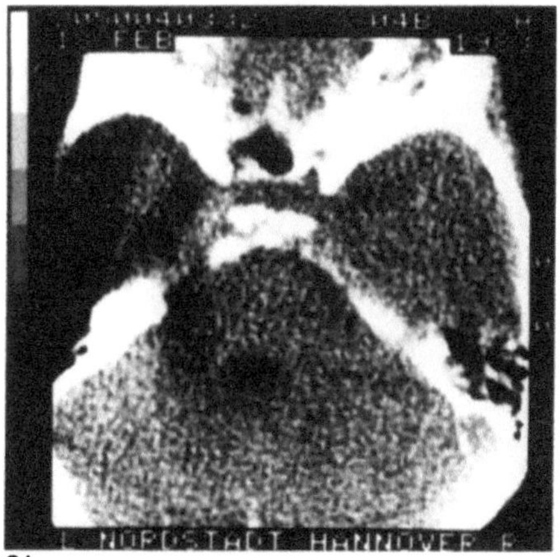

3i

Fig. 3 (Patient 3). Figs. 3 a, b, c, and d are axial CT scans which demonstrate a large medial tentorial notch tumor, extending into the middle fossa, and the petroclival area. Coronal CT scans (Figs. 3 e and f) also reveal the extent of supra and subtentorial tumor. This tumor was resected by a frontotemporal approach, with the drilling of the petrous apex, to reach the petrous ridge and the middle clivus (Fig. 3 g). Note the carotid arteries of both sides (arrows), optic nerves (arrowheads), and the basilar bifurcation (double arrow). Figs. 3 h and i are postoperative CT scans. Note the area of the petrous ridge that has been drilled off.

provided a very flat and unimpeded view of the posterior fossa, and it was easy to dissect the tumor from the midbrain, pons, and the seventh and eighth cranial nerves. Towards the conclusion of the operation, some tumor was also removed from the region of the cavernous sinus. The patient had temporary paralysis of the facial nerve postoperatively, but this has recovered completely, and she is normal on follow-up, two years after the operation (figs. 3 a–h).

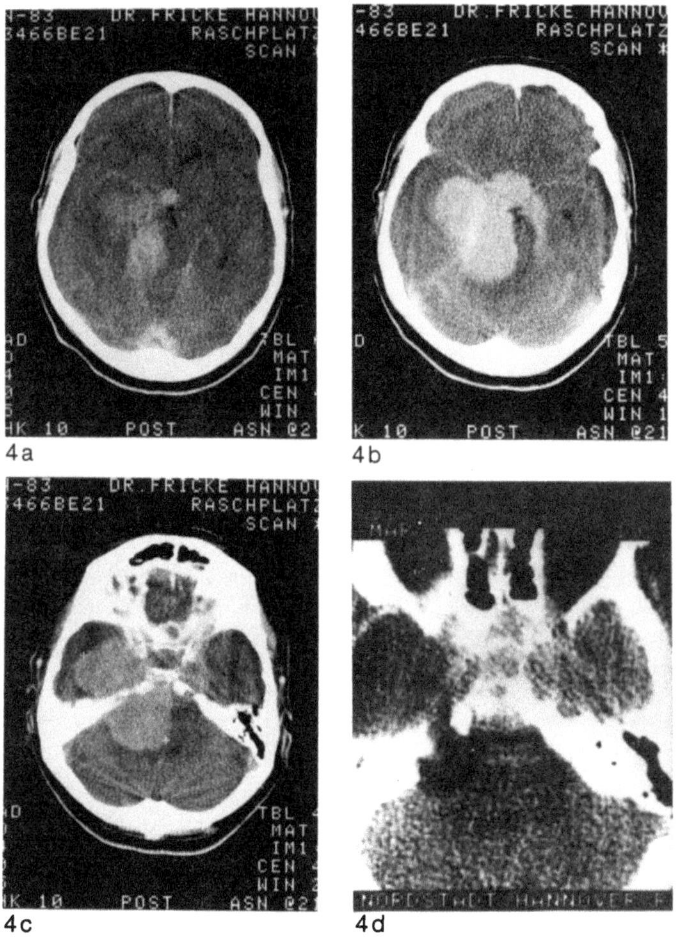

Fig. 4 (Patient 4). Figs. 4a, b, and c are axial enhanced CT scans which revealed a "pan-skull base meningioma" arising from the left petrous ridge, clivus, the left middle fossa, the left cavernous sinus, the tuberculum sella region, and the right parasellar area. The tumor was operated in two stages. The first was a left frontotemporal approach to remove it from the left middle fossa, petroclival area, tentorial notch, and the cavernous sinus. The second was a right frontotemporal approach to remove the tumor from the tuberculum sella and parasellar regions. A postoperative CT scan after the second stage of resection reveals the total excision of the tumor (Fig. 4d).

Patient 4: Surgeon: M. Samii
This man presented with a history of progressive ataxia and the involvement of the third through the ninth cranial nerves on the left side, and mild dementia. CAT scan revealed a giant meningioma of the skull base extending from the petroclival region into the tentorial notch, and the cavernous sinus on the left side, the tuberculum sella area, as well as the parasellar region on the right side. The patient was operated in two stages, the first stage consisted of a left frontotemporal craniotomy with an excision of the tumor from the middle fossa, the left cavernous sinus, the tentorial notch and the petrous ridge areas. The petrous apex was drilled, as described in patient 3. The cavernous sinus was entered, and the third,

fourth, and the fifth cranial nerves were divided on account of their involvement with the tumor. Tumor was removed from around the internal carotid artery from the base of the skull to the supraclinoid area.

At a subsequent operation six months later, the rest of the tumor from the tuberculum sella and the right parasellar region was removed. The patient has also undergone radiation therapy and is being followed (figs. 4a-d).

Discussion

Clusters of meningothelial cells are found in normal individuals around the venous sinuses and around the exit sites of the cranial nerves. Even though basal meningiomas may originate primarily in one site, they soon do spread to involve the adjacent areas. Thus, a lesion originating in the petrous ridge will soon extend into the clival region, the tentorial notch, the Meckel's cave, and the cavernous sinus. Classifications are therefore artificial, however, they do help the surgeon in planning the operative approaches, and in comparing the results of different series.

In considering operations on these lesions, the surgeon should consider the different approaches available [5, 6, 7]. A careful preoperative evaluation with CAT scans and cerebral angiograms is essential. Recently, we have found the use of intraoperative monitoring most useful in reducing the morbidity of these operations. Microsurgical techniques and minimal brain retraction are essential. In addition, increasing operator experience reduces the time required for each operation. Staging of operations should be considered when the operation takes an inordinately long time, or when more than one approach is essential for complete removal of the tumor. As with all other sites, the best time for radical resection of the lesion is the time when the patient first presents to the surgeon. Unfortunately, this is still not possible with some lesions in the petroclival and medial tentorial areas.

The different operative approaches available for excising these lesions are outlined in table 6. The retromastoid approach carries a low morbidity since cerebel-

Table 6 Operative approaches to petroclival and medial tentorial meningiomas

1. Retromastoid, paracerebellar
2. Subtemporal (posterior subtemporal)
3. Combined retromastoid - subtemporal
   with division of sigmoid sinus
4. Frontotemporal
   with sylvian fissure splitting
   with anterior temporal lobectomy
5. Frontotemporal with petrous apex drilling (anterior subtemporal)
6. Transtemporal - infratemporal (transpetrous approach)

lar retraction is benign. In the past, we have used the half sitting position for this approach. Recently, however, we have found the lateral position equally effective. With the majority of the lesions in this area, the seventh and eighth cranial nerves, the ninth, tenth, and eleventh cranial nerves, as well as the fifth cranial nerve, can often be identified early with this approach which is an advantage to the surgeon. However, the surgeon has to work between the cranial nerves in order to remove the tumor. The exposure of the petrous ridge area, as well as the middle and lower clivus on the ipsilateral side is excellent with this approach. However, the exposure of the tentorial notch region, and the contralateral clivus area, may be poor, and dissection of tumor from the brain stem on the other side may be difficult [5].

The subtemporal approach (also, called by us the posterior subtemporal approach) provides an excellent exposure of the tentorial notch region, the upper and the middle clivus area, including the contralateral side. The division of the tentorium is necessary to provide exposure of the cerebellopontine angle and of the middle clivus region. The main drawback of this exposure is retraction of the temporal lobe, which carries a morbidity, even in experienced hands. The vein of Labbé should not be divided and must be protected. The retromastoid and the subtemporal approaches may be combined in stages, or in the same operation. If there is a good communication between the two transverse sinuses, and the drainage is good on both sides, the transverse sinus can be divided at its junction with the sigmoid sinus, distal to the entrance point of the vein of Labbé, and in combination with the division of the tentorium, one can achieve an excellent exposure to the tentorial notch area [1, 2].

The frontotemporal approach with the splitting of the sylvian fissure provides an excellent exposure of the medial sylvian area, as well as the parasellar region. In order to remove tumor from the tentorial notch through this approach, one has to work through a narrow space, and also, the sylvian fissure must be split widely. One can reach the cerebellopontine angle after division of the tentorium, but the depth is great, and the exposure is very restricted. When the tumor has already displaced the temporal lobe from the middle fossa, or after an anterior temporal lobectomy, one can use the frontotemporal approach without splitting of the sylvian fissure, and with the division of the tentorium, to achieve an excellent exposure. This operation does not have the morbidity of the posterior subtemporal approach. As mentioned earlier, the drilling of the apex of the petrous bone with a diamond burr provides an excellent access to the cerebellopontine angle down to the seventh and the eighth nerves. When the tumor involves the region of the cavernous sinus or the Meckel's cave, this approach is ideal. While drilling the petrous apex, one must be careful not to injure the internal carotid artery, which comes close to this area. This can be easily done with the use of the diamond drill, and with repeated irrigation and suction.

Three main adjuvants are available for the resection of the tumor itself. These include the suction irrigation-bipolar combination, the cavitron ultrasonic aspirator, and the laser. Of these, we have found the suction irrigation-bipolar to be the most useful. The debulking of fibrous and vascular tumors can be quite tedious using this technique, however, it can be relatively bloodless, and it is also easy to dissect cranial nerves and blood vessels sharply while using this technique. We have not found a cavitron ultrasonic aspirator useful in removal of vascular basal meningiomas, since this technique only creates more bleeding and is not effective for removal of tough and fibrous tumors. The laser, which has become available recently, is advantageous for the debulking of vascular and fibrous tumors. However, since the surgeon does not have the feel of the instrument, one has to be very careful in dissecting around cranial nerves and blood vessels, or other critical structures, and one must revert to other microsurgical techniques.

The preservation of cranial nerves and vessels is of great importance to minimize the morbidity after removal of these tumors. Dissection of cranial nerves is aided by a knowledge of their anatomy, intraoperative monitoring and the use of microsurgical techniques. Some arteries may run through the tumor and supply the brain distally after providing branches to the tumor, such arteries must be carefully dissected and preserved. On occasion, we have had to perform an arterial anastamosis following injury at operation, with good result. With the exception of the vein of Labbé, most small veins in the vicinity of the tumor can be divided, but attempts must be made to preserve them if possible.

When there is hyperostosis underneath the lesion, it should be drilled using a diamond burr, and the area should be covered with a fascia lata graft and fat.

The continuing unsolved problems in operations on these tumors include cranial nerve and vascular preservation, retraction induced brain injury, inability to resect tumors completely, and the involvement of the cavernous sinus and extradural structures. Recently, progress has been made in the excision of tumors involving the cavernous sinus with cranial nerve preservation [4]. The value of radiation therapy for treatment of subtotally resected lesions remains controversial. Most experienced neurosurgeons, however, have observed some instances of remission of meningiomas following radiation therapy.

References

[1] Decker R. E., Malis L. I.: Surgical approaches to midline lesions at the base of the skull: a review. Mount Sinai J. Med. N. Y. 37 (1970), 84-102

[2] Sekhar L. N., Jannetta P. J.: Cerebellopontine Angle Meningiomas. Microsurgical Excision and Follow-Up Results. J. Neurosurg. 60 (1984), 500-505

[3] Sekhar L. N., Jannetta P. J., Maroon I. C.: Tentorial Meningiomas. Surgical Management and Results. Neurosurgery 14 (1984), 268-275

[4] Sekhar L. N., Moller A. M.: Operative Excision of Intracavernous Tumors with Monitoring and Preservation of Cranial Nerve Function. J. Neurosurg. (in press)

[5] Samii M., v. Wild K.: Operative Treatment of Lesions in the Region of the Tentorial Notch. Neurosurg. Rev. 4 (1981), 3-10
[6] Stein B. M., Leeds N. E., Taveras I.-M., Pool I. L.: Meningioma of the Foramen Magnum. J. Neurosurg. 20 (1965), 740-751
[7] Symon L.: Surgical Approaches to the Tentorial Hiatus. In: Advances and Technical Standards Nr. 9 (ed.) H. Krayenbühl (1982). Springer, Wien - New York
[8] Wond B. G. et al.: Surgical problems of the base of the skull. An interdisciplinary approach. Arch Otoryngol 106 (1981), 1-5

Surgical concepts in malignant tumors of the lateral skull base

O. H. Shaheen

Introduction

Faced with the question of what constitutes the lateral skull base and whether the term literally means the bone to the exclusion of adjacent areas, one may be hard put to provide a specific answer. Clearly the terms of reference of the title are as broad or as restricted as one wishes to make them. But helped by common sense and the desirability of confining oneself to situations born of personal experience, a picture of the subject in question begins to emerge.

Looking at the osseous component of the area, it would seem that one should be directing one's attention at the greater wing of the sphenoid, the pterygoid plates, a small portion of the squamous temporal bone, and the petrous temporal. Any one of these may in fact represent the site of origin of malignant disease, although in the case of the pterygoid plates and the sphenoid this is not common.

The bony lateral skull base forms the roof of two potential anatomical spaces, one clearly much larger than the other, namely the infratemporal fossa and subtemporal space. The former is not uncommonly the repository of disease, although generally this is the result of spread from contiguous areas such as the maxilla, nasopharynx, oral cavity, and the parotid gland. Rarely, the infratemporal fossa is the seat of origin of a primary malignancy. The slit-like space beneath the petrous bone is invaded by malignant disease from the middle ear cleft and by glomus jugulare tumors.

The malignancies with which one deals vary in their degree of invasiveness and lethality and not all are necessarily bound to cause distant metastases. At one end of the spectrum may be found the locally destructive condition of osteoblastoma of the skull base or fibrosarcoma of the infratemporal fossa, and at the opposite extreme is squamous carcinoma of the antrum invading the infratemporal fossa or condrosarcoma of the pterygoid plates (table 1).

Even over a span of many years surgical experience in a major teaching hospital, the number of cases which one eventually accumulates looks unimpressive and relates to malignancies arising in close proximity to the skull base, but not specifically arising from the bone thereof.

Table 1 Swellings of the infratemporal fossa

Primary swellings	
Meningioma	1
Lymphoma	1
Fibrosarcoma	2
Angioma	1
Fibroma	1
Histiocytosis X	1
Secondary swellings	
Carcinoma maxilla	4
Ameloblastoma	1
Chondromo sarcoma	1
Deep lobe mixed tumors of the parotid	9
Angiofibromata of the nasopharynx	9
Carcinoma of oral cavity	(Indeterminate number)

Surgical procedures directed at the lateral skull base

Radical anterolateral approach [1]

The approach required to deal with aggressive malignancies of the greater wing of the sphenoid or those arising from the maxilla and spreading backwards has to be ambitious in terms of surgical exposure. The kind of malignancies which one would be seeking to eradicate by this type of operation are chondrosarcoma of the bony base, malignant ameloblastoma and squamous carcinoma of the maxilla invading the infratemporal and pterygopalatine fossae.

The avenue of access most likely to afford the best exposure for this purpose is the radical anterolateral approach, combined possibly with partial or total maxillectomy, and orbital exenteration when maxillary cancer invades the orbit. The essence of this procedure is an osteoplastic flap of the hemimandible, allowing external rotation of the bone by division of all its muscular attachments.

Superolateral approach [1]

A superolateral approach via the temporal fossa, involving forward and downward retraction of the pinna, outward displacement of the zygomatic arch, and detachment of the upper insertion of the temporalis muscle, provides access to the infratemporal crest of the sphenoid while not endangering the facial nerve. This bony landmark serves as the starting point for drilling the sphenoid bone medially for such conditions as osteoblastoma and histiocytosis x.

Conservative lateral approach [2]

This has been used for the eradication of low grade tumors of the infratemporal fossa. After completing a total conservative parotidectomy the ascending ramus of the mandible is split in a trifurcate manner and the coronoid reflected superiorly inbetween branches of the facial nerve, while the base of the ascending ramus is retracted downwards. Final removal of the tumor may be facilitated by outward pressure effected by the insertion of a finger in the nasopharynx. At the conclusion of the procedure the mandible is rewired in position.

Recurrent pleomorphic adenoma invading the infratemporal fossa may be equated to some extent with malignancies of a low grade type, since the multiplicity of nodules in the recurrence makes the task of eradicating it a formidable one, the more so when the nodules are stuck to the periosteum of the skull base. Resection by total conservative parotidectomy with or without mandibular split and subsequent rewiring may prove to be satisfactory in such cases.

Radical lateral approach

When dealing with frank malignancies of the parotid, such as adenoid cystic or mucoepidermoid carcinoma of the deep lobe, no compromise should be offered in the interests of permanent eradication of the tumor. Radical resection of the ascending ramus is nearly always mandatory as part of a radical parotidectomy, and it may be necessary to include a partial drill-out of the temporal bone if the disease involves the fallopian canal, as can be the case with adenoid cystic carcinoma.

Petrosectomy [3]

Disease involving the petrous bone and invading the subtemporal space is dealt with by petrosectomy. The sort of dissection described by Fisch for glomus jugulare tumors, involving as it does transposition of the facial nerve and forward displacement of the ascending mandibular ramus has shown its worth in practice. An even more radical version, but without the need to conserve the facial nerve may be required for cancers of the middle ear cleft and petrous bone.

Summary

Within the context of a brief discussion of the anatomy and pathology of the lateral skull base, some surgical procedure for dealing with problems on this area have been described.

References

[1] Shaheen, O.H.: Swellings of the infratemporal fossa. J. Laryngol. Otol. **96** (1982) 817-836.
[2] Conley, J.J., G.T.Pack, S.S.Trinidad: Surgical technique for removal of infratemporal meningioma. Laryngoscope **66** (1956) 540-549.
[3] Fisch, U., H.C.Pillsbury: Infratemporal fossa approach to lesions in the temporal bone and base of skull. Arch. Otolaryngol. **105** (1979) 99-107.

Intratemporal neurinomas of the facial nerve and epidermoids of the petrous bone

H. J. Gerhardt

Neurinomas or more exactly neurilemmomas of the facial nerve are rare. Until 1972 not more than a 100 cases had been published. A certain increase of reports came along with the development of the technique of microsurgery on the petrous bone and progress in radiology especially polytomography.

According to its location a neurinoma of the facial nerve can mimic different diseases. A neurinoma originating in the cerebellopontine angle and/or internal auditory meatus may be difficult to distinguish from an acoustic neuroma.

When growing in the tympanic or labyrinthine region of the facial nerve an impairment of hearing, sensorineural, conductive or combined, is usually the first symptom. A loss of vestibular function may also occur but is often not noticed by the patient because of the efficient compensation by the vestibular system when slowly progressing.

Blockage of airways in the middle ear or penetration through the tympanic membrane or the wall of the external auditory meatus may cause chronic inflammation and give also rise to a misinterpretation. On the other hand neurinomas originating in the extratemporal area are hard to distinguish from tumors of the parotid gland before operation.

What may point to the right diagnosis? Our own experiences with intratemporal neurinomas of the facial nerve are based on 6 cases, 3 men and 3 women, from 22 to 71 years, the mean age being 40 years. This is in good agreement with other authors [2, 7]. All of the patients, suffering from an intratemporal neurinoma told us, that an impairment of hearing on the side involved was the first symptom. It preceded symptoms related to the facial nerve function by between one and ten years. When admitted to our hospital three of the six patients were completely deaf on the side involved, one had a sensorineural, two others a combined hearing loss. The patients who were completely deaf also had a loss of vestibular function in the same ear. All the others showed a deficiency in excitability tests.

As regards the first symptom caused by an intratemporal neurinoma of the facial nerve, opinion is divided among the authors. Our findings are in agreement with those of Pearman and Welch [9] and Taguchi et al. [13]. On the other hand Fisch [4] and Miehlke [7] take the view that facial paresis precedes the hearing loss as a rule.

As regards facial nerve function, two of our patients had a sudden onset of facial palsy and had been treated first as Bell's palsy. Two others became aware of a slowly progressing paresis, preceded by a certain spasm and twitching in different

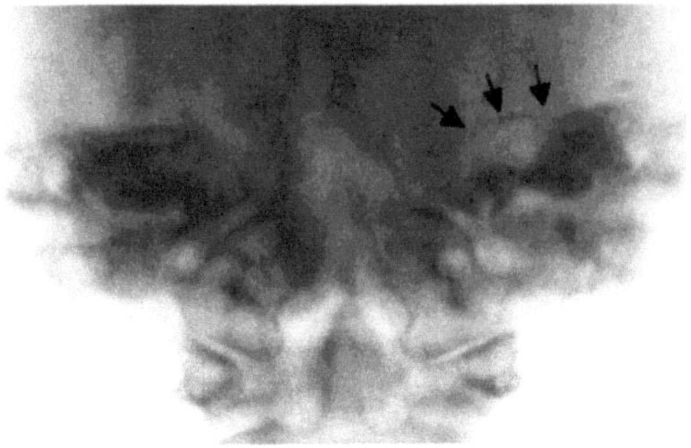

Fig. 1 Defect in the left pyramid caused by neurinoma of the facial nerve.

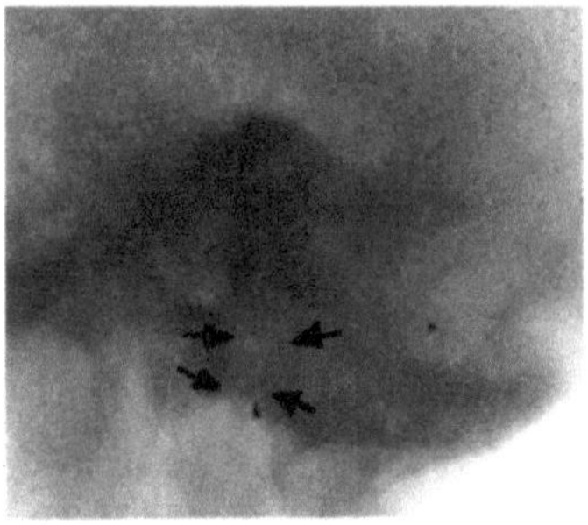

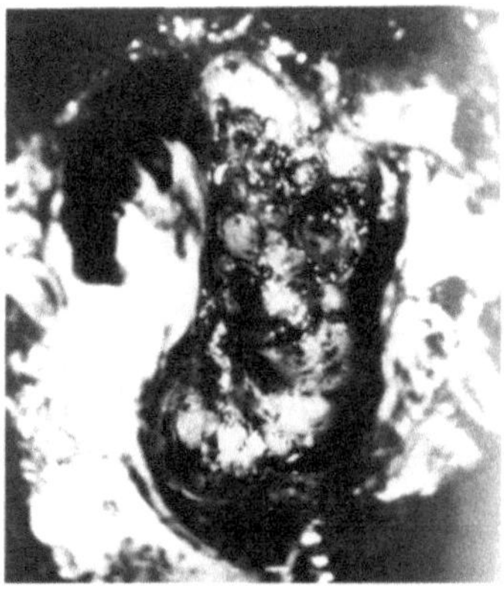

Fig. 2a Widening of the mastoid portion of the Fallopian canal.

Fig. 2b Same patient. Operation finding (mastoidectomy).

regions of the involved side of the face. The last two patients had not noticed any disturbance of the nerve at all. They had been referred to us because of hearing loss.

Different types of onset and course of facial paresis are also reported by others [1, 3-7, 10]. Jackson et al. [5] emphasized, that in acute onset, Bell's palsy is wrongly diagnosed in about 20%. On the other hand especially an intermittent [3, 6, 10] or slowly progressive paresis [1, 4, 5, 10] should arouse suspicion of a tumor.

For the right diagnosis a careful radiological examination of the petrous bone, especially by polytomography, is most informative. In neurinoma it reveals the typical image of a sharply defined bone defect (fig. 1) or often a widening of the Fallopian canal over a long distance (fig. 2). Electrophysiological testing such as EMG and electroneurography gives more information about the functional status of the nerve. Audiometry, if possible, impedance testing and electrogustometry may be of special interest but in general do not contribute much useful information.

The only adequate treatment is complete removal of the tumor and reconstruction of the facial nerve. The approach to the tumor depends on its location and the function of the inner ear and may be translabyrinthine, via the middle cranial fossa or a combined one.

Case reports

Case 1: Young man, 17 years old, complete facial palsy, deafness, large neurinoma of the tympanic and the labyrinthine region of the nerve. Transtemporal approach grafting of the nerve using the greater auricular nerve. Satisfactory result.

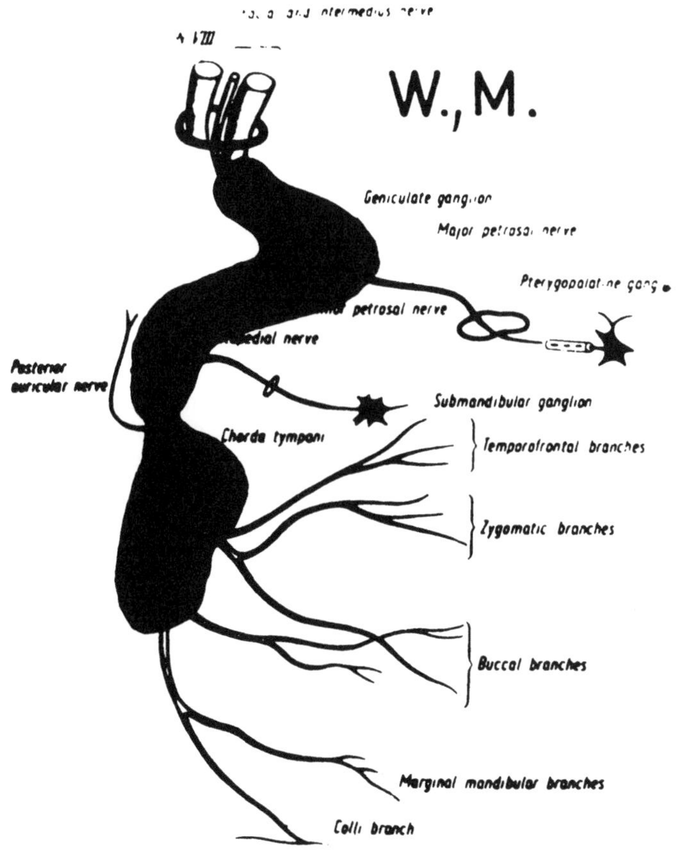

Fig. 3a Very long extension of a neurinoma of the facial nerve. In spite of this only mild paresis of the nerve was present.

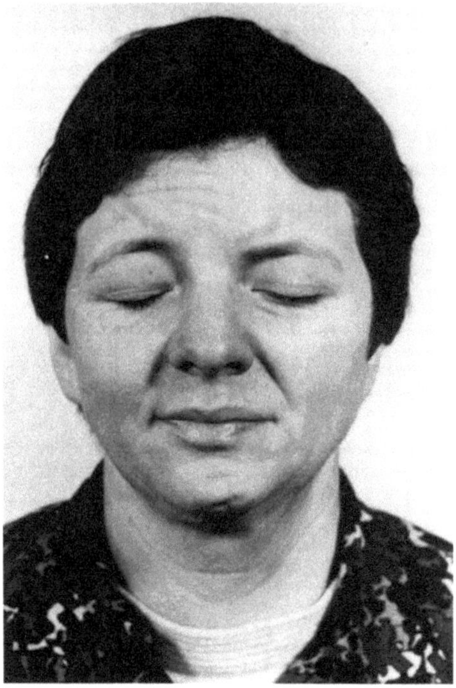

Fig. 3 b Functional result after nerve grafting (7 cm).

Case 2: Woman, 71 years old, chronic discharge from the left ear, slowly progressing facial paresis, deafness. Transmastoid-translabyrinthine approach, chronic mastoiditis, erosion of the labyrinth by a neurinoma of the tympanic and labyrinthine area, nerve grafting. Poor result.

Case 3: Woman, 32 years of age, complete facial palsy within a month. Very large neurinoma of the proximal part of the nerve, broad extension into the cerebellopontine angle. Removal of the tumor by middle cranial fossa approach. Hypoglossus-facial-anastomosis. Satisfactory result.

Case 4: Woman, 34 years of age, very long extensive neurinoma from the fundus of the internal auditory meatus to the parotid gland (fig. 3 a) but only mild paresis. Combined approach, nerve graft 7 cm long, satisfactory result (fig. 3 b).

Epidermoids of the petrous bone originate from ectodermal cells displaced during ontogenesis together with cells developing later on mucosal cells in the temporal bone [8]. Having arrived at their final place those cells according to their genetic imminent behaviour start to multiply and to transform aging cells into keratinised ones. The growing keratinised masses increasingly destroy the adjoining structures mainly by putting pressure on them.

Epidermoids of this region in general are discovered rather late. Apart from irreversible defects on the adjacent structures this may be dangerous to the patient be-

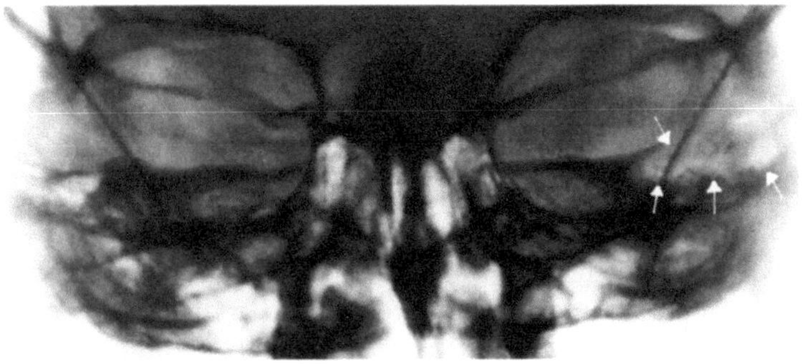

Fig. 4 Large epidermoid in the left pyramid.

cause of threatening intracranial complications, such as meningitis or brain abscess.

Among our twelve patients suffering from epidermoid of the pyramid two got meningitis before the epidermoid has been discovered. A meningitis with a fatal outcome, caused by an epidermoid of the petrous bone in a 71-year-old woman has been reported by Rosen and Vered [11].

Our patients, 7 woman and 5 men, were aged from 14 to 59 years, the mean age being 34.3 years. The symptoms being the cause for referring them to our hospital were meningitis in two, hearing lose and vestibular deficiency in four and facial paresis in six cases. Three of them had a sudden onset of palsy, treated first as Bell's palsy, in two cases with partial improvement. The other three patients became aware of a progressing paralysis that led in one patient within 10 days in another within 4 weeks to a complete palsy.

An attentive inquiry then showed, that all of them had a history of hearing loss for many years. 4 patients were completely deaf in the ear involved when referred to us, 4 had a predominantly conductive hearing loss, 4 a combined one. Caloric vestibular testing revealed a complete loss of excitability in 10 patients, and a deficiency was evident in 2 cases.

Here also the most informative diagnostic method was radiological examination. In epidermoids a sharply defined defect round or polycyclic (fig. 4) is the typical image. Defects of the semicircular canals (12 ×), of the basal turn of the cochlea (6 ×) and penetration into the fundus and meatus internus (10 ×) were clearly visible.

The only adequate treatment in epidermoids also is complete removal. The approach depends on the location of the epidermoid and also on the function of the inner ear. In 7 patients, already deaf, the transmastoid-translabyrinthine approach was performed. In three patients the epidermoid surrounded the seventh and eighth nerves inside the internal meatus. Those nerves had to be severed in the cerebellopontine angle. For reconstruction of the function of facial expression a hypoglossal-facial anastomosis has been performed.

For more medially located epidermoids (5 ×) the middle cranial fossa approach was an advantage [12]. Complete removal of the epidermoid often required extension of erosions on the labyrinth. Therefore in only two patients could useful hearing be still preserved.

Especially delicate was the removal of the very thin matrix from the dura, the facial nerve and from the internal carotid artery (3 ×). In five cases the facial nerve was completely surrounded by the matrix mainly in its labyrinthine region. It was necessary in those cases to sever the greater petrosal nerve and to perform temporarily a rerouting of the facial to get access to the matrix below. In 6 cases with no or only mild facial paresis the continuity of the nerve could be preserved. In 3 cases an extreme atrophy due to pressure was perceptible. In those cases this part was resected. Reconstruction was possible once by rerouting and simple anastomosis and twice by using a nerve graft from the greater auricular nerve. All the patients with the nerve's continuity preserved got a normal or nearly normal function. Even in patients already suffering from facial paralysis before operation an improvement could be achieved.

Case reports

Case 1: A girl, 14 years old, no complaints. During a routine examination a previously unnoticed hearing loss of 40 dB in the left ear was the reason for a closer examination. This revealed a complete loss of vestibular function and by polytomography a bone defect in the pyramid, extending medially to the fundus of the internal meatus.

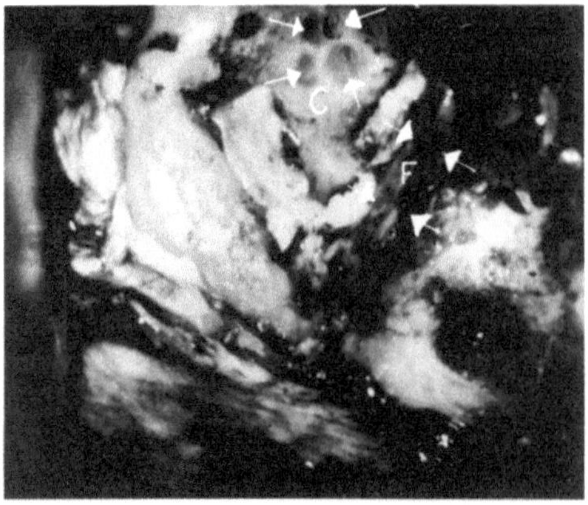

Fig. 5 Erosion of the cochlea (C). F = facial nerve.

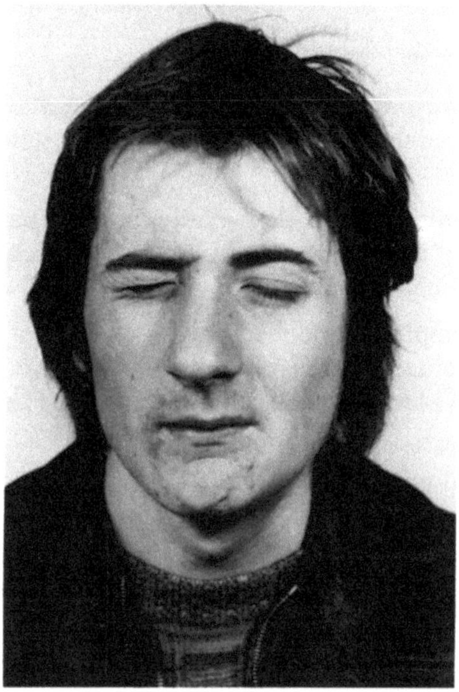

Fig. 6 Same patient. Result of hypoglossal-facial anastomosis.

A middle cranial fossa approach revealed a large epidermoid, erosion of the superior semicircular canal, the facial nerve in the area of the geniculate ganglion completely surrounded by matrix. Malleus and incus were also eroded from medially by lateral extension of the epidermoid. No contact of the matrix with the tympanic membrane. Complete removal of the epidermoid was possible by temporary rerouting of the facial nerve as described earlier. Postoperatively mild facial paresis for 6 weeks, otherwise no complications. Hearing loss diminished to 30 dB. No indication of relapse after 8 years.

Case 2: Boy, 15 years old, hearing loss in the left ear, no treatment. In July 1976, meningitis, cured by treatment with antibiotics. Some months later slowly progressing facial paresis. When admitted to our hospital 4 months later, complete facial palsy, deafness and loss of vestibular function. Radiological examination reveals a large bone defect in the petrous bone (2 × 2 × 2 cm) including the labyrinth and extending from the attic to the medial portion of the pyramid beyond the internal auditory meatus.

Translabyrinthine approach. A wide-spread pneumatised system without any indication of inflammation. Only when exposing the labyrinth, the first parts of the epidermoid became visible, penetrating also into the vestibule and the cochlea (fig. 5). The seventh and eighth nerves in their course in the internal meatus are also in close contact with the matrix. To ensure complete removal of the epidermoid both of them had to be severed in the cerebellopontine angle. The internal carotid artery is covered by matrix 1.5 cm in length but we succeeded in detaching the latter from it. Hypoglossal-facial anastomosis. The functional result is satisfactory (fig. 6).

Conclusions

In general both of these destructive processes in the petrous pyramid are discovered rather late. On the other hand they may become the cause of serious complications.

To achieve an earlier diagnosis requires careful examination in every patient suffering from one-sided hearing loss of unknown origin. Audiometry, vestibular testing and radiological examination is necessary.

Suspicion should be aroused by complaints about spasm or twitching of one side of the face and especially a slowly progressing paresis of the facial nerve, but even in sudden onset of palsy a destructive lesion always should be excluded before taking Bell's palsy for granted.

In all patients suffering from facial palsy without any tendency to improvement during 8-12 months, total exposure of the facial nerve in its intratemporal course should be considered.

References

[1] Charachon, R., O. Roux, G. Dumas: Tumeurs du nerf facial. A propos de trois observations. Ann. Oto-laryng. (Paris) **95** (1978) 777-784.

[2] Conley, J., I. Janecka: Schwann cell tumor of the facial nerve. Laryngoscope **84** (1974) 958-962.

[3] Conley, J., R. W. Selfe: Occult neoplasms in facial paralysis. Laryngoscope **91** (1981) 205-210.

[4] Fisch, U.: Operations on the facial nerve in its labyrinthine and meatal course. In: Surgery of the facial nerve (A. Miehlke, ed.), p. 194. Urban u. Schwarzenberg, München-Wien-Berlin. Saunders Company, Philadelphia-London-Toronto 1973.

[5] Jackson, C. G., M. E. Glasscock, G. Hughes et al.: Facial paralysis of neoplastic origin: diagnosis and management. Laryngoscope **90** (1980) 1581-1595.

[6] Lopes, O., N. Penteado de Castro, F. A. Quantanilha Ribeiro, et al.: Neurinoma of the facial nerve. ORL (Basel) **40** (1978) 254-262.

[7] Miehlke, A.: Surgery of the Facial Nerve, p. 98. Urban u. Schwarzenberg, München-Wien-Berlin. Saunders Company, Philadelphia-London-Toronto 1973.

[8] Otto, H.-D.: Pathogenese der branchiogenen Überschußmißbildungen (Choristien). Teil 1: Epithelversprengungen. HNO-Prax. (Leipzig) **8** (1983) 161-169.

[9] Pearman, K., A. R. Welch: Schwannoma of the intratemporal facial nerve. Case report. J. Laryng. (Lond.) **94** (1980) 779-784.

[10] Portmann, M., J. P. Bébéar: A propos des neurinomas du nerf facial intra-pétreux. Rev. Laryng. (Bordeaux) **98** (1977) 21-29.

[11] Rosen, G., J. Y. Vered: Congenital cholesteatoma causing meningitis and death. J. Laryng. (Lond.) **90** (1976) 1151-1154.

[12] Sterkers, J. M., O. Sterkers: Cholestéatomes congénitaux du rocher. A propos de 5 observations. Ann Oto-laryng. (Paris) **97** (1980) 579-589.

[13] Taguchi, K., T. Ishiyama, K. Higaki, et al.: A case of facial nerve neurinoma in the middle ear. Otol. Fukuoka **26, Suppl. 1** (1980) 321-329.

The intracavernous connective tissue cover of the internal carotid artery – anatomy and surgery

A. Perneczky, E. Knosp

Introduction

The direct surgical management of infraclinoid aneurysms and parasellar tumors poses technical problems on account of their anatomical relationship to the cavernous sinus and surrounding structures. The point where the internal carotid artery passes through the dural plane between its intracavernous and subarachnoidal portion is of specific interest for the neurosurgeon. The direct surgical approach to the intracavernous portion of the internal carotid artery through the lateral wall of the cavernous sinus [1] is hazardous and in most cases of intracavernous vascular lesion it is replaced by methods of the interventional neuroradiology. In our previous reports we described a possible surgical approach to the rostral part of the intracavernous carotid artery because of some anatomical details [2, 3]. Our anatomical studies presented here show that following dissection of a tight fibrous ring the internal carotid artery is surrounded by loose connective tissue, which allows blunt mobilisation along the vessel wall without opening the cavernous sinus itself.

Anatomy

The intracavernous portion of the internal carotid artery is loosely, covered by connective tissue. Only at the level of the roof of the cavernous sinus (transversal plate), a solid radial attachment of the carotid wall to the dura can be seen (fig. 1). If this attachment is sharply dissected, the loose layer of connective tissue is reached, where blunt exposure of the anatomical specimen can be undertaken along the entire wall of the intracavernous carotid artery without opening the sinus (fig. 2).

In the intraoperative dissection, anatomical factors have to be considered as well. On the one hand, the anterior siphon knee is very rarely surrounded by venous canals of the cavernous sinus (fig. 3). On the other hand, the level of the transversal plate is located deeper than the anterior clinoid process, planum sphenoidale and tuberculum sellae. Thus, in the surgical approach to the fibrous ring the anterior clinoid process and the tuberculum sellae have to be resected.

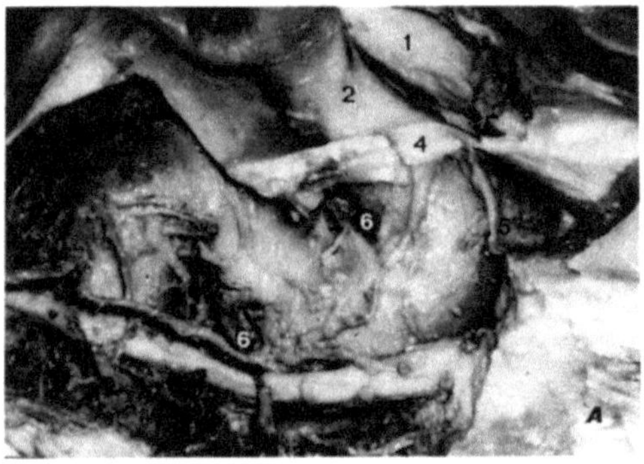

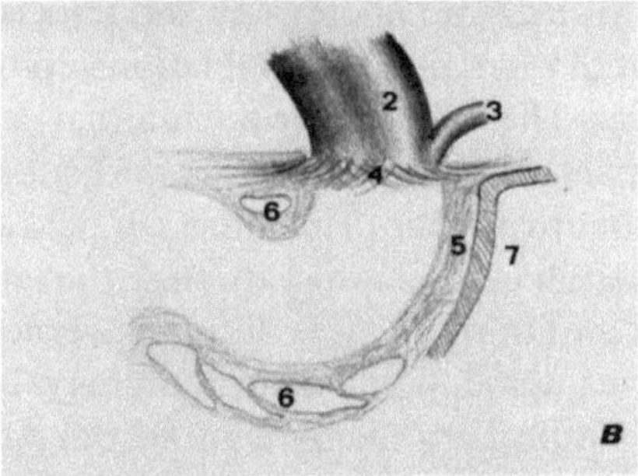

Fig. 1 (A) Anatomical specimen demonstrating the fibrous ring at the level of the roof of the cavernous sinus. Lateral view. (B) Diagram of the same region. 1 = right optic nerve; 2 = subarachnoid part of the internal carotid artery; 3 = ophthalmic artery; 4 = fibrous ring around the carotid artery at the level of the transversal plate; 5 = soft connective tissue layer along the intracavernous carotid artery; 6 = venous channels of the cavernous sinus; 7 = sphenoid sinus.

Surgery

By way of illustration a case of direct operation on an infraclinoidal aneurysm will be presented. By a right pterional craniotomy the optic nerve is exposed. After removal of the anterior clinoid and opening the optic canal the optic nerve is slightly elevated and the fibrous ring around the carotid artery at the level of the transversal plate sharply dissected. The entire anterior siphon knee can be subsequently inspected with a dissector. In a case where an aneurysm is present, a clip may be placed infraclinoidally without tearing the cavernous sinus (figs. 4 and 5).

In cases of parasellar and intracavernous tumors the above described connective tissue cover of the carotid artery makes possible a gentle dissection of the artery during tumor removal. In such cases we prefer the approach through the lateral wall of the cavernous sinus because the sinus is occluded by tumor tissue. Here the only difficulty is if the carotid wall infiltrated by the tumor. We usually open the lateral wall of the cavernous sinus in the triangle of Parkinson.

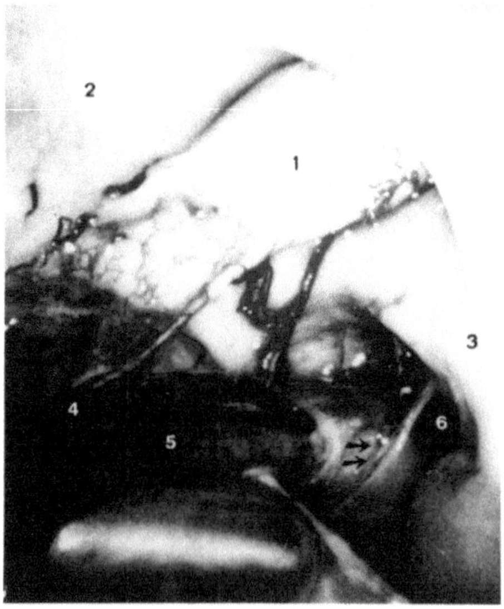

Fig. 2 Anatomical dissection of the connective tissue layer covering the intracavernous portion of the internal carotid artery (view of the right pterional approach). 1 = right optic nerve; 2 = planum sphenoidale; 3 = anterior clinoid process; 4 = dissector retracting the internal carotid artery; 5 = internal carotid artery; 6 = the loose connective tissue layer; arrows = the fibrous ring cut.

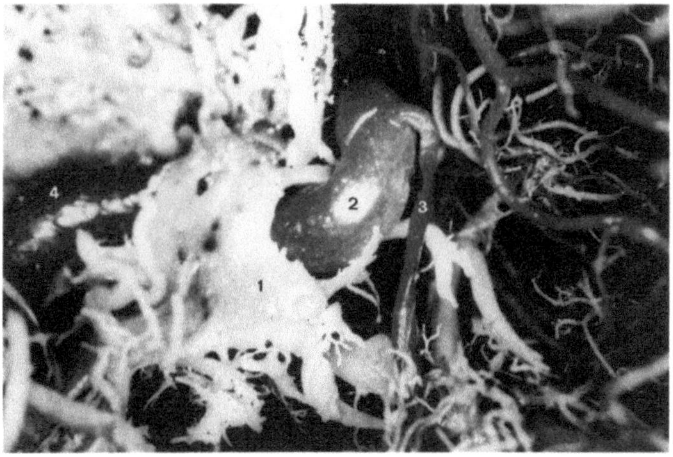

Fig. 3 Corrosion speciment of the intracranial vessels. Arteries dark, veins light. 1 = cavernous sinus; 2 = anterior knee of the carotid siphon; 3 = ophthalmic artery; 4 = intrapetrous portion of the internal carotid artery. Note there are no venous canals surrounding the anterior siphon knee of the internal carotid artery.

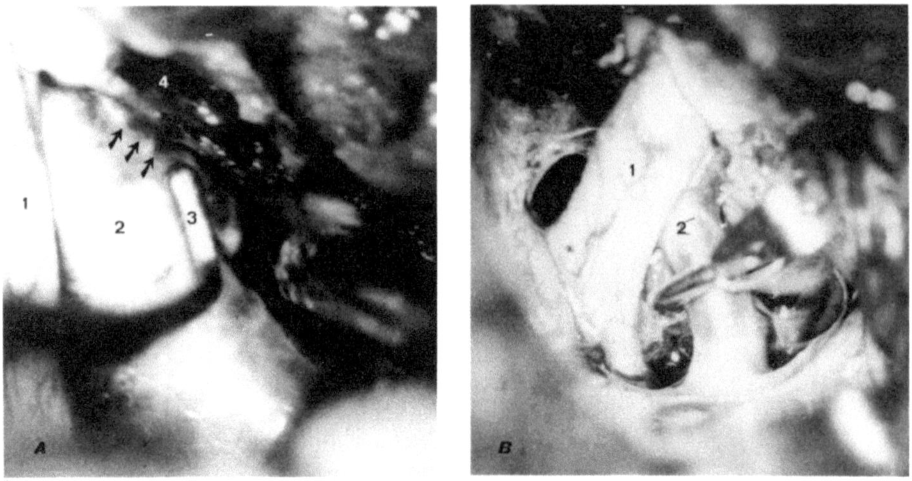

Fig. 4 Intraoperative photographs in a case of infraclinoid aneurysm of the right internal carotid artery. (A) Opening of the fibrous ring with a sharp dissector; (B) clipping of the aneurysm with a tunnel clip where the carotid artery is running through the clip. Note the opened optic canal and the removal of the anterior clinoid process. 1 = right optic nerve; 2 = carotid artery; 3 = sharp dissector; 4 = resected anterior clinoid process; arrows = fibrous ring at the level of the transversal plate.

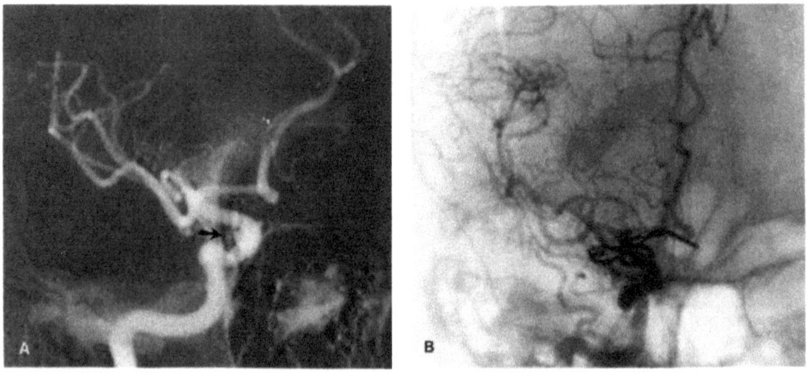

Fig. 5 Angiograms of the demonstrated case. (A) Pre-operative angiogram of the right internal carotid artery, oblique view. Arrow = infraclinoid aneurysm, posteromedially located. A second aneurysm of the anterior communicating artery is also shown. (B) Postoperative angiogram, AP view.

Conclusion

Our anatomical investigations suggest that the anterior knee of the carotid siphon does not run in the cavernous sinus. Rather, a loose connective tissue layer surrounds the vessel and permits blunt dissection. At the level of the transversal plate, the internal carotid artery is fixed by a tight fibrous ring.

Summary

The internal carotid artery in its intracavernous position is covered by a slack connective tissue layer. At the entrance of the artery into the subarachnoid space there is a very dense fibrous ring fixing the artery wall at the roof of the cavernous sinus. After cutting of the fibrous ring it is possible to dissect along the artery wall without opening the cavernous sinus. The anatomical details are described. On the basis of different surgical examples in the region of the cavernous sinus (tumor and vascular surgery) the significance of these findings is demonstrated.

References

[1] Parkinson, D.: A surgical approach to the cavernous portion of the carotid artery. Anatomical studies and case report. J. Neurosurg. **23** (1965) 474–483.

[2] Perneczky, A., E. Knosp: The intracavernous portion of the internal carotid artery. American-European Neurosurgical Winter Conference on Cerebrovascular Disease and Posterior Fossa Pathology. Obergurgl (Austria), March 1982.

[3] Perneczky, A.: Direct surgical approach to infraclinoidal aneurysms. 2nd American-European Neurosurgical Winter Conference St. Anton (Austria), March 1984.

Rare lesions of the parasellar area

W. J. Bock, N. Roosen

Introduction

The syndrome of ophthalmoplegia, due to involvement of one or more of the cranial nerves to the extraocular muscles, associated with trigeminal nerve dysfunction, most often of its ophthalmic or maxillary division, points towards the parasellar region or slightly more anterior towards the superior orbital fissure (syndrome of Foix), although not all parasellar lesions cause this syndrome. The most frequently encountered diseases in this area of the skull base are pituitary adenomas, meningiomas, craniopharyngiomas, germinomas and aneurysms [19]. Some of the more uncommon parasellar lesions are presented in this paper: metastasis, epidermoid cyst, chordoma, sarcoidosis, neurinoma.

Case reports

Case 1: Chordoma (R. A.). A 68-year-old woman had complained of progressive visual loss and temporal hemianopia on the right eye for four years. At the age of 65 years a nasopharyngeal polyp was resected, but was not examined microscopically. At that time she complained also of transient diplopia. Presenting signs now were a blood-stained nasal discharge, amaurosis and bulbar protrusion on the right, as well as an inferior nasal quadrantic field defect on the left. A voluminous, nasopharnygeal growth was found on clinical examination. X-rays showed extensive sellar destruction and erosion of the apex of the right petrous pyramid. Angiography outlined an avascular, space-occupying lesion. The tumor was subtotally resected in three sessions: the first approach was through the nose and the others were subfrontal and temporal. The postoperative course was complicated and death ensued after a few weeks.

Case 2: Chordoma (M. E.). A 58-year-old man presented with progressive, right ptosis and visual loss. For a few months he had also suffered minor headaches. Clinical examination demonstrated a partial external ophthalmoplegia on the right. Sellar erosion and slight calcification in the right middle fossa were seen on radiographs. Angiography showed an avascular tumor. It was subtotally resected by a subfrontal approach. A second operation for recurrence was performed one year later. However, at the age of 60 years the patient had a right amaurosis, complete ophthalmoplegia and trigeminal hypesthesia. Two courses of radiotherapy were given (30 and 40 Gy). After one year nasopharyngeal and anterior skull base infiltration was treated by an ethmoidal approach in the ENT-department. Hemiparesis developed a few months later, and regressed after the fourth operation. 40 Gy of radia-

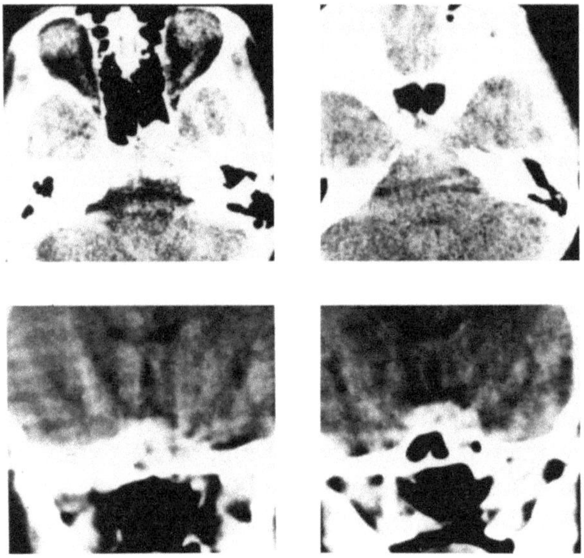

Fig. 1 Chordoma case 4. Axial and coronal CT demonstrating the extent of the tumor and the skull base infiltration.

tion were given, but at the age of 62 years symptoms further progressed. Because of severe headache palliative radiotherapy (30 Gy) was then started. Three months later the patient died.

Case 3: Chordoma (P. H.). A 35-year-old man had complained of diplopia for four years, right facial numbness for two years and then developed a right facial nerve paresis. Skull X-rays demonstrated extensive destruction of the sella and right petrous apex. Angiography showed an avascular lesion. Symptoms regressed after subtotal extirpation by a temporal approach. Two years later the tumor recurred with signs of posterior fossa involvement. At the age of 38 years right hemianopia and visual loss appeared. Middle and posterior cranial fossa exploration was performed. Death followed postoperative complications.

Case 4: Chordoma (E. I.). A 62-year-old woman presented with blood-stained nasal discharge and a left abducens paresis. Bony destruction of the left middle fossa, parasellar area and sphenoid sinus was revealed by radiography. The extent of the tumor was clearly outlined by CT (fig. 1). Angiography showed a rather intense tumor blush (fig. 2). Because of the poor general condition of the patient only a biopsy was performed by a transnasal approach. During the two year follow-up the symptoms slowly progressed.

Case 5: Chordoma (H. G.). A 59-year-old woman had complained of transient diplopia for more than ten years and an abducens paresis as well as facial numbness on the right for one year. Radiologically a large avascular tumor destroying the sella and eroding the right petrous pyramid was present. A subtotal resection was done by a temporal approach. No signs of recurrence developed during one year after which she was lost to follow-up.

Case 6: Neurinoma of the sphenoid and posterior ethmoid sinuses (M. L.). A 31-year-old woman had severe diffuse headaches of many years duration, left facial numbness for three years and a blood-stained nasal discharge as well as left-sided proptosis and visual loss for one year. X-rays showed destruction of the left optic canal, sphenoid sinus and sella by an avascular tumor. An ethmoidal operation was then performed in the ENT-department, and

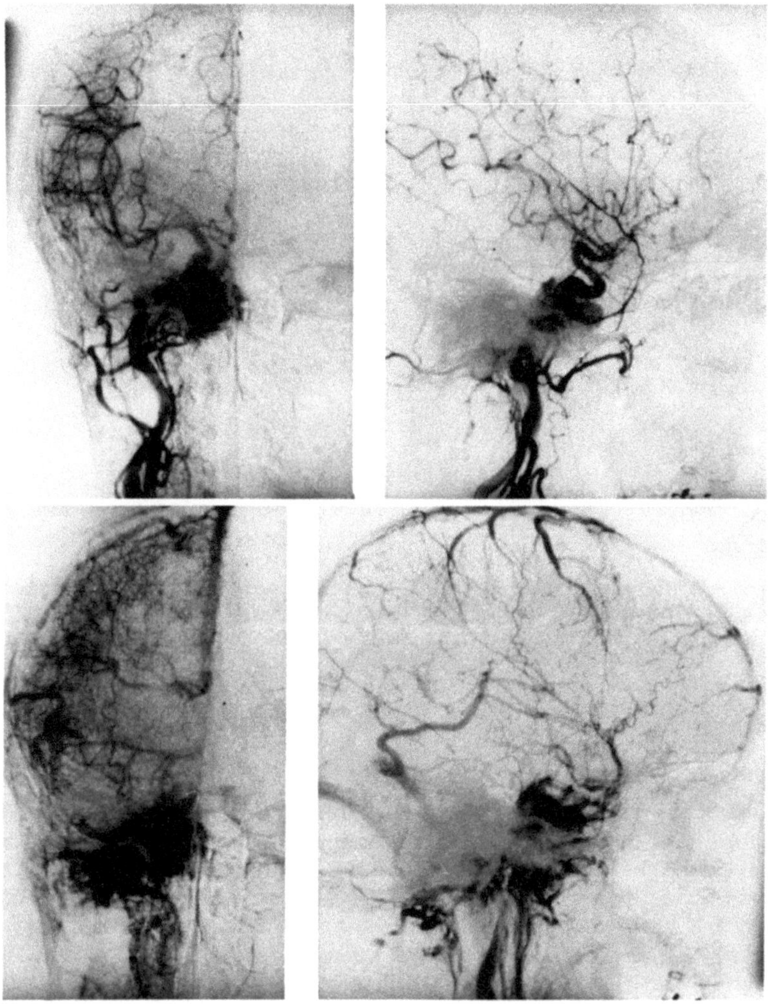

Fig. 2 Chordoma case 4. Arterial and venous phases of carotid angiogram showing the dark tumor staining, especially marked in the venous phase.

again three years later for a recurrence. Two years after the last operation she was last seen for follow-up, and up till then had no signs of recurrence.

Case 7: Trigeminal nerve neurinoma (W. W.). A 59-year-old man presented with a history of progressive left external ophthalmoplegia and trigeminal paresthesiae of three years duration. Pathological vascularization was not demonstrated angiographically. X-rays revealed bony destruction in the left middle cranial fossa. The tumor was completely extirpated. Follow-up until 64 years of age showed no recurrence.

Case 8: Sarcoidosis (O. I.). A 35-year-old woman developed right amaurosis and one year later visual loss on the left. Enlargement of the right optic canal was shown on radiographs. No other abnormalities were found. Surgical exploration revealed an infiltrated, thickened perichiasmatic dura and swollen optic nerves. Pathological tissue extended into the sella

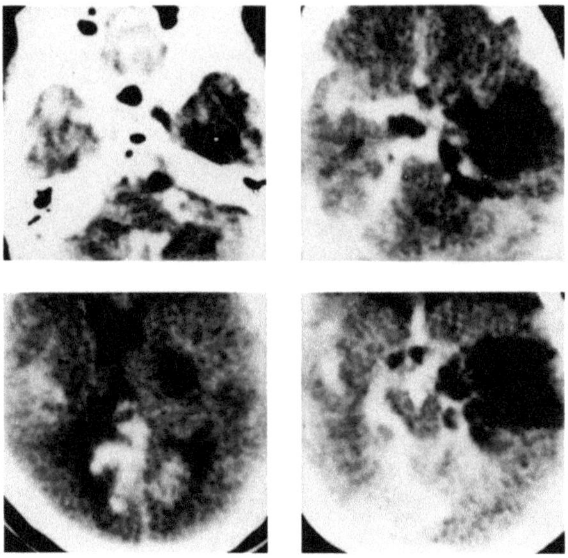

Fig. 3 Epidermoid cyst. Positive contrast CT cisternogram outlining the hypodense tumor extending from the skull base into the temporal lobe. The displacement of the brain stem is seen.

and the right parasellar area. No other signs of sarcoidosis were present at that time. Steroid treatment was begun. Three years later hilar, pulmonary sarcoidosis developed. Death ensued from an unrelated cause.

Case 9: Epidermoid cyst (A. C.). A 53-year-old man had suffered from left-sided trigeminal neuralgia for five years and hypacusis with tinnitus for three years. Clinical examination further showed a right homonymous hemianopia, left trigeminal hypo-esthesia and facial nerve paresis. Extensive erosion of the apex of the left petrous bone was demonstrated by tomography and a large avascular space-occupying lesion by angiography. The hypodense lesion seen on CT was diagnostic of an epidermoid cyst and positive contrast CT cisternography clearly outlined the tumor (fig. 3). The tumor was totally extirpated without neurological deficit. Unfortunately, the patient died of pulmonary embolism.

Case 10: Bronchial carcinoma metastasis (D. W.). A 51-year-old man presented with complete left ophthalmoplegia and trigeminal hypo-esthesia of rapid onset. The patient was in a poor general condition and showed typical signs of neoplastic disease. X-rays of the lungs were diagnostic of bronchial carcinoma. Radiological studies of the skull were normal. After radiotherapy the cranial nerve functions improved. Six months later the patient died of multiple metastases.

Case 11: Prostatic carcinoma metastasis (P. P.). A 58-year-old man developed slowly progressive right ophthalmoplegia, amaurosis, proptosis, trigeminal hypo-esthesia and masticatory paresis. There were no signs of neoplastic disease. X-ray examinations were within normal limits. In the right parasellar area, the middle cranial fossa and the chiasmatic cistern an infiltrated, thickened leptomeningitis was found, which proved to be metastatic in origin. Two weeks postoperatively the patient died of pneumonia. Autopsy revealed multiple bony and hepatic metastases.

Table 1 Presenting clinical signs in eleven cases of rare parasellar lesions

	headache	involvement of cranial nerves					blood-stained nasal discharge
		II	III	IV	VI	V	
I. Metastasis							
- Bronchial carcinoma	+	−	+	+	+	+	−
- Prostatic carcinoma	+	+	+	+	+	+	−
II. Epidermoid cyst	++++	+	−	−	−	+	−
III. Chordoma							
- Case 1	−	+	−	−	−	−	+
- Case 2	+	+	+	+	+	−	−
- Case 3	−	−	−	−	+	+	−
- Case 4	(+)	−	−	−	+	−	+
- Case 5	−	−	−	−	+	+	−
IV. Sarcoidosis	−	+	−	−	−	−	−
V. Neurinoma							
- Trigeminal nerve	−	−	+	+	+	+	−
- Sphenoid and posterior ethmoid sinuses	++++	+	+	−	−	+	+

Discussion

The presenting clinical features of our cases of rare, parasellar lesions are shown in table 1. Six patients had tumor-related headaches. These were most severe in the case of the epidermoid cyst with trigeminal neuralgia and in the patient with neurinoma of the sphenoid and posterior ethmoid sinuses, who had a diffuse type of headache. The parasellar metastases caused minor headaches in both patients. Although very extensively infiltrating into the skull base, the chordomas were not characterized by pain as a presenting sign. Some sign of cranial nerve involvement, e.g. visual loss, reduced visual fields, diplopia, facial numbness, was present in every patient. Noteworthy is the absence of strabismus in three patients despite the parasellar location of the disease. As expected, blood-stained nasal discharge was only present in those tumors extensively invading the skull base, vi. chordoma and neurinoma of the sphenoid and posterior ethmoid sinuses.

On the basis of radiological examinations (table 2) our patients can be separated in two groups. Metastases did not show any pathological changes and sarcoidosis produced unilateral optic canal enlargement as a minor but important finding. Most reported cases of parasellar metastasis, however, have abnormal plain skull radiograms or tomograms [8]. In intracerebral or meningeal sarcoidosis plain radiological studies usually do not demonstrate any change [4, 18]. The second group consists of epidermoid cyst, chordoma and neurinoma, which cause extensive

Table 2 Radiological features in eleven cases of rare parasellar lesions

	Skull X-ray	X-ray of optic canals	Tomography	Angiography
Group I				
I. Metastasis				
- Bronchial carcinoma	nil	nil	nil	nil
- Prostatic carcinoma	nil	nil	nil	nil
II. Sarcoidosis	nil	path.	nil	nil
Group II				
III. Epidermoid cyst	nil	–	apical erosion of pyramid	avascular mass
IV. Chordoma				
- Case 1	apical erosion, sellar destruction	–	apical erosion sellar destruction	avascular mass
- Case 2	apical erosion, sellar destruction	–	apical erosion tumor calcification	avascular mass
- Case 3	apical erosion, sellar destruction	–	apical and sellar erosion	avascular mass
- Case 4	sellar erosion	–	sellar and pyramid erosion	vascularized mass
- Case 5	nil	nil	nil	avascular mass
V. Neurinoma				
- Trigeminal nerve	pyramid erosion	–	pyramid erosion	avascular mass
- Sphenoid and posterior ethmoid sinuses	sellar destruction, sphenoid and ethmoid sinus destruction	path.	sellar and sphenoid sinus destruction, ethmoid sinus destruction, orbital wall destruction	avascular mass

bone erosion and displacement of intracranial vessels. CT and determination of density values are diagnostic in the case of epidermoid cyst (fig. 3), although sometimes other unusual features have been noted [2, 10]. In the other cases it is not, but CT demonstrates the volume of these tumors very well. Using a wide window the extent of bone destruction and skull base infiltration is clearly demonstrated.

As regards operative treatment we divided our patients into three groups (table 3),

Table 3 Classification of rare parasellar lesions according to malignity and local invasiveness

		Malignity	Invasiveness
I.	Epidermoid cyst (1 case)	benign	0
II.	Sarcoidosis (1 case)	benign	+
	Neurinoma (2 cases)	benign	+/++
	Chordoma (5 cases)	benign	++/+++
III.	Metastasis (2 cases)	malignant	+++

according to their nature and local invasiveness. In groups I and III it is evident that an epidermoid cyst should be completely removable in all cases [2] and that operation is futile in metastatic disease [8, 9, 31]. Radiotherapy, however, is a valuable alternative in malignant neoplasms.

The group of benign lesions with more or less pronounced local invasiveness (group II) requires a more sophisticated therapeutic policy. Sarcoidosis presented to us as a rather diffuse dural thickening as well as swelling of the optic nerves, without other signs of systemic disease. Infiltrative meningeal disease is the most common way of presentation of neurosarcoidosis, whereas the nodular intracerebral type is less frequent [18].

Among sarcoidosis patients 1.5% have CNS involvement and one third of those have neurological dysfunction as the only clinical manifestation, with the hypothalamus, the pituitary gland and the meninges as the most frequently involved areas of the intracranial nervous system [4]. Operation is necessary to obtain a tissue diagnosis if sarcoidosis is not made obvious by other manifestations of the disease. However, steroids remain the main treatment in neurosarcoidosis [14, 20].

Neurinomas displace neighbouring structures and erode the bones. They are not infiltrating in the histological sense, but grow through natural foramina and along anatomical planes, as seen classically in hour-glass tumors [29]. Trigeminal nerve neurinomas constitute less than eight per cent of intracranial neurinomas and are most often located in the middle cranial fossa, originating from the Gasserian ganglion (52%, type A of Jefferson), and less frequently in the posterior fossa (24.5%, type B of Jefferson) and in both locations with a dumb-bell shape (23.5%, type C of Jefferson) [13, 24, 29, 33]. In Jefferson's type A the involvement of one or more cranial nerves to the extraocular muscles is a common presenting sign, whereas symptoms of trigeminal nerve dysfunction are not [22, 27]. These tumors can be removed completely in most cases [26, 27, 31].

Very rarely, neurinomas in the skull base have been reported without any obvious connection to a nerve. Some of these tumors originated in the olfactory groove [32], some in the pituitary fossa [7, 28] and our case was located in the sphenoid sinus and posterior ethmoid cells. The neurinomas of the skull base located outside the

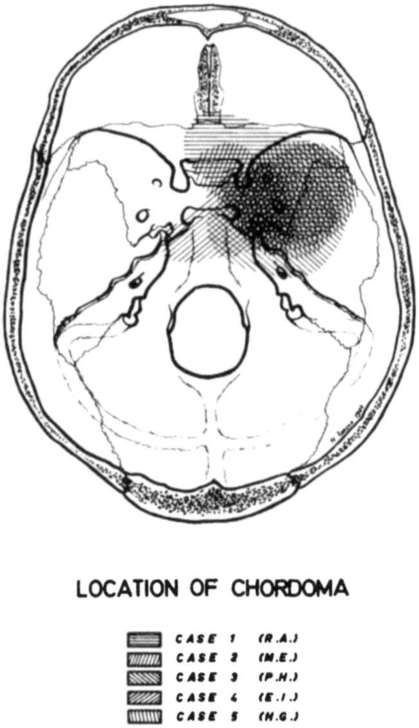

Fig. 4 The extent of the chordomas reported in this paper is seen on this diagram as it was at initial diagnosis. All tumors involved the parasellar area. All cases were drawn as if they were located on the right side.

sella are already rather voluminous tumors, by the time patients seek medical care, because neurological or nasal symptoms develop late. The tumors have eroded the bones of the paranasal sinuses, sometimes the medial orbital wall. Thus, complete extirpation can be very difficult and extensive surgery may be required.

Chordomas are found in 0.2% of intracranial tumors, but if only skull base tumors are considered, this percentage rises [3]. These essentially benign tumors are regionally very invasive, infiltrating the bones of the skull base, growing into the nasopharyngeal cavity and the infratemporal space. Malignant degeneration is rare, as is distant metastasis [11, 21]. The expansion at the skull base is depicted in figure 4 for our five cases of predominantly parasellar location. Skull X-rays and tomography, and CT in even more detail, outline the extent of these tumors [1, 15, 17]. Angiographic features have been described in detail and include narrowing and displacement of major arteries, as well as only faintly visible or absent pathological vascularization [15, 16]. Sometimes a very dense tumor stain is shown, as in our chordoma case 4 (fig. 2). Treatment of chordoma requires operation and radiotherapy, but these measures are only palliative in the great majority of cases [11, 23, 25, 34]. The tumors are usually too large at the time of diagnosis, and subtotal excision is the most that can be accomplished by the usual transcranial, trans-sphenoidal or trans-ethmoidal operative approaches [21, 30]. In case of unilateral involvement of the skull base the infratemporal approach, as described by Fisch [5, 6], can be more successful.

Cooperation between the disciplines of neurosurgery, ENT-surgery and maxillofacial surgery is essential in developing a treatment policy for the individual patient [12]. After careful and thourough work-up of the patient, a decision has to be made about the extent of the operation to be performed. Radical operations should be planned accordingly: combined craniotomy and ENT-approaches should both be incorporated from the beginning and not be decided during the operation. Since these procedures can be mutilating the readiness of the patient to accept this, should be ascertained. If radical therapy is not possible, most authors advocate irradiation of any residual tumor, although it is known that they are relatively radioresistant and require extremely high doses of radiation [21, 25, 34].

Summary

Eleven cases of rare parasellar lesions are presented: metastasis, epidermoid cyst, chordoma, neurinoma, sarcoidosis. The clinical signs and radiological features found in these patients are described. They indicate the location of the disease, so that in combination with the evolution of the symptomatology, the extent of the lesion and the general examination, a pre-operative diagnosis can be made. The results of therapy are reported and combined neurosurgical, ENT and maxillofacial treatment is advocated. This allows a more radical operative policy to be adopted, since technics in all three disciplines are much more advanced than in earlier years. Patients will benefit by longer and qualitatively better survival. Our prime efforts, however, should now be directed towards earlier diagnosis as the tumors are still too large at the time of initial diagnosis.

References

[1] Banna, M., H. L. jr Baker, O. W. Houser: Pituitary and parapituitary tumours on computed tomography. A review article based on 230 cases. Br. J. Radiol. **53** (1980) 1123-1143.

[2] Cobb, C. A., J. R. Youmans: Brain tumors of disordered embryogenesis in adults. In: Neurological surgery, 2nd ed. (J. R. Youmans, ed.), pp. 2899-2935. W. B. Saunders Company, Philadelphia 1982.

[3] De Cremoux, P., G. Turpin, P. Hamon, et al.: Les chordomes intrasellaires. Principaux aspects cliniques, biologiques, radiologiques, évolutifs et histologiques. A propos de deux observations. Sem. Hôp. Paris **56** (1980) 1769-1773.

[4] Delaney, P.: Neurologic manifestations in sarcoidosis. Review of the literature with a report of 23 cases. Ann. Intern. Med. **87** (1977) 336-345.
[5] Fisch, U.: Infratemporal fossa approach to tumors of the temporal bone and base of the skull. J. Laryngol. Otolaryngol. **92** (1978) 949-967.
[6] Fisch, U., H.C. Pillsbury, C.T. Sasaki: Infratemporal approach to the skull base. In: Surgery of the skull base (C.T. Sasaki, B.F. McCabe, J.A. Kirchner, eds.), pp. 141-160. J.B. Lippincott Company, Philadelphia 1984.
[7] Goebel, H.H., K. Shimokawa, T. Schaake, et al.: Schwannoma of the sellar region. Acta Neurochir. **48** (1979) 191-197.
[8] Greenberg, H.S., M.D.F. Deck, B. Vikram, et al.: Metastasis to the base of the skull: clinical findings in 43 patients. Neurology **31** (1981) 530-537.
[9] Hall, S., L. Carlin, E.S. Roach, et al.: Pupillary sparing oculomotor palsy from metastatic carcinoma. Surg. Neurol. **19** (1983) 363-364.
[10] Handa, J., K. Okamoto, Y. Nakasu, et al.: Computed tomography of intracranial epidermoid tumours with special reference to atypical features. Acta Neurochir **58** (1981) 221-228.
[11] Heffelfinger, M.J., D.C. Dahlin, C.S. MacCarty, et al.: Chordomas and cartilaginous tumours at the skull base. Cancer **32** (1973) 410-420.
[12] Hybels, R.L., S.R. Freidberg: Combined otolaryngologic and neurosurgical approaches to tumors of the temporal bone and skull base. Surg. Clin. North Am. **60** (1980) 609-628.
[13] Jefferson, G.: The trigeminal neurinomas with some remarks on malignant invasion of the Gasserian ganglion. Proc. Congr. Neurosurg. **1** (1955) 11-54.
[14] Karnik, A.S.: Nodular cerebral sarcoidosis simulating metastatic carcinoma. Arch. Intern. Med. **142** (1982) 385-386.
[15] Kendall, B.E., B.C.P. Lee: Cranial chordomas. Br. J. Radiol. **50** (1977) 687-698.
[16] Krayenbühl, H., M.G. Yasargil, P. Huber: Cerebral angiography. 2nd ed., pp. 61, 139, 140, 169. Georg Thieme Verlag, Stuttgart 1982.
[17] Krol, G., N. Sundaresan, M. Deck: Computed tomography of axial chordomas. J. Comput. Assist. Tomogr. **7** (1983) 286-289.
[18] Kumpe, D.A., C.V.G.K. Rao, J.H. Garcia, et al.: Intracranial neurosarcoidosis. J. Comput. Assist. Tomogr. **3** (1979) 324-330.
[19] Landolt, A.M., C.B. Wilson: Tumors of the sella and parasellar area in adults. In: Neurological surgery, 2nd ed. (J.R. Youmans, ed.), pp. 3107-3162. W.B. Saunders Company, Philadelphia 1982.
[20] Lazarus, A.A.: Sarcoidosis. Otolaryngol. Clin. North Am. **15** (1982) 621-633.
[21] Long, D.M., S.A. Kieffer, S.N. Chou: Tumors of the skull. In: Neurological surgery, 2nd ed. (J.R. Youmans, ed.), pp. 3227-3268. W.B. Saunders Company, Philadelphia 1982.
[22] Menegalli-Boggelli, D., Y. Lajat, R. Robert, et al.: Neurinome du trijumeau chez l'adolescent révélé par une paralysie du droit externe. Rev. Ontoneuroophthalmol. **53** (1981) 271-277.
[23] Miller, R.H., G.E. Woodson, J.G. Neely, et al.: A surgical approach to chordomas at the base of the skull. Otolaryngol. Head. Neck Surg. **90** (1982) 251-255.
[24] Montaut, J.: Les neurinomes du trijumeau. Thèse de Médicine, Nancy 1962. Nr. 75.
[25] Müller, R.P., M. Wannenmacher, K. Rieck, et al.: Beitrag zur Strahlentherapie der Chordome anhand eigener Fälle und im Vergleich der Literatur. Strahlentherapie **156** (1980) 92-96.
[26] Olive, I., H.J. Svien: Neurofibromas of the fifth cranial nerve. J. Neurosurg. **14** (1957) 484-505.

[27] Paillas, J. E., F. Grisoli, P. Farnarier: Neurinomes du trijumeau. Neurochirurgie **20** (1973) 41-54.
[28] Perone, T. P., B. Robinson, S. M. Holmes: Intrasellar schwannoma: case report. Neurosurgery **14** (1984) 71-73.
[29] Russell, D. S., L. J. Rubinstein: Pathology of tumours of the nervous system, 4th ed., pp. 372-401. Edward Arnold (Publishers), Ltd., London 1977.
[30] Sasaki, C. T., B. F. McCabe, J. A. Kirchner (eds): Surgery of the skull base, pp. 63-93, 113-124. J. B. Lippincott Company, Philadelphia 1984.
[31] Thomas, J. E., R. E. Yoss: The parasellar syndrome: problems determining etiology. Mayo Clin. Proc. **45** (1970) 617-623.
[32] Ulrich, J., A. Lévy, C. Pfister: Schwannoma of the olfactory groove. Case report and review of previous cases. Acta Neurochir. **40** (1978) 315-321.
[33] Vaquero, J., J. M. Cabezudo, G. Leunda, et al.: Simultaneous posterior and middle cranial fossa neurinomas. Acta Neurochir. **55** (1981) 321-327.
[34] Vollrath, M.: Das Chordom - eine Übersicht: ergänzt durch zwei eigene Fallbeobachtungen. HNO **27** (1979) 41-49.

The fate of glomus tympanicum tumors after surgical and radiological treatment

M. Strohm

Glomus tumors or chemodectomas are benign tumors derived from the glomus organs, which are encountered along the carotid artery, the jugular bulb and the tympanic plexus. The skull base is involved by these tumors when they grow in the middle ear cleft where in most cases they originate from Jacobson's nerve in the inferior tympanic canaliculus or from the apex of the jugular bulb. Usually the onset of these tumors is insidious. In spite of their histologically benign characteristics they may have a destructive growth pattern and destroy surrounding bone and invade the soft tissue, mimicking a malignant tumor thus creating great surgical problems.

As suggested by Fisch, we have classified these tumors according to their size and location: stage A tumors are limited to the middle ear cleft; a stage B tumor is in contact with, or originates from, the jugular bulb; stage C has a sublabyrinthine extension with bone destruction and stage D tumors grow medial to the labyrinthine block into the cranial cavity.

From 1968 to 1984, 61 patients with glomus tympanicum tumors were diagnosed at the ENT-clinic in Tübingen. There were 52 female and 9 male patients. The age ranged from 25 to 81 years with a median of 54 years (females 56 years, males 48 years). 6 patients had previous treatment elsewhere, therefore the findings at the time of the primary diagnosis are unknown. In the remaining 55 patients pulsating tinnitus and unilateral hearing loss - or a combination of both - were the most common symptoms (42 patients). A discharge, which was occasionally bloody, was present in 6 cases. 7 patients suffered from cranial nerve palsies; most commonly they complained of hoarseness due to vagus nerve damage (5 cases), which was associated with glossopharyngeal and accessory nerve damage in 2 patients. 2 patients presented with facial weakness and 3 patients complained of dizziness. The tumor could be seen in 50 cases. It presented as a bluish pulsating mass behind the

Table 1 61 glomus tympanicum tumors

Stage	A	B	C	D
No treatment	2	1	1	2
Operation	26	9	6	4
Radiotherapy	–	2	–	1
Operation + Radiotherapy	1	3	2	1
n=	29	15	9	8

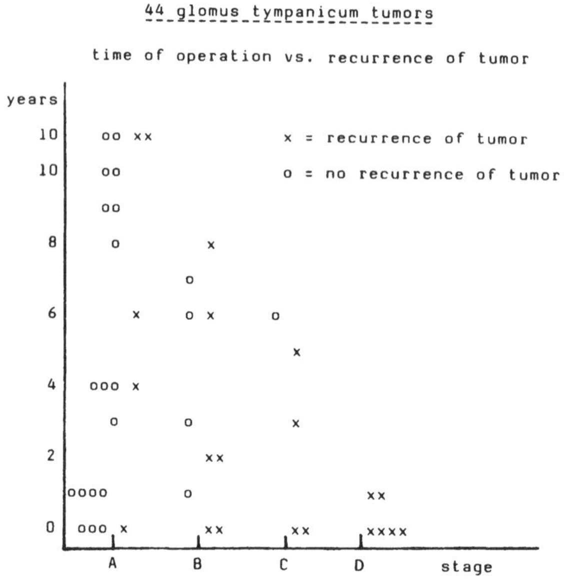

Fig. 1 Synopsis of the results of treatment in the different tumor stages. Crosses at the abscissa (0 years) indicate persistent tumors.

eardrum or actually invading it. The fact that in most cases the interval between the first symptoms and the diagnosis was very long (from 2 weeks up to 20 years with a median of 3.5 years) emphasizes the slow and insidious growth of these tumors.

When they presented, nearly half of our patients had stage A tumors (tab. 1). One stage D patient had an associated glomus caroticum tumor; another stage D case had a possible familial predisposition, because his brother also suffered from a glomus tympanicum tumor. 6 patients refused treatment. In the treated patients, operation was the treatment of choice. Radiotherapy alone was rarely given. It was used in old patients with advanced tumors or when the patients refused operation. Irradiation was more often given as secondary treatment when a previous operation had failed.

11 of our 55 treated patients were lost to the follow-up. In 3 cases the follow-up is less than one year, so we cannot seriously state that these patients are tumor-free. Among the patients who had a longer follow-up, only the majority of the stage A patients remained tumor-free (fig. 1). In this stage one persistent and 4 recurrent tumors were seen whereas 15 patients were successfully treated. 4 patients initially with stage B tumors were tumor-free for a longer period, whereas 2 had persistent and 4 had recurrent tumors. Of the stage C tumors only one patient remained tumor-free (2 had persistent and 2 had recurrent tumors). For stage D, only 2 patients had a radical operation and both developed recurrences. Some of the recurred tumors were found after more than 10 years. Therefore even a long-term follow-up

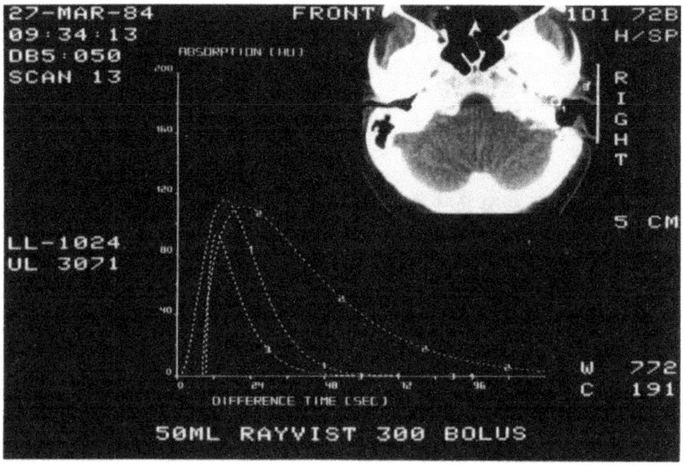

Fig. 2 Example of a dynamic computerized tomogram. The enhancement after an intravenous bolus of 50 ml contrast medium is measured at the tumor site (1), the sigmoid sinus (2) and the temporal artery (3) every 5 seconds. The time-enhancement curves are harmonized by calculation of the regression curves.

does not give absolute certainty that the patient is tumor-free. 9 patients underwent secondary treatment for a recurred tumor. Two of them (stage A and B) were disease-free after 2 and 4 operations respectively (follow-up: 4 and 7 years). 3 patients (1 stage A, 2 stage C) who had several operations as well as radiotherapy remained tumor-free (follow-up: 3.3 and 6 years). 4 other patients (2 stage A, 1 each stage C and D) who were operated on several times, but who did not have radiotherapy, developed recurrences after 4, 11, 5 and 1 years respectively.

The follow-up examinations of glomus tympanicum patients and the detection of a recurrence are essentially based on the clinical symptoms. Computerized tomography does not allow one to differentiate between a recurrence and postoperative scarring. Arteriography which is the most accurate investigation is not routinely indicated and should be used only in cases with clinical symptoms or signs of a recurred tumor. In the pre-operative evaluation regarding the size and site of a glomus tympanicum tumor and especially for the evaluation of its blood supply, arteriography is essential. However, we are of the opinion that for the routine follow-up dynamic tomography (angio-CT) is a very accurate investigation with a minimal risk to the patient. The principle of this investigation is to make serial computerized tomograms of the suspected region at 5 second intervals after the intravenous administration of a contrast medium. When a vascular tumor with an arterio-venous shunt is present, a transient marked enhancement can be seen. The time-enhancement curve of the tumorous region is established and is then compared with the curve of a large artery (the internal carotid in most cases) and that of a central vein or sinus. Typically, the peak of the tumor curve lies between those of the artery and the vein and the shape of the curve is similar to that of the artery

Table 2 Clinical symptoms related to angio-CT in the follow-up of 19 patients

Stage	A	B	C	D
clin Ø/CT Ø	7	1	1	–
clin +/CT Ø	1	–	–	–
clin Ø/CT +	–	clin A/CT D	–	clin?/CT D
clin +/CT +	2	4	–	1
n=	10	6	1	2

(fig. 2). After radiotherapy the time-enhancement curve of a glomus tumor is flattened, indicating fibrosis of the tumor vessels. A post-operative scar without tumorous vascularization is characterized by a time-enhancement curve which is nearly parallel to the abscissa.

19 patients who had had glomus tympanicum tumors of different stages were investigated by means of angio-computerized tomography after operation and/or radiotherapy. In 16 cases the results of the clinical examination and those of the dynamic computerized tomography were comparable: 9 patients were found to be tumor-free; in 6 cases the clinical diagnosis of a persistent or recurred tumor was confirmed by angio-CT (tab. 2). In one case, however, a clinically suspected tumor could be excluded by this radiological examination. In two other cases, the clinical signs were doubtful or in favour of a small recurrence, whereas the dynamic computerized tomography revealed the existence of large tumors extending into the cranial cavity. 4 patients who were examined by angio-CT had had previous radiotherapy. All of them showed flattened time-enhancement curves indicating tumor fibrosis. Pre-therapeutic computerized tomograms are not available in these cases, so we cannot confirm a non-progression of tumor growth, but we are of the opinion that a vascular tumor should stop growing, when its vessels become fibrotic. This is supported by the fact, that no recurred tumor was found in patients where a second operation was combined with radiotherapy. These findings verify our therapeutic concept, that operation is the treatment of choice for small glomus tympanicum tumors, but that large stage C and D tumors and recurred tumors are best treated by a combination of operation and radiotherapy.

Recommended Literature

Axel, L.: Cerebral blood flow determination by rapid-sequence computed tomography. Radiology **137** (1980) 679–686.

Graf, K., U. Fisch: Geschwülste des Ohres und des Felsenbeins. In: Hals-Nasen-Ohren-Heilkunde in Praxis und Klinik (J. Berendes, R. Link, F. Zöllner, eds.). Thieme Verlag, Stuttgart 1979.

Hildmann, H.: Die Glomustumoren des Mittelohres. HNO (Berlin) **21** (1973) 344–346.

Phleps, P. D., G. A. S. Lloyd: Glomus tympanicum tumors: demonstration by high resolution CT. Clin. Otalaryngol. **8** (1983) 15-20.
Plester, D.: Das operative Vorgehen bei Tumoren des Mittelohres. Arch. Ohr.-Nas.-Kehlk.-Heilk. **175** (1959) 517-519.
Sharma, P. D., A. P. Johnson, A. C. Whitton: Radiotherapy for jugulo-tympanic paragangliomas. J. Laryng. Otol. **98** (1984) 621-629.
Spector, G. J., J. Compagno, C. A. Perez et al.: Glomus jugulare tumors: effects of radiotherapy. Cancer **35** (1975) 1316-1321.

The place of "salvage" petrosectomy

P. M. Stell, J. B. Miles

Introduction

The main forms of treatment advocated for carcinoma of the middle or external ear are primary petrosectomy (with or without post operative radiotherapy), and radical mastoidectomy followed by radiotherapy. Lewis [1] has been the main proponent of the former policy whereas several English authors notably Lederman [2] have advocated the second policy. Others, particularly the Manchester School [3, 4] advocate primary radiotherapy alone.

Whatever method of treatment is used the cure rate is no more than 30%. Clearly many patients suffer primary recurrence, and it is curious that salvage surgery in these circumstances has scarcely been discussed in the literature.

If a patient suffers a recurrence of his disease after radical mastoidectomy and radiotherapy petrosectomy may be considered, as indeed it may be if a patient is treated primarily by radiotherapy. The descriptions of the technique of petrosectomy appear to confine themselves to the procedure as a primary form of treatment, and its place in "salvage" has not been defined.

The purpose of the present paper is to try to define the place of salvage surgery after failed radiotherapy.

Patients

This paper is based on 49 patients with carcinoma of the middle or external ear seen between 1963 and 1983. 33 patients were treated initially by radiotherapy. The details of the primary site, histology, age, sex, T and N stage are shown in table 1.

The tumors were staged using a system suggested by the author [6] as follows:
T_1 Tumor limited to site of origin, i.e. with no facial nerve paralysis and no bone destruction on radiology.

T_2 Tumor extending beyond the site of origin indicated by facial paralysis or radiological evidence of bone destruction, but no extension beyond the organ of origin.

Table 1 Details of patients

	Ext. auditory meatus	Middle ear
Age and sex		
Men	7	9
Mean age	60.9	63.1
Women	15	2
Mean age	57.3	62.5
Histology		
Squamous carcinoma	20	11
Basal cell carcinoma	1	0
Adenoid cystic carcinoma	1	0
T Stage		
T_1	10	5
T_2	2	1
T_3	1	3
T_x	9	2
N Stage		
N_0	13	9
N_1	2	0
N_x	7	2

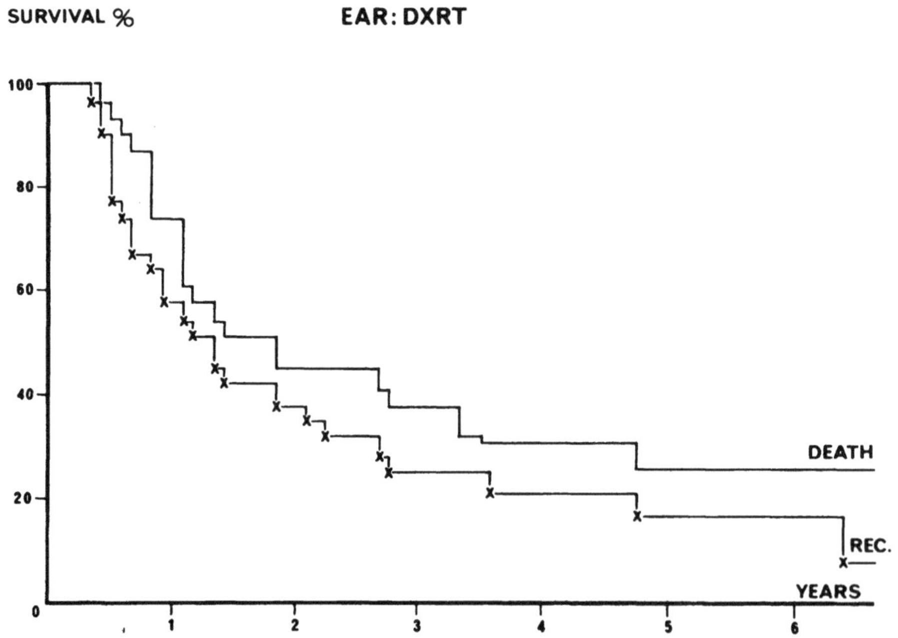

Fig. 1 Actuarial recurrence rate after radiotherapy.

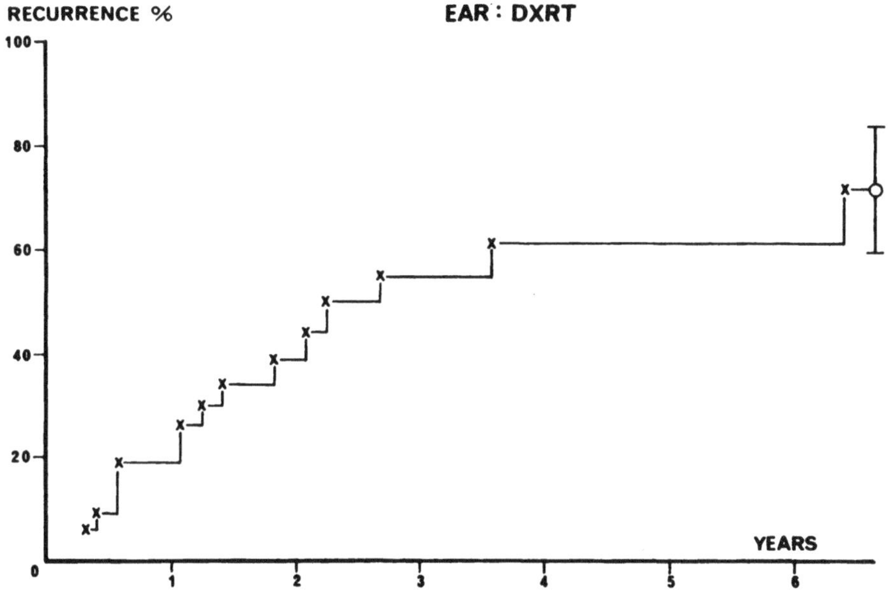

Fig. 2 Actuarial curves of time to recurrence and to death.

T_3 Clinical or radiological evidence of extension to surrounding structures (dura, base of the skull, parotid gland, temperomandibular joint, etc.).
T_x Patients with insufficient data for classification, including patients previously seen and treated elsewhere.

Results

The time to recurrence is shown in figure 1 using the actuarial method. 11 of 22 patients with carcinoma of the external auditory meatus suffered a primary recurrence, and nine of these have been treated by petrosectomy. In the other 2 patients the recurrence was too extensive or associated with inoperable neck disease to allow surgery to be carried out. The subsequent fate and other details are shown in table 2.

8 of 11 patients with carcinoma of the middle ear suffered a primary recurrence, one died of intercurrent disease and 2 are alive. Of the 8 patients who suffered a primary recurrence, the recurrence was deemed to be too advanced for surgery in 6; a salvage petrosectomy was attempted but abandoned in the other 2.

The survival using the life table method shown in figure 2, which shows 2 curves: one for time to death and one for time to recurrence.

Table 2 External auditory meatus: Survival after petrosectomy

Histology	Survival (months)	Fate
SCC	24	alive
BCC	18	alive
ACC	50	alive with disease
SCC	1, 2, 5, 6, 10, 18	dead

Discussion

Briefly, the above results show that a primary recurrence of a carcinoma of the middle ear in a patient previously treated by radiotherapy was either too advanced for petrosectomy, or the operation had to be abandoned if it was attempted. Recurrent carcinoma of the external auditory meatus was usually operable, but the subsequent course of these patients was far from happy. Most were dead within one year, and the few long-term survivors seem to be those patients with non-squamous carcinomas. Similar unfortunate experiences have been shared by Harrison (Tucker [5]): 7 patients were submitted to petrosectomy and none survived more than ten months.

Summary

33 of 49 patients with carcinoma of the external auditory meatus and middle ear were treated by radiotherapy. 19 patients suffered a recurrence. This proved to be unsuitable for petrosectomy in all patients with tumor of the middle ear. A few patients with tumours of the external auditory meatus, usually of non squamous variety, have survived for a reasonable period after "salvage" petrosectomy.

References

[1] Lewis, J.S.: Surgical management of Tumors of the Middle Ear and Mastoid. Jour. Laryngol. Otol. **97** (1983) 299-311.
[2] Lederman, M.: Malignant Tumours of the Ear. Jour. Laryngol. Otol. **79** (1965) 85-119.
[3] Holmes, K.S.: Carcinoma of the middle ear. Clin. Radiol. **16** (1965) 400-404.
[4] Boland, J., R. Paterson: Cancer of the Middle Ear and External Auditory Meatus. Jour. Laryngol. Otol. **69** (1955) 468-478.
[5] Tucker, W.N.: Cancer of the Middle Ear. **Cancer** (1965) 642-650.
[6] Stell, P.M., M.S. McCormick: Carcinoma of the middle ear: prognostic factors and a suggested staging system. Jour. Laryngol. Otol. (in press).

Transtemporal-infratemporal approach to the skull base

L. N. Sekhar, R. Estonillo

Introduction

The increasing collaboration between neurosurgeons and otolaryngologists in recent years has enabled the radical resection of some tumors of the skull base, previously considered inoperable. An awareness of what can be achieved by approaches commonly used by the other discipline have also fostered some new applications of preexisting surgical techniques. Operative approaches to the clivus area have been developed by Fisch, particularly for dealing with glomus tumors (infratemporal fossa approach) and by House for other lesions of this area (transcochlear approach) [1, 2]. We undertook the following anatomical work to study the structures of the clivus that could be exposed by a modification of these approaches, and to explore the advantages and disadvantages. Two examples of the clinical application of such an approach are also provided.

Material and methods

Ten cadaver heads were used for the purpose of the study. The specimens were fixed in alcohol, the cranial arteries were perfused with formalin, and were subsequently injected with latex rubber. These specimens were placed in a three point pin fixation device, and between dissections were kept frozen. This technique allowed the brain and cerebral blood vessels to maintain an relatively firm consistency for up to a month. Regular macrosurgical instruments, microsurgical instruments, a Stryker drill, a suction irrigation set-up, and the operation microscope were used during these dissections. Thirty-five millimeter micro and macro photographs were taken. Anatomical drawings were made to illustrate details of this approach since the depth of the exposure did not permit an overview of all the structures in photographs.

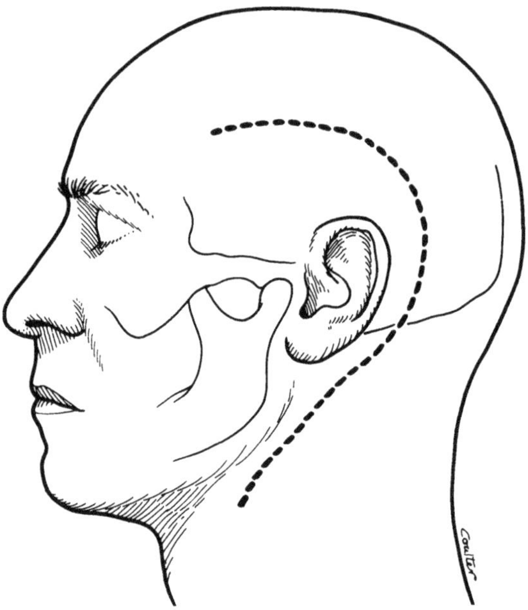

Fig. 1 Incision used for transtemporal-infratemporal approach to the skull base.

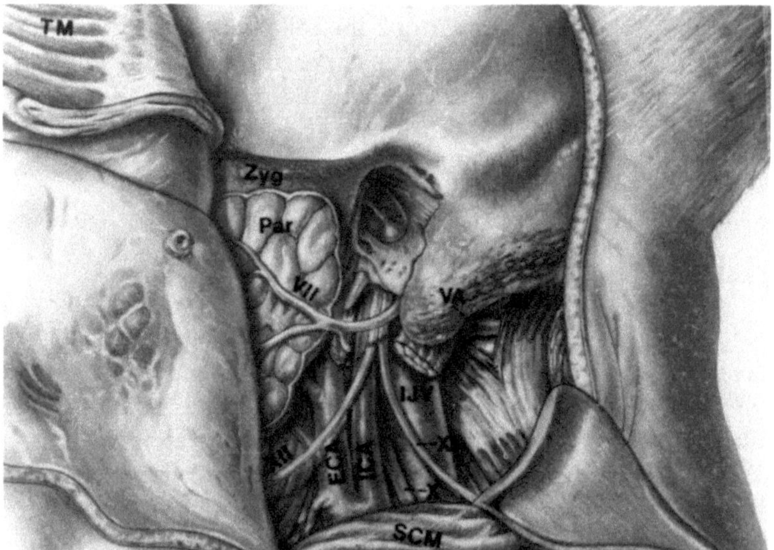

Fig. 2 Illustration of the extracranial exposure achieved. Notice the position of the vertebral artery. TM = Temporalis muscle; Zyg = Zygoma; Par = Parotid gland; VA = Vertebral artery; IJV = Internal jugular vein; ECA = External carotid artery; ICA = Internal carotid artery; VII, X, XI, XII = Cranial nerves.

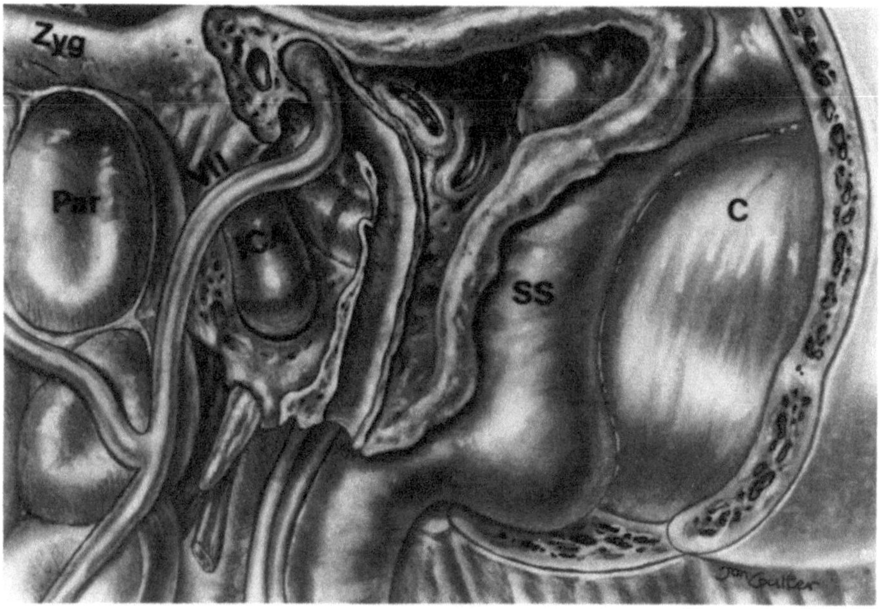

Fig. 3 The facial nerve has been exposed from the stylomastoid foramen through the middle ear to the geniculate ganglion. The semicircular canals are exposed prior to opening of the internal auditory canal. The internal carotid artery has also been exposed partially. Zyg = Zygoma; Par = Parotid gland; ICA = Internal carotid artery; SS = Sigmoid sinus; C = Cerebellum; VII = Cranial nerve.

Procedure

A question mark incision was made starting in the temporal area extending behind the ear and the mastoid region and down in front of the sternomastoid behind the angle of the jaw (fig. 1). The external ear canal was divided at the junction of the cartilaginous and bony parts and the pinna was reflected anteriorly along with the skin flap. The posterior portion of the temporalis muscle was reflected forwards and preserved for subsequent reconstruction. The sternomastoid muscle was disconnected from the mastoid process and reflected downwards and laterally taking care to preserve the accessory nerve which traversed the muscle. The posterior belly of the diagastric was divided and reflected downwards. Following this, the facial nerve was dissected from the stylomastoid foramen through the proximal portion of the parotid gland exposing its major divisions, simultaneously performing a superficial parotidectomy. The external and internal carotid arteries, the internal jugular vein, the ninth, tenth, eleventh, and twelfth cranial nerves were dissected and entirely exposed extracranially (fig. 2). A simple mastoidectomy was then performed. With the aid of the operation microscope, the drill and the suction irrigation, the facial nerve was unroofed in a stepwise fashion from the stylomastoid fo-

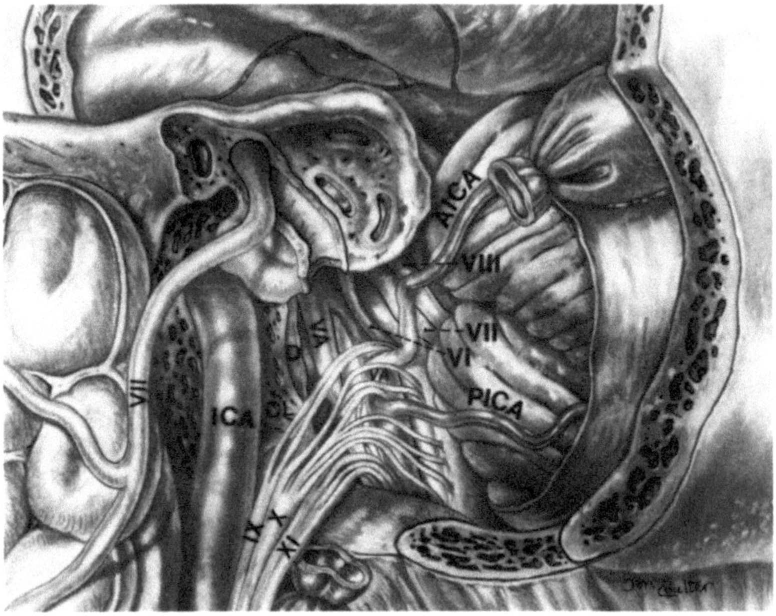

Fig. 4 Illustrates the displacement of the facial nerve and the exposure of the lower clivus. The sigmoid sinus and the internal jugular vein have been ligated and divided. The ninth, tenth, and eleventh nerves have been dissected from the brainstem all the way through the jugular foramen. Both vertebral arteries and the vertebral basilar junction are exposed. The drilling of the semicircular canals indicated here is not necessary for this exposure and sensorineural hearing can be preserved if such drilling is avoided. AICA = Anterior inferior cerebellar artery; VA = Vertebral artery; D = Dura; ICA = Internal carotid artery; CL = Clivus; PICA = Posterior inferior cerebellar artery; VI, VII, VIII, IX, X, XI = Cranial nerves.

ramen up through the middle ear to the geniculate ganglion. The labyrinth was then drilled to expose the facial nerve within the internal auditory canal and the nerve was followed from here all the way to the geniculate ganglion. The cochlear and vestibular nerves were divided (fig. 3). After division of the superior petrosal nerve beyond the geniculate ganglion, the facial nerve could be mobilized entirely and displaced as needed for further exposure. The transverse and sigmoid sinuses were completely unroofed through the jugular bulb area. Bone removal was then accomplished to expose a small portion of the dura in the retromastoid area as well as in the temporal area above the transverse sinus region. After the displacement of the facial nerve backwards and downwards, the internal carotid artery was unroofed entirely from its entrance into the carotid canal to its exit from the temporal bone to enter the cavernous sinus, drilling off the tympanic bone and the cochlea in order to do so. After the complete removal of the cochlea, the clival bone was identified by its soft and crumbly nature, in contrast to the hard petrous bone. A portion of the clival bone was also removed.

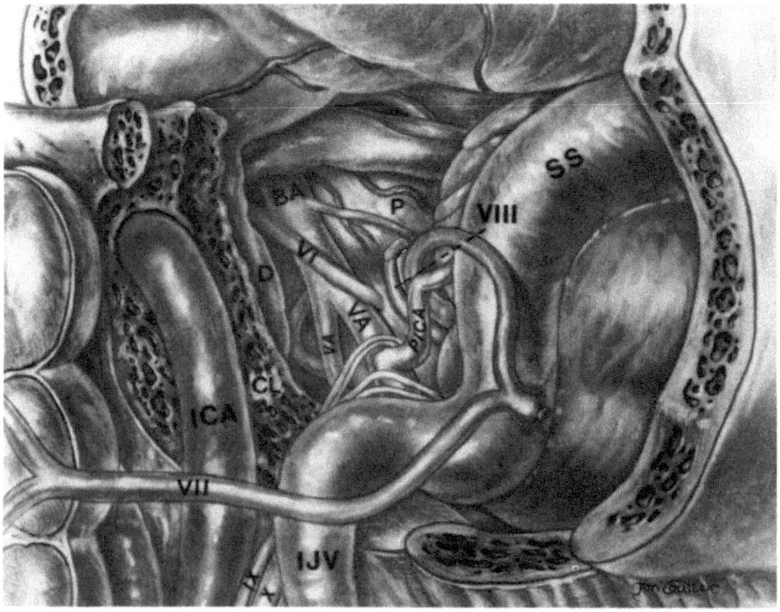

Fig. 5 Exposure of the middle clivus. Note that the exposure becomes limited above the region of the trigeminal nerve. In order to expose the contralateral side, the internal carotid artery has to be completely unroofed and displaced anteriorly. BA = Basilar artery; P = Pons; SS = Sigmoid sinus; D = Dura; VA = Vertebral artery; PICA = Posterior inferior cerebellar artery; CL = Clivus; ICA = Internal carotid artery; IJV = Internal jugular vein; VI, VII, VIII, IX, X = Cranial nerves.

For the exposure of the lower clivus, the seventh cranial nerve was displaced forwards and upwards. The drilling of the cochlea, the labyrinth, and the destruction of the eight nerve could be avoided. The sigmoid sinus had to be ligated and divided (fig. 4).

For the exposure of the middle clivus, the seventh cranial nerve was displaced backwards and downwards and the drilling and destruction of the labyrinth and cochlea was an essential part of the procedure (fig. 5).

The dura was opened in a cruciate fashion. Reconstruction was accomplished by dural closure, followed by occlusion of the eustachian tube with bone, packing of the cavity with fat, and suturing the sternomastoid muscle to a portion of the temporalis muscle that was rotated backwards and downwards. The external ear canal was closed carefully.

Results

Lower clivus exposure (fig. 4)

The lower pons, the origin of the seventh and eighth cranial nerves, the medulla, the spinal medullary junction, the ipsilateral ninth, tenth, eleventh, and twelfth nerves, the ipsilateral posterior inferior cerebellar artery, both vertebral arteries, and sometimes, the vertebral basilar junction were exposed. The ipsilateral aspect of both medulla and pons were exposed without any retraction. A portion of the anterior surface of the contralateral aspect of the brainstem was also exposed. The lower cranial nerves could be dissected entirely through the jugular foramen and reflected backwards in order to avoid having to work between these cranial nerves. Hearing could be preserved with this approach, the ligation and division of the sigmoid sinus and sometimes, the ligation of the internal jugular vein, were essential for this exposure.

Middle clivus (fig. 5)

In order to expose the middle clivus, the seventh cranial nerve was displaced backwards and downwards. The sigmoid sinus did not have to be divided, but such division improved the exposure. The seventh and the divided eighth cranial nerves, the sixth and fifth cranial nerves, the basilar artery and its branches, and the vertebral basilar junction were well exposed. The pons and the pontomedullary junction were exposed just beyond the midline. When the internal carotid artery was displaced anteriorly after drilling, even the contralateral anterior surface of the brainstem was partly exposed. The superior limit of this exposure was just above the origin of the trigeminal nerve from the pons.

Upper clivus

As mentioned, exposure above the trigeminal root entry zone was limited by this approach. For exposure of the upper clivus, the midbrain, and the basilar junction, a subtemporal transdural exposure was essential.

Clinical application

This approach has been used by the senior author (LNS) in the operative treatment of petroclival meningiomas as well as some vertebrobasilar aneurysms. This approach is also applicable to chordomas and chondromas of the clivus, temporal bone carcinomas, neurinomas of the cranial nerves eroding the bone, to cranial nerve reconstruction, and to vertebrobasilar reconstructive procedures.

Case reports

Case 1: This 51-year-old lady presented with subarachnoid hemorrhage secondary to a large vertebral aneurysm arising at the origin of the posterior inferior cerebellar artery (PICA). In addition, she had aneurysms at the left internal carotid PCom, left basilar-superior cerebellar, and right middle cerebral locations. At operation, the PICA aneurysm was exposed by a standard retromastoid approach with the patient in the lateral position. During the dissection of the aneurysm, we were unable to visualize the vertebral artery distal to the aneurysm and the distal aspect of the neck of the aneurysm. The aneurysm was located very medially in front of the hypoglossal nerve. In order to visualize the vertebral artery in a better fashion, the transtemporal approach to the lower clivus was utilized and the aneurysm was clipped uneventfully.

Case 2: This 50-year-old man had a history of a left-sided posterior fossa meningioma being resected subtotally about two years previously. He presented to us with severe left-sided headaches. A CAT scan revealed a very large meningioma arising from the petrous ridge occupying almost one-half of the posterior fossa, going up through the tentorial notch, and down through the foramen magnum to the level of the atlas. An arteriogram revealed that the left transverse sinus was draining the vein of Labbe, but did not communicate with the opposite transverse sinus at the torcula.

The tumor was operated in two stages. In the first stage, the lesion was exposed by a retromastoid approach, unroofing the foramen magnum and unroofing the atlas. After a tedious dissection, a very vascular tumor was removed. The predominant attachment of the tumor was to the petrous ridge behind and inferior to the internal auditory canal, and around the ninth, tenth, and eleventh nerves, with the invasion of the left jugular bulb. The PICA was large and coursed through the tumor, but could be preserved after careful dissection. The superior cerebellar artery and a branch of the anterior inferior cerebellar artery ended in the substance of the tumor and were divided at the point of entry into the lesion. At the conclusion of the operation, the posterior fossa portion of the mass was entirely removed but tumor extension remained in the region of the sigmoid sinus, the jugular bulb, and around the caudal cranial nerves. The pathology was angioblastic meningioma.

Because of the nature of the pathology, and the rapidity of recurrence, it was felt that a radical resection was essential. The patient was reoperated two weeks later. At this time, a saphenous vein graft was performed from the sigmoid sinus to the internal jugular vein, to preserve the drainage from the vein of Labbe. Using a transtemporal and infratemporal approach, the lesion was excised radically from within the sinus and the jugular bulb, with the preservation of the ninth, tenth, and the eleventh cranial nerve function. The patient has also received postoperative radiation therapy.

Discussion

The operative approaches available to the clivus are summarized in table 1. Among the extradural approaches, the transoral, the transsphenoidal, and the transethmoidal invade the mucosal plane of the pharynx or the sinuses. They provide a limited exposure of the midline clivus. The bifrontal transbasal approach of

Table 1 Operative approaches to the clivus

Extradural approaches	Area exposed	Advantages	Disadvantages
Transoral	Lower clivus	No brain retraction	Septic spaces traversed
Transsphenoidal	Upper clivus		
Transethmoidal	Upper and lower clivus	Good exposure of midline	Great depth of work Limited to midline by carotids
Bifrontal transbasal (Derome)	Upper and lower clivus		Vital structures at end of resection Dural repair difficult
Transtemporal-infratemporal	Middle and lower		
Intradural approaches			
Frontotemporal sylvian	Upper clivus	Limited brain retraction	Great depth of work
			Narrow field Limited exposure
Subtemporal	Upper and middle clivus	Excellent for tentorial notch	Temporal lobe retraction
			Limited exposure of lower clivus
Retromastoid	Middle and lower clivus	Cerebellar retraction is less morbid	Exposure beyond midline poor
			Upper clivus not exposed

Derome is submucosal but if there is a cerebrospinal fluid fistula, the mucosal plane does not provide a major barrier. All of these approaches are limited to the midline by the two internal carotid arteries on either side.

On the other hand, the transtemporal infratemporal approach provides a good exposure of the middle and lower clivus with excellent visualization of the structures and no retraction. The septic spaces of the mouth or the pharynx are not transgressed. The depth of exposure is small compared to the anterior approaches. The cranial nerves and vessels are identified early in the dissection in contrast to the anterior approaches where they are identified at the very end of tumor resection making it difficult for the surgeon to be entirely sure of where they are situated. This approach can also be easily combined with a retromastoid or subtemporal transdural approaches at the same sitting.

The disadvantages of the transtemporal and infratemporal approach include lengthy bone drilling to expose the seventh nerve completely, a temporary postoperative paralysis of the seventh cranial nerve, destruction of hearing when the middle clivus has to be exposed, poor exposure of the upper clivus, and the possibility of cerebrospinal fluid leakage. The length of bone drilling can be considerably shortened when the neurosurgeon is working with an experienced otologist. Facial paralysis is temporary when it occurs and usually recovers within six months. Exposure across the midline can be achieved by drilling and displacement of the internal carotid artery. However, one may need to open into the temporomandibular joint and retract the condyle of the mandible in order to gain this exposure. Dural repair can be performed easily with the use of dura graft and tissue adhesive followed by packing of the cavity with fat and muscle repair, and the occlusion of the eustachian tube. If the mucosa of the sphenoid sinus is exposed at the anterior limit of the tumor resection, care must be taken to place a lot of fat in this area as well.

The anatomy of these dissections in cadaver specimens is pertinent to operations for glomus tumor, clivus chordoma, petroclival meningiomas, vertebral basilar aneurysms, and radical temporal bone resection. Following radical temporal bone resection, it may be necessary to close the area with a pectoralis myocutaneous flap. For clivus chordoma, this approach may be combined in stages with the transbasal approach. If surgical vertebrobasilar reconstruction becomes possible, this approach will be ideal because the depth of the exposure is small, and there is no brain retraction.

References

[1] Fisch, U., H.C. Pillsbury: Infratemporal fossa approach to lesions in the temporal bone and base of the skull. Arch. Otolaryngol. **105** (1979) 99-107.

[2] House, W.F., W.E. Hitselberger: The transcochlear approach to the skull base. Arch. Otolaryngol. **102** (1976) 334-342.

Acknowledgements

Jon Coulter made the drawings. The difficulties encountered during the operation of Mr. John Lavra stimulated the senior author to study this approach.

Mary Ann Polakovic prepared the manuscript. Jan Hart of the Department of Anatomy prepared the specimens.

Skull base chordoma – neurosurgical problems

H. Arnold, H.-D. Herrmann

Skull base chordoma derives from the vestigia of the notochord situated in the clivus. It is a rare tumor. Among 1100 tumors of the sella region treated in our department between 1971 and 1983 there were only 8 cases of chordoma. They amount to 0.7% compared to 79% of pituitary adenomas and 8% of craniopharyngiomas.

The tumor is characterized by 2 cell types: little stellate cells with single mitoses, and bigger necrobiotic vacuolated cells, so-called physalipherous cells, which appear to be degenerated stellate cells. The validity of the tumor is a point of discussion. According to Saeger et al. [4], chordomas are potentially malignant, whereas Derome and Guiot [3] consider them histologically benign tumors. Morphological differentiation between choriod sarcomas, myxoid chondrosarcomas and chordomas can be difficult. Skull base chordomas are reported to metastasize in about

Table 1 Skull base chordoma: Signs and symptoms

Case	Age sex	Cranial nerve deficit	Pituitary deficit	Seizures
1	66 f	R I, II, III, V_2 L I, II, III, IV	+	
2	60 f	R III, V_1, VI L		
3	51 f	R II, III, VI L (amaurosis since 20 y.)		+
4	68 m	R II, III, VI L		
5	29 m	R II L II	+	
6	67 m	R II, III L (anophthalmia)		+
7	61 m	R II, III, IV L	+	
8	41 f	R L II, III, IV, V1+2, VI		

Cranial nerve impairment predominated. Pituitary deficit or seizures never represented the predominant symptoms.

Table 2 Skull base chordoma: Extent of tumor

Case		Clivus	Sella	Parasell.		Suprasell.	Ethmoid	Nasal Cavity	Base of skull laterally	
1	pr.	+	+							
	rec.	+	+	R	L	+				
2	pr.	+	+	R	L				R	
	rec.									
3	pr.	+	+	R					R	
	rec.	+	+	R		+	+		R	
4	pr.	+	+	R	L	+				
	rec.									
5	pr.	+	+	R		+				
	rec.	+	+	R	L	+			R	L
6	pr.	+	+	R	L	+				
	rec.	+	+	R	L	+	+	+	R	L
7	pr.	+		R		+			R	
	rec.									
8	pr.	+	+	(R)	L	+				L
	rec.	+	+	R	L	+	+	+		L

pr. = primary tumor extent; rec. = extent of tumor recurrence. Parasell. means parasellar region, it is almost always identical with invasion of the cavernous sinus by tumor. R = right; L = left.

20% [1]. In contrast to the literature, however, we never found any metastatic spread.

In our cases, the predominant symptoms were deficits of the second to the sixth cranial nerves. Thus, impaired vision and diplopia represented the most common signs. Reduced activity due to hypothalamic-hypophyseal impairment, and epileptic seizures were occasionally observed (see table 1). Spastic pareses appeared only in advanced cases. For determination of the nature of the tumor, skull base X-rays and computerized tomography were essential. Skull base destruction involving the clivus, the sphenoid, the apex of the petrous bones and, depending on the extent of the tumor, other skull base regions were visualized. By chance, irregularly shaped calcifications were demonstrated, which were considered to be remnants of the skull base dislocated by tumor growth. The most complete information concerning the extent of the tumor was given by computerized tomography. All but one tumor had invaded at least one cavernous sinus (see tab. 2). Angiograms showed the internal carotid artery stretched and occasionally stenotic. In all cases, the tumor

Table 3 Skull base chordoma: Treatment

Case	Op. approach	Date of op.	Radiation	Follow up
1	trans-sphenoidal	2/1972		died 1973
2	fronto-temporal	4/1973	50 GY 1973	died 1976
3	fronto-temporal	7/1980	50 GY 1981	
	fronto-temporal	3/1981		died 1982
4	trans-sphenoidal	10/1975		died 1977
5	trans-sphenoidal	10/1976		
	trans-sphenoidal	1/1978		
	right fronto-temporal	11/1978		
	right fronto-temporal	6/1979	55 GY 1979	
	left fronto-temporal	7/1982		died 12/1983
6	trans-sphenoidal	11/1981		
	bifrontal ethmo-sphe-noidal	2/1982		
	bifrontal→palate clivus	8/1982		died 12/1982
7	right frontotemporal	7/1982		died 7/1982 (gastric ulcer, hem-orrhage)
8	left subtemporal	6/1980		left ophthalmople-gia, slight r. hemi-paresis
	left subtemporal	9/1983	1984	

In case 6, the third operation was performed *via* a bifrontal transethmosphenoidal approach; it included resection of the nasal septum down to the palate and of the clivus. - In cases 5 and 8 the left frontotemporal and subtemporal approaches included attack through the left cavernous sinus region, severing the II., III, IV. and VI. nerves as well as the first and second divisions of the trigeminal nerve. The intracavernous part of the internal carotid artery could be retracted after cutting the ophthalmic artery. In this way an attack on the posterior ethmoid, medial sphenoid and clivus was rendered possible.

vasculature was sparse. Blood supply derived from thin arteries of the skull base as well as from tentorial branches of the carotid. Only in a single case, branches of the ophthalmic artery contributed to tumor vascularisation.

In 4 cases, the tumor was primarily attacked by the trans-septal sphenoidal route. In the remaining 4 cases, the transcranial approach was used according to tumor extent and location. 4 patients needed further operations. In 6 cases the first operation was performed with the aim of preserving vision and oculomotor function. Consequently, tumor removal was incomplete, and more or less extensive tumor remnants were left *in situ*. Recurrence inevitably followed. Only in 1 case, the function of one eye, that was impaired by the tumor, was primarily sacrificed.

During the early days after operation one patient died of gross hemorrhage from gastric ulcer. A second one deteriorated to an apallic state after his third operation and died 3 months later. Another 5 died 1 to 7 years after the diagnosis had been established. The seven year survival period of one patient was purchased by 5 operations, 3 of which were transcranial, and radiation. One female patient whose tumor was operated on in 1980 and 1983 is living with left ophthalmoplegia and slight right hemiparesis (tab. 3).

Case reports

Two case reports may illustrate the problems of the operative approach.

Case 6: After 2 palliative operative interventions that gave only transitory improvement, the patient had eventually put up with loss of sight. He returned to hospital, when the tumor had obstructed his nose and began to cause headache and vomiting. In between the chordoma had occupied his skull base extensively from anterior ethmoid to clivus and both petrosal tips, both cavernous sinus regions, and supra- and retrosellar region as well as his nose. A bifrontal combined extra- and intradural approach was used and ethmoid resection performed. Both orbits were widely opened and the septum nasi, that could be merely identified in big masses of tumor, was resected down to the hard palate. Both carotids including the cavernous segments were exposed. The tumor was also removed from the sphenoid and clivus region, but the rim of the skull base defect could not be rendered completely free of tumor. The skull base defect was closed by a calvarian flap with a big pericranial pedicle after it had been closed off from the nasopharyngeal cavity by using fascia lata with adhesive and pieces of muscle. For the first two postoperative days things seemed to run a favourable course, but during the subsequent period, recurring meningitis produced deterioration of neurological state; presumably spasm of internal carotid branches developed additionally, resulting in multifocal brain edema. The patient became apallic and died 3 months after operation.

Comment

In this advanced case, the tumor could not be readily removed using the bifrontal transbasal approach, because it had already extended to regions lateral to the internal carotid arteries. Although the patient was already blind and the function of the first to the sixth cranial nerves could be disregarded, the mobilization of the carotids could not be performed to the extent, that would have been needed to attack the lateral tumor masses in both posterior cavernous sinus and petrosal apex regions. CSF fistula and meningitis could not be avoided since the pedicled flap finally bordered on remnants of tumor.

Case 8: This 37-year-old woman was admitted because of left-sided blindness and incomplete ophthalmoplegia. The tumor had occupied the intra- and suprasellar space, sphenoid sinus, clivus, both parasellar regions, and a large part of the left middle fossa. (figs. 1 a and

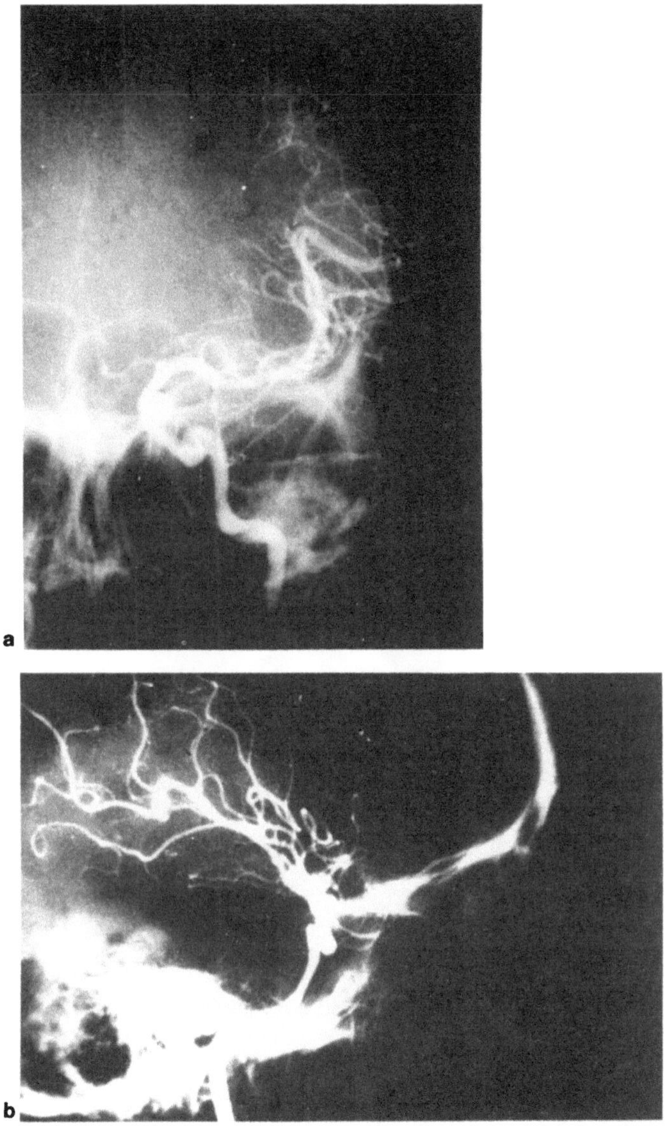

Fig. 1 Case 8, 1. angiogram: the internal carotid artery is stretched and narrowed. Accessory finding: ophthalmic artery aneurysm. a) AP view, b) lateral view.

b). She was operated on by a left frontotemporal approach. Incidentally, an ophthalmic aneurysm was clipped after the left optic nerve had been servered. The ophthalmic artery was clipped and transected, and large masses of tumor were removed from the middle fossa, sphenoid sinus, clivus, sella, and suprasellar region. The third, fourth and sixth cranial nerves as well as the first and second divisions of the trigeminal were cut. The internal carotid artery beginning at its bifurcation down to petrous bone was detached from surrounding tumor, but remnants of tumor were left. It was intended to give radiation, but for various reasons, radiotherapy was delayed, and 4 years later the patient was admitted again, after

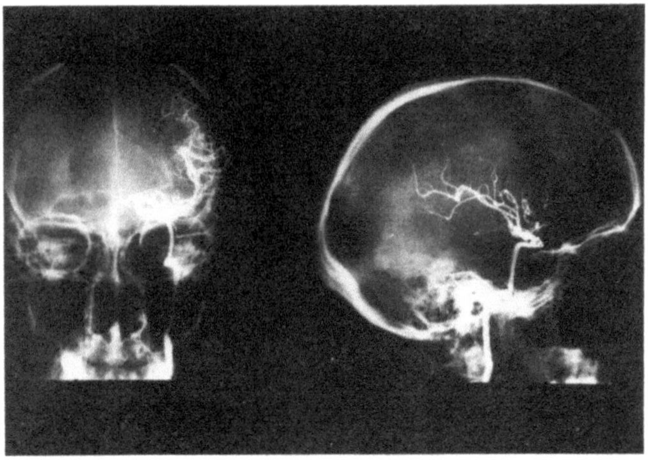

Fig. 2a Case 8, angiogram before second operation: Stretching and dislocation of the cavernous part of the internal carotid artery. The ophthalmic aneurysm was clipped during the first operation.

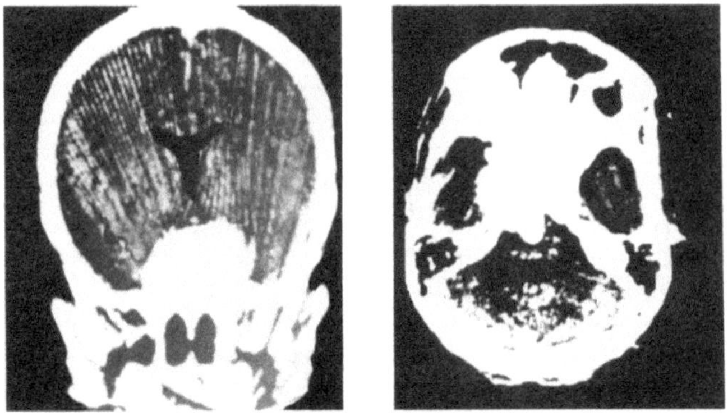

Fig. 2b CT before second operation. Extent of the tumor recurrence in skull base and cranial cavity is visible.

computerized tomography had demonstrated a very large recurrence (figs. 2a and b). Another operation was done by the same approach. The internal carotid as well as posterior communicating and anterior choroid arteries had to be carefully dissected from the tumor. In the mean time the chordoma had invaded the ethmoid and the left orbit. The apex of the left orbit was broadly resected, the ethmoid was removed including the medial wall of right orbit and the optic canal. The left maxillary sinus was opened, and both petrosal tips and the clivus were resected. In spite of this extensive procedure it is questionable, whether we succeeded in radical tumor removal, since the dura in the upper clival region, that might have been invaded by the tumor, was left *in situ* and the resection of left petrosal apex was not as complete as desirable. However, the operation had to be stopped at this point, because of diffuse bleeding due to a coagulation deficit. A part of the tumor cavity was filled with palacos, and the connections to the paranasal sinuses were closed by fascia lata, adhesive, pieces of muscle, and a pericranial flap. The postoperative course was complicated by

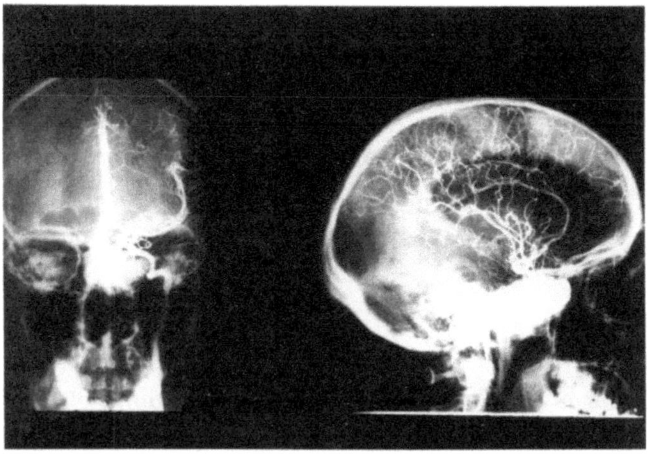

Fig. 3 a Case 8, angiogram after second operation. The tumor has been removed and partially replaced by palacos. The course of the internal carotid artery is now normal.

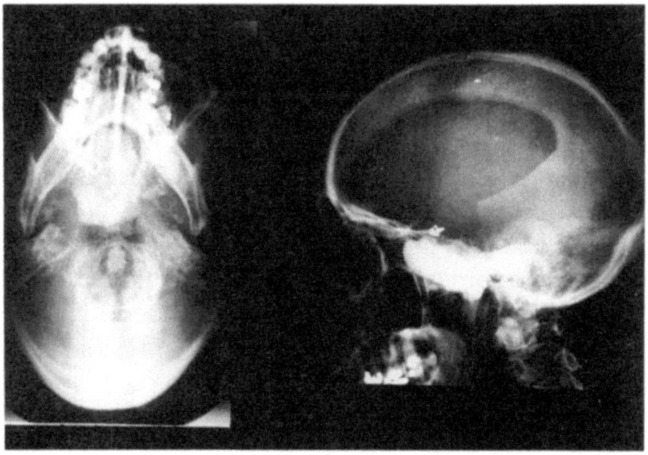

Fig. 3 b Skull base and lateral X-rays demonstrate the extension of the piece of plastic in the skull base. The ethmoidal defect in front of the hyperdense plastic was closed by fascia lata, pieces of muscle and a pericranial flap fixed by fibrin adhesive.

an epidural hematoma and spasm of the anterior choroid artery. The patient is now doing well and is self-supporting, with left ophthalmoplegia and minimal right hemiparesis (figs. 3 a and b). Radiotherapy has now been given.

Comment

Retrospectively, a more radical procedure ought to have been performed during the first operation. However, it has been demonstrated that a chordoma involving the cavernous sinus and even a huge chordoma recurrence can be attacked by a frontotemporal-subtemporal approach. Transsection of the second to sixth cranial nerves must not be avoided, if the corresponding eye is always blind, and may need to be considered, if only one cavernous sinus is invaded by the tumor. In this way, ethmoid, sellar and sphenoid region, clivus and both petrosal tips can be approached, and the internal carotid artery is preserved.

Discussion

The biological behavior of the tumor is illustrated by the course of the illness in those patients, who were initially or exclusively treated by palliative operative measures and radiation; - unfortunately, our radiotherapists were not as successful in combatting chordomas as Cummings and co-workers, who found 5 out of 9 patients living 5 or more years after tumor biopsy or incomplete tumor resection and megavoltage radiation.

From our observations it seems wiser - in spite of the high risk - to try radical tumor removal as soon as the diagnosis of chordoma is established rather than to be content with short-lived improvements in the patient's state, which of course may be achieved by cautious partial tumor resection. Unilateral involvement of cavernous sinus should not be a reason for avoiding operation. Since the tumor inevitably will kill the patient within a comparatively short period of time, even the loss of function of one eye can be taken into the bargain. It is a matter for discussion, whether a frontal transbasal approach as proposed by Derome and Guiot [3], in combination with a subtemporal approach will primise preservation of the three oculomotor nerves (III, IV and VI) in cases where one cavernous sinus is invaded by the tumor.

References

[1] Chambers, P. W., Ch. P. Schwinn: Chordoma. A clinicopathologic study of metastasis. Am. J. Clin. Pathol. **72** (1979) 765-776.
[2] Cummings, B. J., St. Esses, A. R. Harwood: The treatment of chordomas. Int. J. Radiat. Oncol. Biol. Phys. **9** (1983) 633-642.
[3] Derome, P. J., G. Guiot: Surgical approaches to the sphenoidal and clival areas. In: Advances in Technical Standards in Neurosurgery, vol. 6 (H. Krayenbühl, ed.), pp. 101-136. Springer Verlag, Wien-New York 1979.
[4] Saeger, W., D. K. Lüdecke, D. Müller, et al.: Chordome des Clivus. Histologie, Ultrastruktur und Klinik. Tumordiagn. Therap. **4** (1983) 74-79.

Transclival transcervical approach to the upper cervical spine and clivus

F. Lesoin, M. Jomin, P. Pellerin, G. Lozes, S. Carini, R. Servato

Introduction

The approach to lesions of the cranio-cervical junction remains tricky. Several approaches have been suggested: transbasal, transoral, rhinoseptal, combination of the transbasal and rhinoseptal approaches or combination of the transoral and submandibular approaches [2, 5, 6, 7, 9, 10]. The work done by Derome [3] showed that only the transbuccal approach could give access both to the lower part of the clivus and to C1-C2. This approach involves two risks however: the first is of an infectious nature since it establishes communication between a septic cavity and the operative zone; the second is due to the difficulties encountered in getting the pharyngeal mucosa to heal. Following Stevenson's first publication in 1967 [11] we have used the transclival transcervical approach in order to overcome these two disadvantages. We propose to report on our experiences with this approach in 6 patients. We will then discuss its various advantages and disadvantages.

The transclival transcervical approach

In 1967, Stevenson [11] described this approach which he used successfully to deal with a chordoma of the clivus. Nagashima [8] used it in the treatment of a metastasis of C1 and C2. Wiessenger [12] used this same approach in 1969 to operate on an aneurysm of the lower third of the basilar artery.

The purpose of this approach is to expose the lower third of the clivus and the upper cervical spine by pushing back the retropharyngeal space and the roof of the cavum on which the aponeuroses of the pharynx are attached. The obstacles in the way of this route are vascular, nervous and muscular. The facial nerve is easily pushed upwards out of the way with the parotid gland; the hypoglossal nerve projects into the center of the approach zone and must be pushed inwards out of the way. The second obstacle is vascular and comprises the anterior collateral veins of Faraboeuf's venous trunk, the facial artery, the lingual and thyroid arteries.

There is also a muscular barrier composed of the muscles stretched in an oblique manner between the middle fossa of the base of the skull and the hyoid bone: the digastric and styloid muscles.

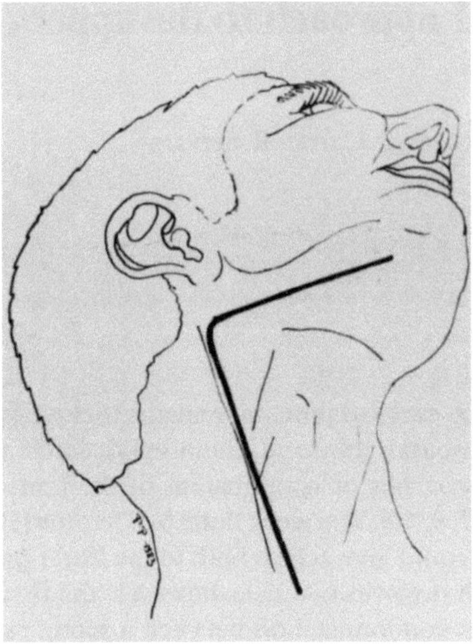

Fig. 1 L-shaped skin incision.

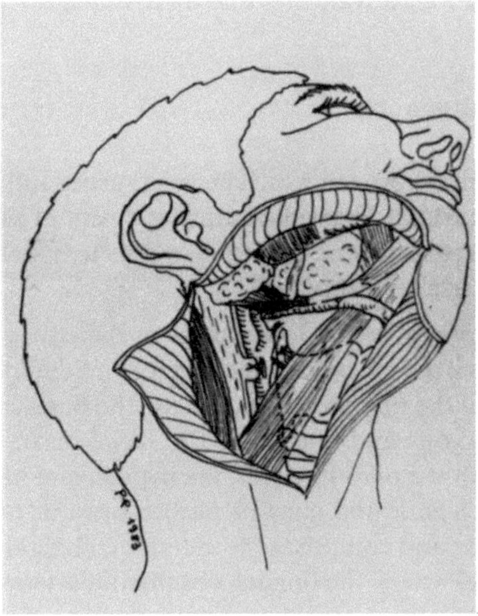

Fig. 2 Ligation of the facial, thyroid, lingual and pharyngeal venous trunk which provides access to the branches of the external carotid artery.

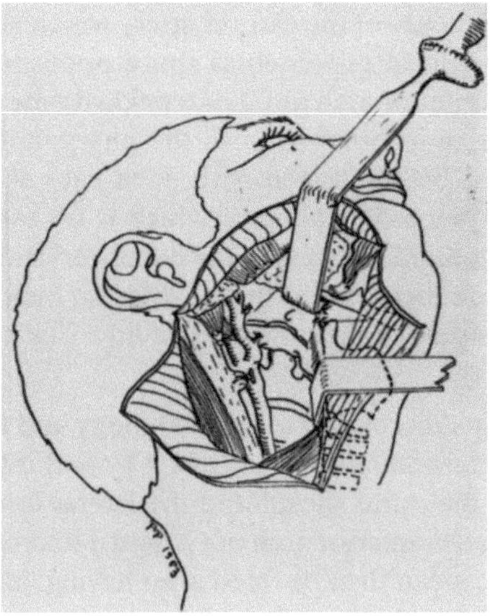

Fig. 3 The dissected retropharyngeal space provide access to the cranio-cervical junction.

The approach is performed with the patient in the supine position and under general anesthetic. The head is slightly hyperextended and turned slightly away from the point of incision [15]. Tracheotomy was performed on the first patient in order to be able to keep the bottom jaw closed and through fear of respiratory difficulty following the operation caused by the retropharyngeal dissection. Subsequently this was abandoned in favor of nasal intubation using a reinforced tube. An L-shaped skin incision is made starting under the symphysis mandibulae and working towards the angle of the jaw. It is then taken down the anterior edge of the sternomastoid muscle (fig. 1). Provided a curvilinear incision is made under the angle of the jaw, there is less risk of skin necrosis than with the incision recommended by Stevenson [11], which is T-shaped and goes from the symphysis mandibulae to the mastoid bone with a vertical incision going down from the middle of the horizontal incision in front of the sternomastoid muscle. The platysma is incised and the external jugular vein which crosses the incision obliquely in the vicinity of the maxillary angle is ligated. Next the aponeurosis is cut opposite the anterior edge of the sternomastoid. The incision along the anterior edge of the sternomastoid muscle is carried upwards from the bottom as far as the parotid gland. The inferior pole of the gland is pushed upwards with great care in order to protect the facial nerve. Dissection is continued by ligating the Faraboeuf trunk (fig. 2). Under the parotid gland, the posterior belly of the digastric muscle is located, this going forwards and downwards and passing 1 cm above the greater horn of the hyoid bone. The twelfth nerve passes behind the belly of the digastric muscle. The intermediate tendon is cut and the belly pushed backwards out of the way. The superior thyroid, lingual and facial arteries are ligated and divided.

It is the intersection of the anterior branches of the carotid artery which constitutes the point of entry into the retropharyngeal prevertebral space opposite C2, C3. The approach to the clivus, from the anterior arch of C1, is a ticklish time requiring dissection of the retropharyngeal space in order to push the pharynx out of the way. This part of the operation must be performed with great care as to avoid creating a breach in the pharyngeal mucosa, healing of which is no easy matter. The dissected retropharyngeal space provides access to the craniocervical junction (fig. 3). The anterior arch of C1 is then located and this enables an incision to be made in the prevertebral aponeurosis strictly along its median line. The aponeurosis is pushed to the side out of the way.

Bone resection is performed as required according to the pathology and the osteosynthesis selected. It comprises the excision of the body of C2 by first intention in order to control the anterior face of the dural sheath and the lateral limits of the resection. It is continued by abrading the anterior arch of C1 und a microscope using a rotary burr. The odontoid process can then be freed after having cut the ligaments and any adhesions to the dural sheath. Resection of the clivus may be necessary and involves an area approx 2.5 cm wide X 3.5 cm high. Its lateral and upper limits are the internal carotid artery and the inferior petrous sinus. We have never attempted reconstruction through the use of a bone graft. The technique used by Stevenson [11] is that of a bony inlay between the clivus and the body of C3. Our fixation technique involves the insertion of metal pins. The pin is forced into the clivus and the body of C3 or of a lower vertebra if a broad-based body excision has been required, an image intensifier being used to do this. In the case of our last two patients, this fixation was reinforced with 2 pins positioned laterally in the occipital condyles using the technique described by Fang [5]. The metal assembly is then embedded in methyl methacrylate. The solidity of the set-up is increased by the fitting of one or more metal loops which provide a greater surface of contact between the methyl methacrylate and the metal reinforcement. In order to avoid the risk of erosion or of posterior pharyngeal necrosis resulting from contact with the prosthesis, a flap of fatty tissue is inserted between the pharynx and the methylmethacrylate before closing up.

Postoperatively, a gastric tube is sometimes required for a few days because of pharyngeal edema or an accidental breach in the mucosa which will have been carefully closed up in order to prevent septic contamination of the operative zone through the pharyngeal cavity.

Clinical material

Over the last 18 months, six patients have been operated on using this technique. The average age of the 4 male and 2 female patients was 68.

One patient presented with rheumatoid disease together with a subluxation of C3/C4 and an upward dislocation of the odontoid process. The neurological symptoms had been developing for a period of 3 years. The rheumatoid disease had been known about for 8 years. Examination of the patient revealed a spastic tetraparesis. The paraclinical assessment brought to light compression of the brain stem through the displaced odontoid process, compression of the upper cervical spinal cord through dislocation of C1/C2 and subluxation of C3/C4. The dual character of the nervous damage was confirmed by a study of the somatesthetic evoked responses (SER's). Operation involved excision of C2, C3 and C4 bodies, excision of the anterior arch of C1 and of the bottom part of the clivus, followed by excision of the odontoid process which had been forced up into the posterior fossa in front of the brain stem. This excision was followed by the insertion of a pin between the clivus and C5 bedded in methylmethaycrylate.

2 patients had developed a malunion of the odontoid process after an upper cervical trauma that had been neglected. Subsequent of this a progressive spastic tetraparesis developed over a period of 3 months. The paraclinical assessment showed that the site of the compression was at C1/C2, opposite the bony compression created by the anterior fixation of the fractured odontoid process. Operation involved the resection of the body of C2, the anterior arch of C1 and the odontoid process. An acrylic prosthesis was put in place between the clivus and the body of C3.

1 patient aged 80 developed a spastic tetraparesis related to a pseudarthrosis of the odontoid process which had been tipped forward. After an attempt at immobilization with a Minerva jacket, then with a Halo brace for a period of 6 months, the patient finding it hard to accept this type of fixation, an anterior approach was performed especially as there was a subluxation of C2/C3 with discopathy responsible for an additional anterior compression. Operation involved the resection of the body of C2 and the degenerated C2/C3 disc. After intraoperative reduction with monitoring of the somatesthetic evoked responses (SER's), a metal pin was fixed in the odontoid process and the clivus as far down as the body of C3. The assembly was set with methylmethacrylate after the insertion of two additional pins in the occipital condyles.

1 patient presented a secondary slipping of the odontoid process. The instability of the lesion was responsible for a dislocation of the odontoid process, easily reducible, and the progressive development of a spastic tetraparesis. This, together with the absence of any evidence of a primary neoplasm, made us decide to operate. Operation involved the resection of the body of C2, the anterior arch of C1, the odontoid process and the bottom part of the clivus. A reinforced acrylic prosthesis was then put in place between the clivus and C3. The histopathological examination showed that it was a solitary plasmacytoma.

Finally, the last patient presented with a cervical chordoma which had already been operated on twice and had been brought to light initially by a dysphagia. A

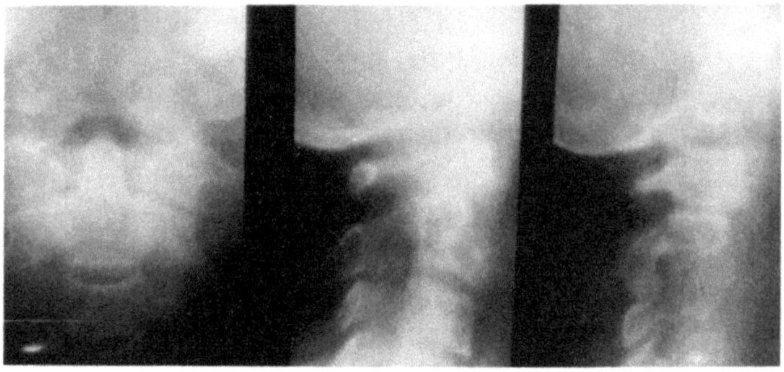

Fig. 4a Lysis of C2 and C3.

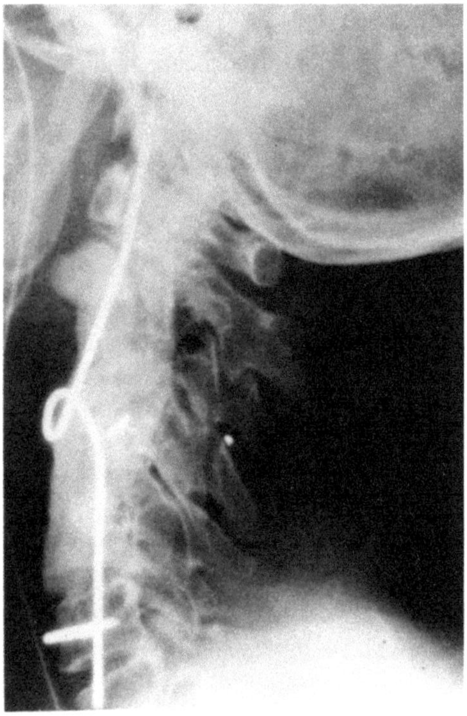

Fig. 4b Acrylic prosthesis between the clivus and C5 for cervical chordoma.

retropharyngeal lateral cervical mass had been resected initially in an E. N. T. department. As the pathological examination revealed that it was a chordoma, the patient was then transferred to the Neurosurgery Department, especially as the CT scan revealed a posterolateral extension which was operated on using a posterolateral approach. The appearance of upper cervical pain and a spastic tetraparesis six months later called for a further extensive assessment which revealed the collapse of C2 and C3. Operation consisted of a broadbased resection, because of considerable bone infiltration, including the bodies of C2, C3, C4, resection of the anterior arch of C1, abrasion of the odontoid process. A reinforced acrylic prosthesis was put in place between the clivus and C5 (figs. 4a–b).

Results

These must be studied as a function of the pathology responsible from the neurological and orthopedic standpoints. From the neurological point of view, all the patients showed improvement. Recovery occurred over periods varying from 3 weeks to 6 months and was complete in 5 of the patients and partial in the other patient, this probably being due to the great length of the period of development (3 years) before operation and the associated rheumatoid disease, resulting in a handicap through the existence of the articular deformities alone. The stability of the set-up was checked for all the patients. No external retention was required, even temporarily.

The following gave us cause for regret: a retropharyngeal wound made when a pin was put in place which was sutured immediately. Healing was no easy matter and required insertion of a gastric tube throughout its entire duration of 4 weeks.

One death occurred 3 weeks after operation in a patient who had previously been operated upon for a chordoma. This patient's postoperative course was very tedious and was marked by pulmonary infection probably caused by prolonged intubation required because of an extensive edema, as the patient's general condition was poor. Death was sudden and was probably caused by a massive pulmonary embolism despite the fact that the repeat X-rays showed the fixation to be stable. As regards this patient, the tumorous infiltration appeared at operation to be considerable, even laterally opposite the articular masses of the foramen transversarium and that an ischemia due to compression of the vertebral arteries could not be ruled out, as a post-mortem examination was not carried out.

Comments

The transclival transcervical approach described by Stevenson [11] has as its main interest an extrapharyngeal exposure. This approach therefore enables reconstruction work to be performed using bone or reinforced methyl methacrylate without any risk of infectious contamination of the material implanted. Control of the lower part of the clivus and of C1 and C2 is easy to obtain. The L-shaped incision reduces the risk of necrosis and facilitates the pushing back of the various elements towards the midline. The exposure of the clivus, the anterior arch of C1 and the body of C2 by pushing the loop of the hypoglossal nerve downwards also provides control of the anterior surface of the underlying spine. Through this approach the surgeon, by resecting the disc C2/C3, can gain perfect in-depth control when removing the body of C2 and at the same time of the resection of the odontoid process and the anterior part of the clivus, by following the spinal dural upwards. This appears to be an important point when faced with lesions which readily alter the various relationships between the bony structures and the dura. Laterally, control is satisfactory since the surgeon locates the midline and can if he desires identify the vertebral arteries in the foramina transversaria. The danger comes from the loop of the vertebral artery between C1 and C2. Resection of the clivus upwards is limited by the inferior petrosal sinus and it is limited laterally by the carotid arteries.

This approach does however have certain limitations:
- it only provides exposure of the lower part of the clivus;
- it is rather deep, but the use of an operating microscope enables this disadvantage to be overcome;
- the dissection of the retropharyngeal space must be done carefully and we think that by inserting a flap of fatty tissue at the end of the operation, it is possible to reduce the risk of necrosis of the wall as a result of direct contact with an acrylic prosthesis or bone graft;
- lastly, the postoperative pharyngeal edema sometimes means prolonging the period of intubation and also necessitates a gastric tube.

This approach can be used to treat primary or secondary bone tumors of the clivus and of the upper cervical spine. As Stevenson [11] and Nagashima [8] have shown, it enables lesions to be treated which affect not only the lower part of the clivus but also C1 and C2. We have used it twice for such cases. Malunions and pseudarthrodeses of the odontoid process are an excellent indication. For such cases this approach seems to us to be superior to the approach described by several authors in dealing with these lesions. Actually, these authors make an incision which starts opposite the mastoid bone and goes down anterior to the sternomastoid muscle. They recommend pushing the loop of the hypoglossal nerve upwards. This approach only allows satisfactory control of the disc C2/C3 and is only compatible with a bony inlay. We have used the transclival transcervical approach to treat 7 patients who had a fracture of the pedicles of C2 with compound dislocation of C2/C3 through an associated disc lesion. With this approach it proves to be relatively easy, after discectomy, to insert not only a bone graft but also a Senegas plate with 4 screws fixed in C2 and C3. This approach can also be considered in the event of setbacks associated with a posterior approach to the upper cervical spine, when the occipitovertebral graft does not take or the osteosynthetic plate is a failure.

Although we have no experience of this approach for malformations of the hinge-joint, it would probably be worth considering here. In point of fact, our case report may be likened to those cases of upward dislocation of the odontoid process following rheumatoid disease. Moreover the deformities produced by this at the upper cervical level can be treated by using this approach. Lastly, and somewhat audaciously, we must mention the usefulness of this approach in the treatment of aneurysms of the lower third of the basilar trunk as described by Weissinger. Despite the exceptional nature of this location, it seems that even for Drake his treatment poses a few problems hitherto poorly resolved.

References

[1] Bohler, J.: Anterior stabilization for acute fracture and non-unions of the dens. J. Bone Joint Surg. **64 A** (1982) 18-28.

[2] Delandsheer, J. M., M. Jomin: Voie transbucco-pharyngée et malformations de la charnière cervico-occipitale. Neurochirurgie **23** (1977) 276-281.

[3] Derome, P., J. P. Caron, M. Hurth: Indication de la voie trans-bucco-pharyngée et malformations de la charnière crânio-vertébrale. Neurochirurgie **23** (1977) 282-286.

[4] Fang, H. S. Y., G. B. Ong: Direct anterior approach to the upper cervical spine. J. Bone Joint Surg. **44 A** (1962) 1588-1604.

[5] Jomin, M., J. M. Delandsheer: Possibilités de la voie trans-bucco-pharyngée dans les lésions traumatiques anciennes des deux premières vertèbres cervicales. Neurochirurgie **23** (1977) 271-275.

[6] Jomin, M., J. M. Delandsheer, J. de Rougemont: Possibilités de la voie trans-bucco-pharnygée dans les lésions traumtiques anciennes des deux premières vertèbres cervicales. Neurochirurgie **23** (1977) 271-275.

[7] Nagashima, C., T. Iwasaki, K. Okada et al.: Reconstruction of the atlas and axis with wire and acrylic after metastatic destruction. J. Neurosurg. **50** (1979) 668-671.

[8] Rougemont, J. de, M. de Abada, M. Barge: Les possibilités de la voie d'abord antérieure dans les lésions des trois premières vertèbres cervicales. Neurochirurgie **12** (1966) 323-336.

[9] Southwick, W. O., R. A. Robinson: Approaches to the vertebral bodies in the cervical and lumbar regions. J. Bone Joint Surg. **39 A** (1957) 631.

[10] Stevenson, G. C., R. J. Stoney, R. K. Pekking et al.: A transcervical transclival approach to the ventral surface of the brain stem for removal of a clivus chordoma. J. Neurosurg. **24** (1966) 544-551.

[11] Weissinger, J. P., D. Danoff, E. S. Wisiol et al.: Repair of an eneurysm of the basilar artery by a transclival approach. Case report. J. Neurosurg. **26** (1967) 417-419.

Interdisciplinary approach to benign tumors of the lateral skull base

J. Helms, K. Schürmann

The medical profession and its specialities have evolved *pari passu* with the development of surgical and medical knowledge, and in accordance with the results of treatment of various diseases. The disciplines of today developed as a result of the requirements of the majority of patients within a certain medical sector.

However, the originally somewhat unattractive boundary areas in some of these fields have recently gained combined interest, thanks to a reduction in political interest and an increase in theoretical and practical activities e. g. at the lateral skull base.

Refined experience in one area can enhance and support the adjoining one, thus improving the results of treatment. Following this concept neurosurgeons, neuroradiologists, neurologists, maxillofacial surgeons and otorhinolaryngologists commenced closer cooperation e. g. in Mainz.

In order to illustrate these activities it is not our aim to discuss the data of 196 acoustic neurinomas and increased success in the preservations or improvement of hearing. Interest is focussed on the more infrequently appearing lesions (tab. 1).

A previously described purely otological series of glomus tumors showed that the size of the tumor does not always determine the difficulty and extent of an operation, for example, the involvement of the jugular bulb depends primarily more on the origin than the size of an ear tumor. Because the origin is initially unknown, expert neuroradiology is necessary before all operations on glomus tumors of the ear. This particularly includes subtraction angiography, even in apparently small tu-

Table 1 Benign “tumors” of the lateral skull base

Acoustic neurinoma	196
Glomus tumor	23
Genuine cholesteatoma (epidermoid)	7
Meningioma	7
Brain prolapse	6
Facial nerve neuroma	5
Angioma	4
Chondroma	3
Arachnoidal cyst	2
Mucocele	1
Aneurysmal bone cyst	1
Cholesterol granuloma of pyramid	1

mors. These small ones seem to grow only in the middle ear space, behind the translucent ear drum.

Treatment may include embolization, as well as neurological and otolaryngological operations. If the jugular bulb is involved and has to be excised partially or totally the transverse or sigmoid sinuses are preferably occluded by neurosurgical ligation techniques rather than by otosurgical packing. The internal carotid artery is freed in the temporal bone until all tumor invasion is visible beneath the Eustachian tube and medially at the horizontal part of the vessel or at the cavernous sinus. The neurosurgical position of the head has the advantage of a lower venous blood pressure resulting in a smaller blood loss and reduced filling of the tumor.

If the vagus and glossopharyngeal nerves cannot be preserved Denecke's deglutition reconstruction operation is indicated. The desired functional improvement was achieved in all 7 of our cases. Out of 23 glomus tumor operations during the last 5 years one case illustrates combined team work.

Epidermoids or primary cholesteatomas develop from epidermal tissue which is wrongly incorporated into the neural tube and its surrounding during ontogenesis. These malformations are a neurosurgical problem when located purely intradurally, but they may grow in the pyramid extradurally. In this case oto-neurosurgical cooperation serves for the benefit of the patient if combined experience is applied in this problematic area. Facial nerve or cochlear problems always warrant careful examination of Stenvers X-rays. Bony defects with sharp edges and some signs of displacement are frequently observed.

Further surgical cooperation included 7 meningiomas, 3 chondromas, 1 cholesterol granuloma and an aneurysmal bone cyst of the pyramid protruding into the cerebellum. This case was treated together with neurosurgeons of Freiburg University.

In some of these patients a staged operation was performed. First of all, neurosurgeons removed the intradural part of the tumors, resected the dura and preserved it for reconstruction. In the second stage the disease was removed from the temporal bone by oto-surgical techniques, including facial nerve repair where necessary. Under these conditions the neurosurgeon had anastomosed centrally in the posterior fossa and left the peripheral end of the nerve transplant free extradurally for the peripheral connection (Samii's technique). In other cases the hypoglossal nerve was anastomosed.

If possible a one stage combined neck-, neuro- and otosurgical intervention is performed for removal of tumors involving the tip of the pyramid and adjacent intradural spaces. If facial function is still present this nerve is reflected anteriorly to enlarge the access to the deep parts of the temporal bone (Fisch). It finally runs from the geniculate ganglion over the Eustachian tube and the medial and posterior aspect of the mandibular joint to the parotid gland. The external auditory canal, middle ear and labyrinth are removed.

Larger intradural tumors may cause involvement not only of the eighth but also of seventh and other cranial nerves passing the pyramid. In this cases extensive pyramid removal with planned primary or second stage facial nerve repair offers advantages. The internal carotid artery is identified and therefore not inadvertently injured. Transverse, sigmoid and superior petrosal sinuses are dissected free of bone and easily handled if bleeding. Ligation if necessary is performed in the usual manner when the intracranial supratentorial and/or infratentorial area is to be exposed. These procedures are carried out without retraction of the cerebellum or temporal lobe, because of the space gained by removal of the pyramid. Mobilization of a tumor near the brain stem is thus possible with wider exposure and less brain retraction. The angle of access is more anterior than if one tries to preserve the temporal bone, which is useless for the patient. Experience with 7 such cases is most encouraging. These otosurgical possibilities might also add positive variations to the field of modern neurosurgical operations at the anterior part of the tentorial hiatus.

A particular patient is at present recovering from her first stage operation and might benefit from the discussion of this meeting.

A right vagal glomus tumor was removed from the neck, with resection of vagus and glossopharyngeal nerves. It had been shown pre-operatively that neither the internal carotid artery nor the jugular vein on this side were of any hemodynamic relevance. Both had been compressed by the tumor over decades and had lost function. It was planned to preserve both of these vessels uninjured, and this was successfully achieved at the operation.

Deglutition was restored by Denecke's technique. Conservation of the larger vessels seemed desirable because of her second glomus tumor on the other side. This is an extensive jugular foramen chemodectoma. The inferior border of the tumor is situated in the foramen magnum, the main mass involves the pyramid with the jugular bulb and internal carotid artery, as well as the posterior cranial fossa, and the tip is estimated to be in direct contact with the cavernous sinus. After the course of diagnostic and initial therapeutic measures so far it is hoped that the greater vessels on the operated side may recover with some restoration of patency. The decision about further intervention has still to be made.

Vascular problems of the carotid artery and reconstructive procedures

J. F. Vollmar

For tumor surgery in the neck and skull base recent progress in vascular surgery may be helpful and important in making the procedure Simpler, Safer and Shorter; following the three S-principle. This is specially true for two complicating situations:

1. *Control of intraoperative bleeding* and
2. *preservation of the carotid arteries* and the *jugular vein* when the tumor mass is in close anatomical relationship to these vessels.

The *carotid body tumor* is a typical example. It arises from the glomus caroticum and is a relatively rare condition. Its clinical picture and the various patho-anatomical patterns have been well described for more than one century [2, 3, 7]. A true malignancy of the tumor has been proved in only 5% to 10%.

The *clinical picture* is characterized by a slowly growing indolent tumor at the lateral aspect of the neck, frequently misinterpretated as a lymph node or cervical cyst. It is a remarkable phenomenon that only 20% of carotid body tumors are correctly diagnosed pre-operatively. The classical *clinical tests* described by Fontaine and Kocher at the beginning of this century are still of unequivocal diagnostic value [8]. The definitive diagnosis is made by computer tomography (CT) and carotid *arteriography*. Of our last 20 patients in 16 there had been a previous surgical exposure by general surgeons or otolaryngologists resulting twice in severe bleeding and ligature of the common carotid artery with persistent neurological deficit.

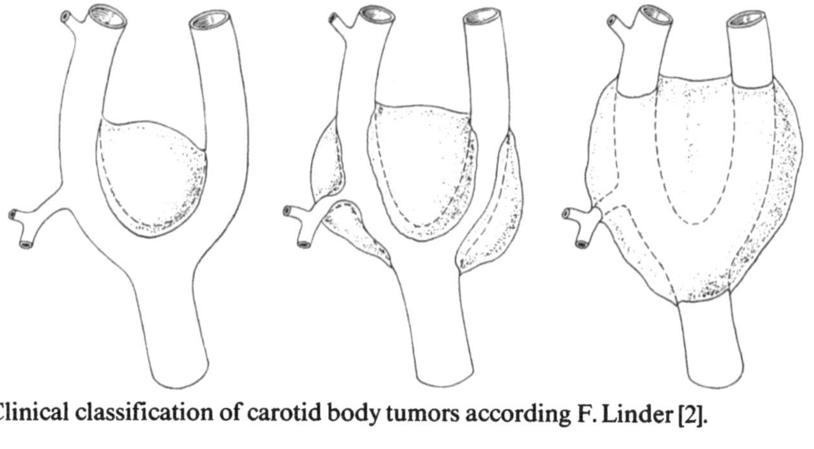

Fig. 1 Clinical classification of carotid body tumors according F. Linder [2].

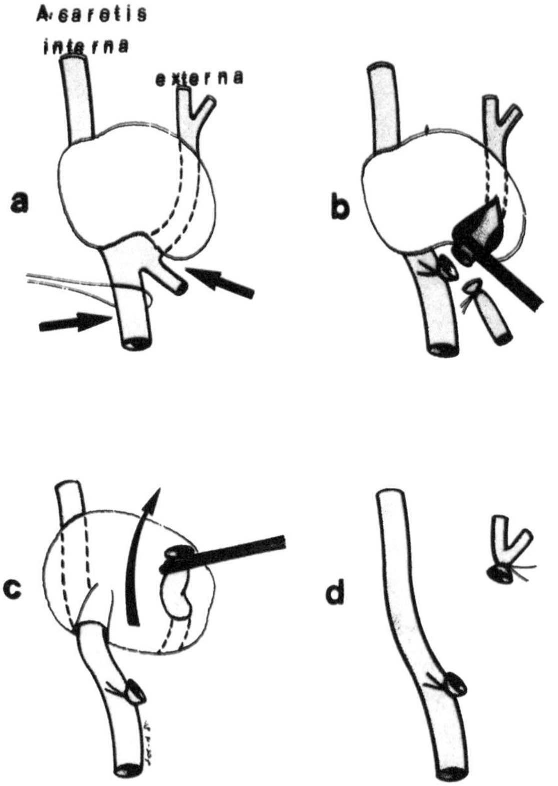

Fig. 2 Operative procedure (transection technique): a) Exposure of the common carotid artery (A) and isolation of the origin of the external carotid artery (B); b) Ligation and division of external carotid artery at its origin followed by transection of the tumor; c) Lifting up of the tumor anteriorly and dissection of the wall of the internal carotid artery; d) Operative site after local excision of the tumor with the internal carotid artery left intact (from: J. Vollmar, E. U. Voss and W. Mohr [7]).

Cure of a carotid body tumor can only be achieved by a total surgical excision. In relation to the extent of tumor growth three clinical types may be differentiated (figs. 1 and 2). In Type III the tumor sometimes extends up to the skull base, displacing the pharynx to the contralateral side. This is best seen in the CT scan. Until quite recently carotid artery resection was considered as clearly indicated in Type II and III lesions. In the last ten years a *changed surgical technique* was used even at this advanced stage, enabling the continuity of the common and internal carotid artery to be preserved.

1. After exposure of the common carotid artery for central vascular control the first segment of the external carotid artery is exposed if necessary by splitting the tumor down to the arterial wall (fig. 2) [6, 8]. By ligation and division of the external carotid artery the blood supply of the tumor is interrupted.
2. As the next step the distal stump of the external carotid artery is grasped in a

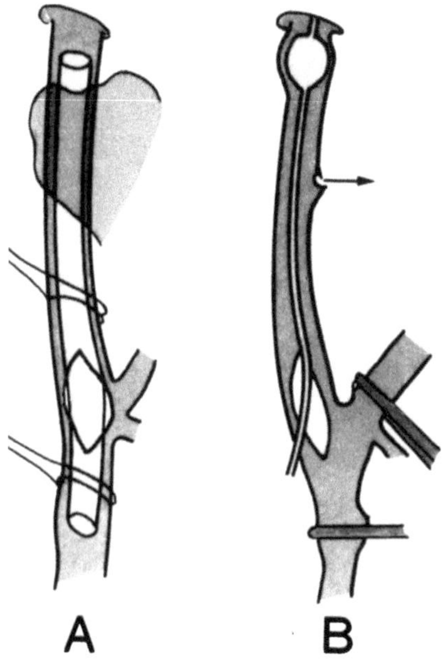

Fig. 3 Carotid body tumors. Types of repair Ulm 1970–1984 (n = 22).

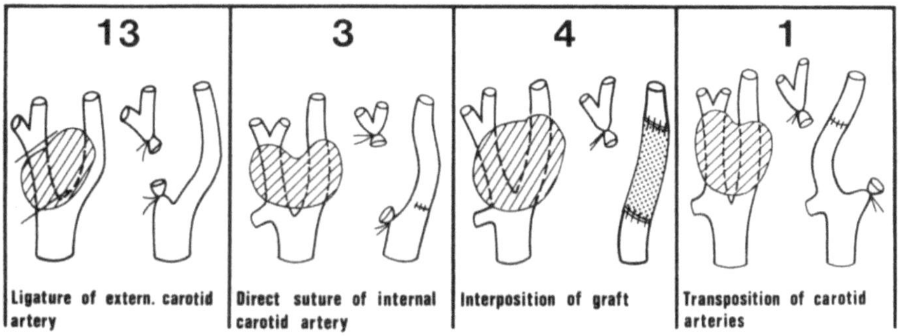

Fig. 4 Surgical techniques for protection or control of bleeding of the main neck vessels.

clamp and lifted anteriorly. This maneuver allows the surgeon to dissect the tumor free from the carotid bifurcation and from the internal carotid artery. In the presence of partial or total inclusion of the arteries by the tumor mass, the tumor is divided and the vessel is freed by sharp dissection.

Only if the transection results in an arterial lesion is an arterial clamp put on the common carotid artery. If the integrity of the internal carotid artery could not be preserved an arterial reconstruction has to be done. Several types of *arterial repair* may be used: Lateral direct suture, patch graft, interposition of a venous graft or transposition of the internal carotid artery to the stump of the external carotid artery. In 12 of 13 patients, even in Stage II and III the tumor could be removed with-

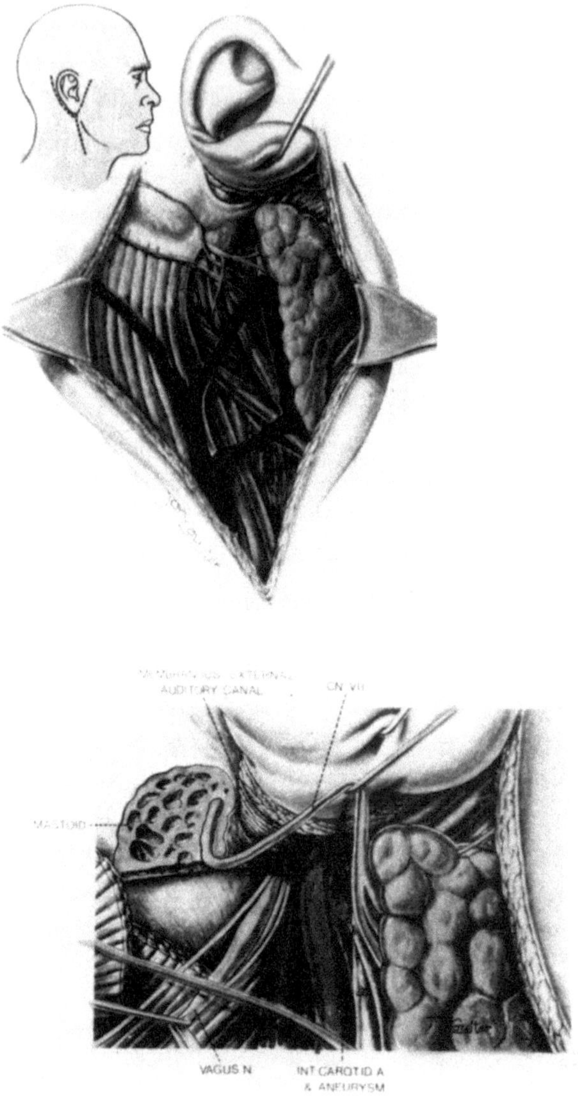

Fig. 5 a + b Modified approach for the exposure and repair of high located lesions to the internal carotid artery or the jugular vein, according S. Arena et al. [1, 4, 5].

out any damage to or clamping of the internal carotid artery. Before using this dissecting technique an interposition of a venous graft was necessary in only 4 patients (fig. 3).

There was one death in a 30 year old patient with bilateral body tumors from cerebral infarction due to secondary thrombosis of his left internal carotid artery.

None of the 13 patients operated on for carotid body tumor with transection of the tumor mass developed a tumor recurrence or deposits in the following 5 to 10 years. This operative technique as presented contradicts the oncological principle of taking out the tumor *en bloc.* On the other hand the absence of any tumor recurrence in the follow-up seems to justify such a simple approach preserving the continuity of the common and internal carotid artery in the most cases. As an additional help especially in extensive tumor masses up to the skull base it has proved a useful adjunct to insert an *intraluminal shunt* in the internal carotid artery for easier identification of this important vessel and the avoidance of any traumatic vascular lesion (fig. 4).

Recently, a *modified surgical exposure* (fig. 5) offers a quite satisfactory approach to the distal part of the internal carotid artery and the jugular vein [1, 4, 5]. Especially for the repair of high lesions of the internal carotid artery this technique also offers a good exposure for graft insertion, which is best done under the protection of an intraluminal shunt. Concomitant tumors arising from the *jugular body* should be kept in mind if the tumor mass extends to the level of the skull base. Here also a cervical approach usually allows the removal of both tumors in one stage. We have done this on two occasions.

Control of intraoperative *bleeding* during the removement of high located tumors is best achieved by the following techniques:
1. Preliminary *exposure of the carotid bifurcation,* i.e., temporary clamping of the carotid arteries;
2. the availability of an *intraluminal shunt* for the protection of the brain;
3. *balloon catheter blockage* of the internal carotid artery or else the internal jugular vein at any level up to the skull base.

Any *iatrogenic lesion* to the carotid artery should be repaired immediately. The era of ligature of the common or internal carotid artery should be considered as definitely over. Even in younger persons the outcome is not predictable.

Summary

1. The surgical removal of carotid body tumors requires a considerable degree of *knowledge* and *technical training* in *vascular surgery* because all these tumors have a very close relationship to vascular structures. Primary interruption of the external carotid artery inflow represents an important technical step for bleeding control and for dissection of the tumor from the internal carotid artery. Preserving the continuity of the internal carotid artery may be realized even in Type II and III lesions by using the transection technique.

2. Any *blind exposure,* for the biopsy of undiagnosed tumors near the carotid artery *should be avoided.* Control of bleeding may be difficult and a second intervention for total extirpation of the tumor is usually a surgical procedure with increased risk. Therefore any surgical approach to the tumors should be undertaken with the goal of *primary total excision.* Every effort must be made pre-operatively to clear up the type and extent of the tumor by *arteriography* in combination with *computerized tomography.* Extension of the tumor up to the skull base should be considered as a challenge for a close cooperation between neurosurgeon and the vascular surgeon.

References

[1] Arena, S.: Tumor surgery of temporal bone. Laryngoscopy **84** (1974) 645-670.

[2] Linder, F.: Tumoren der Karotisdrüse. Langenbecks Arch. Klin. Chir. **276** (1953) 156.

[3] Linder, F., M. Wagner, I. J. Allenberg et al.: Tumoren des Glomus caroticum. Chirurg. **55** (1984) 19-24.

[4] Pellegrini, R. V., G. W. Manzetti, R. F. DiMarco et al.: The direct surgical management of lesions of the high internal carotid artery. J. Cardiovasc. Surg. **25** (1984) 29-35.

[5] Purdue, G. F., R. V. Pellegrini, S. Arena: Aneurysms of the high internal carotid artery: A new approach. Surgery **89** (1981) 268-270.

[6] Vollmar, J.: Rekonstruktive Chirurgie der Arterien, 3rd ed. Thieme, Stuttgart-New York 1982.

[7] Vollmar, J., E. U. Voss, W. Mohr: Carotid body tumors - diagnostic and surgical aspects -. Angéiologie **22** (1980) 253-270.

[8] Voss, E. U., J. Vollmar, H. Meister: Tumoren des Glomus caroticum. Thoraxchirurgie **25** (1977) 1-12.

The diagnosis and operative strategy of large glomus tumors

M. Samii, W. Draf

Introduction

Glomus jugulare tumors are classified by the pathologists as chemodectomas or non-chromaffin paragangliomas. In a study made by Van Baars [1] a high familial incidence was observed; he stated the incidence of two or more glomus tumors in members of the same family to be as high as 38%. Glomus tumors may arise from the carotid body in the neck or higher up in the jugular foramen. The tumors may vary in size, and in the case of a large tumor it may not be possible to determine the point of its origin. The tumor growth, though largely spread over the length of the neck, may extend further up to the skull base and even infiltrate it [8, 11, 12, 14, 15].

Investigative methods are not merely aimed at diagnosing the obvious, but also to detect hidden pheochromocytomas, the evidence of which would help the surgeon to avert, anticipate or overcome a possible intra-operative hypertonic crisis. Dynamic angioscintigraphy, in this context, is an extremely valuable method of investigation [13].

The evolution of surgery of glomus tumors has been greatly influenced by Denecke [2-6]. We share his view with regard to the futility of radiotherapy for the treatment of these tumors. However large the tumor be, the goal should be its total extirpation and this must be attempted in all cases. This holds true particularly in the case of younger patients who are otherwise in a good physical condition. Ungerecht [16], Kleinsasser [9], and Mündnich [12] have elaborated on the difficulties of the operative approach. Whichever it may be, and in certain cases a two-stage removal may in fact be recommended, the ultimate goal is to achieve a total removal [10].

Diagnosis

A reddish, pulsating tumor within the middle ear and often appearing out of the external auditory meatus is pathognomonic of a glomus tumor. It may bleed to touch. If there is bulging of the pharyngeal wall, then the tumor has not only invaded the skull base but has also extended down into the neck. Signs relating to

Table 1 Radiological methods of evaluating the size and feeding vessels of a glomus tumor

Mapping of the tumor
1. Routine skull films
2. Tomography of the skull base, AP Towne's projection, Stenver's projection
3. Computed tomography with and without contrast medium
4. Angiographic studies with ipsilateral compression of the carotid arteries
5. Venography of the jugular vein, when required
6. Orbital phlebogram, also when necessary

the ninth, tenth and the twelfth cranial nerves are strong evidence of tumorous destruction of the jugular foramen. This indicates a very high probability of actual tumor extension into the cranium itself.

In order to map out the extent of the tumor all the possible tools of modern radiology need to be employed (tab. 1)*. Apart from skull films and tomographical studies of the skull, a CT scan with and without contrast medium, as well as complete angiographic studies of all cerebral vessels are required. Selective angiography of the external and internal carotid arteries on both sides as well as of the vertebral arteries helps to demonstrate tumor vessels and collateral channels, the size of the tumor and its blood supply. By compression of the ipsilateral common carotid artery, while selectively catheterising the internal carotid artery of the opposite side, the potential of the opposite carotid artery in maintaining the function of the circle of Willis should be evaluated. The surgeon will thus be cautioned against being too radical while removing tumor of the internal carotid artery, especially when a sufficient cerebral blood supply from the opposite side has not been demonstrated angiographically.

The patient ought to be informed about the risks of additional impairment of the cranial nerves, risk of aspiration and the potential necessity of a second surgical procedure either to do a complete removal of the tumor or for the repair of a pharyngeal paresis as described by Denecke [7]. If the paresis of the ninth, tenth and twelfth nerves has come on over the years, there is an altered mechanism of swallowing which has been well compensated, leaving the patient without significant complaints. In the postoperative course these patients are spared from the problems which usually arise if the ninth and tenth nerves cannot be preserved at operation. A surgical attempt should then be made to facilitate a safe act of swallowing as well as to correct vocal impairment.

* We thank Prof. Haas (Radiology Department of Fulda) for sharing some of his material.

Operative management

The surgeon undertaking the operative management of glomus tumors at the base of the skull has to be prepared to encounter specific problems:

1. *Bleeding:* This occurs from the tumor tissue itself; from the adjacent bone whose vascular supply is highly arterialized; and from the sigmoid and transverse sinuses when involved by the tumor growth. In addition Denecke [3, 4] emphasized that the tumor spreads along the basal venous pathways from the jugular bulb along the jugular rete to the carotid artery; along the accessory inferior petrous sinus to the horizontal part of the internal carotid artery; and along the inferior petrous sinus to the cavernous sinus. There is a fairly high risk of hemorrhage from tumor vessels arising from the common and the internal carotid arteries as well as from the vertebral arteries; in very rare instances a malignant tumor will actually erode the walls of these vessels.
2. Despite the above mentioned difficulties of achieving hemostasis the surgeon must set out to preserve the caudal cranial nerves in the jugular foramen, the facial nerve and the hypoglossal nerve.
3. If a huge tumor has invaded the middle and the posterior fossa, the dura is infiltrated and warrants resection, and in that case, duraplasty.
4. In the final stage of the operation attention has to be paid to the external auditory meatus and to the eustachian tube. Both of them should be sealed in order to prevent infection.

A combined otological-neurosurgical management is advised. The modern techniques of anesthesia have also contributed to the successful surgical treatment of glomus tumors. The surgeon is therefore not confronted with a time-limit for these generally very long operations; the blood pressure is well controlled and can be lowered if required. Special attention should be paid to the proper positioning of the patient so that decubitus ulcer is avoided.

Case report

The following case report demonstrates the operative steps.

In this 24-year-old patient the tumor arose from the jugular bulb, as is demonstrated on vertebral angiography. It was broadly covering the skull base posteriorly, crossing the sigmoid and the transverse sinuses and then extending forward to the cavernous sinus while reaching caudally as far as the clavicle (fig. 1). The CT scan shows the intracranial portion of the tumor (fig. 2).

The skin incision was Y-shaped so that the outer ear lay between its arms. This, of course, may be modified.

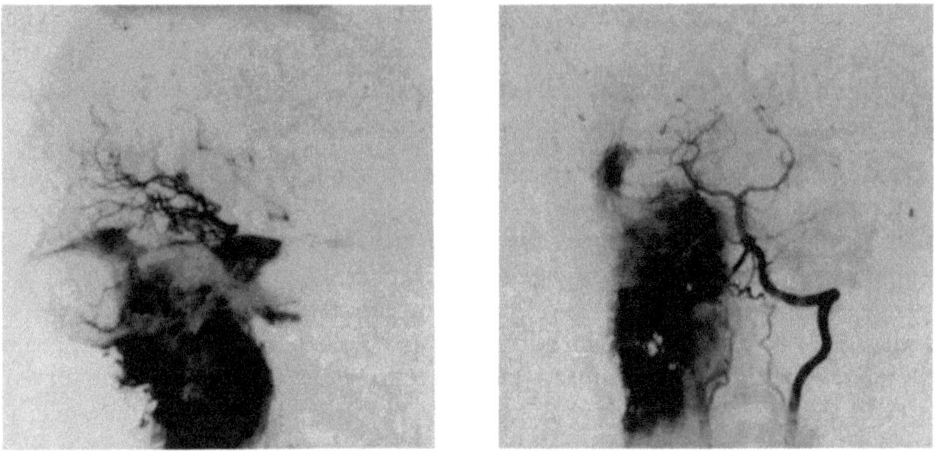

Fig. 1 Subtraction views of a vertebral angiogram of the contralateral side; by reflux the right vertebral artery and a huge glomus tumor are opacified.

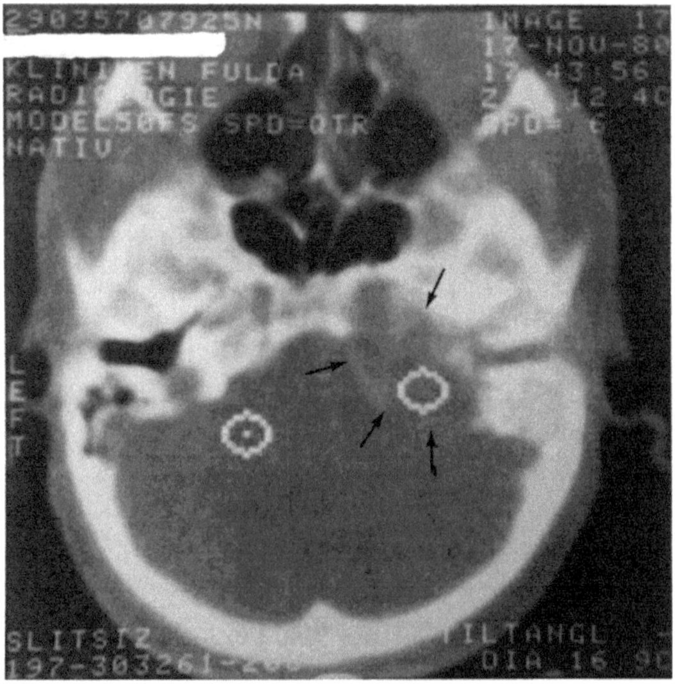

Fig. 2 Axial CT scan. The intracranial extension of the tumor is outlined (arrows).

Caudally the incision ran along the posterior border of the sternomastoid muscle down to the clavicle. In doing so, the tumor may be freed from the adjacent tissues (fig. 3), but its direct handling must be avoided.

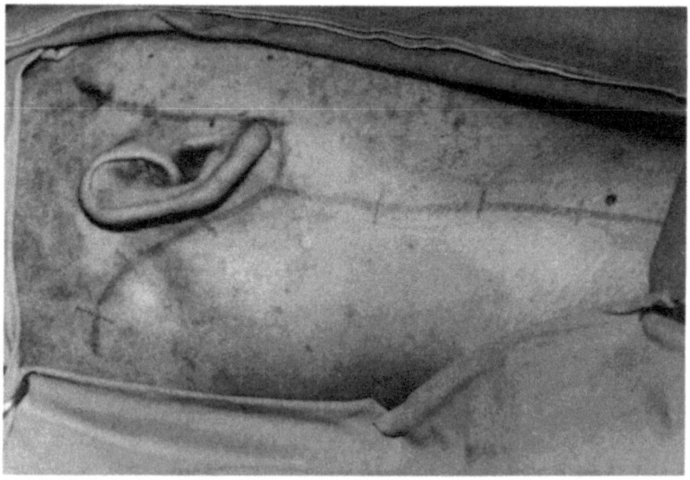

Fig. 3 Skin incision.

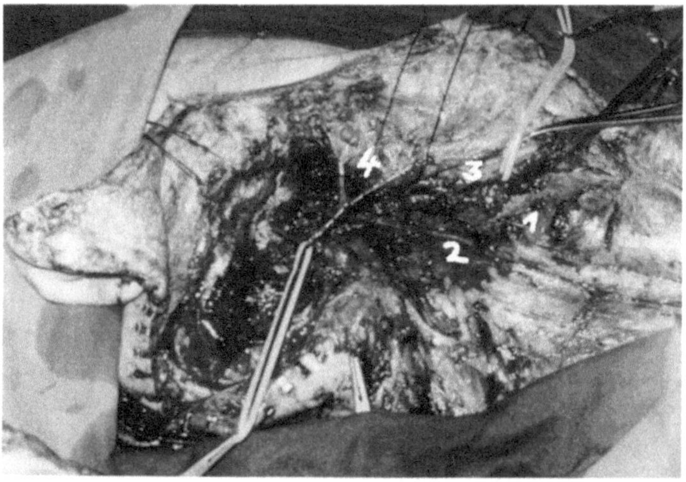

Fig. 4 Dissection of the cervical portion of the tumor. 1 = ligated branches of the external carotid artery, 2 = internal carotid artery, 3 = XII nerve, 4 = facial nerve.

In the next step a craniectomy of the middle and posterior fossae was carried out. The carotid artery was exposed above the clavicle. It is advisable to resect a part or the whole of the parotid gland and of the temporo-mandibular joint if there is evidence that the upper cervical and the petrous portions of the carotid artery are surrounded by tumor. This procedure is not only time-saving, but also permits an excellent view of the facial nerve and the carotid artery. While raising the skin flap the sternomastoid muscle is mobilized over two thirds of its length and resected from the clavicle. The cranial portion is also freed, but remains attached to the skin

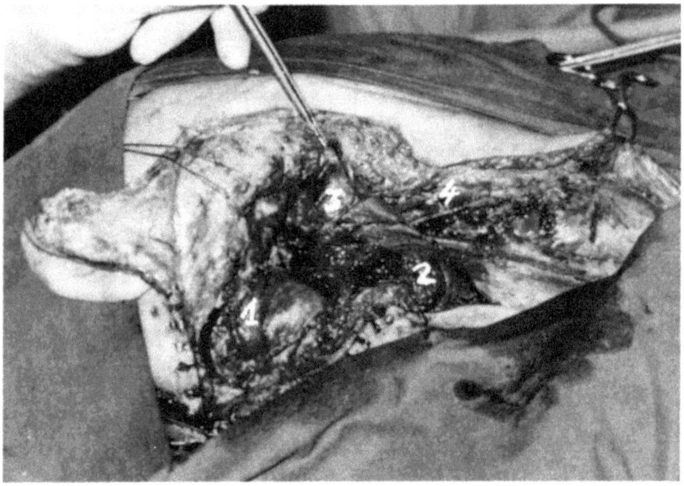

Fig. 5 Final stage of operative removal. 1 = duraplasty, 2 = mobilized and cranially rotated sternocleidomastoid muscle, 3 = VII nerve, 4 = XII nerve.

of the mastoid. In this manner the muscle can later on be used to fill the dead space of the operative cavity and to improve hemostasis (Denecke).

Exposure of the tumor in the neck was continued. In our experience this is achieved best by sharp dissection and by bipolar coagulation. The carotid artery and the cranial nerves can easily be identified. Stepwise the tumor was mobilized, always moving from a caudal to a cranial direction. The feeding vessels arising from the external carotid artery were ligated. In some cases the pharyngeal artery is hyperplastic; it has to be kept in mind that it may originate from the medial aspect of the carotid bifurcation (fig. 4). The tumor covering the internal carotid artery was completely removed including the adventitious layer. When freeing its petrous portion a diamond drill is employed for bone removal. Resection of the petrous bone is also necessary in order to achieve free access to the venous vessels. An attempt to preserve the facial nerve should be made. The transverse sinus was occluded at some distance from the sigmoid sinus. The internal jugular vein could then be ligated. Doing this procedure in this order prevents venous engorgement. Thereafter the dura was excised, carrying the incision from behind forwards. The medial portion of the tumor vessels was easily identified. The rest of the tumor adjacent to the cavernous and petrous sinuses can then be removed at the end. Sometimes major venous bleeding is encountered. Initially it may be controlled by using gelfoam. In the case demonstrated above (fig. 4) the vagus nerve had to be excised because only a blind stump ending in the tumor could be identified; it was possible to save the seventh, ninth and twelfth nerves. The dural defect measuring 12 × 10 cm was closed by lyophilized dura (fig. 5). The operative cavity and the tube was filled with the already prepared portion of the sternomastoid muscle receiving its feeding vessels from the remaining skin of the mastoid portion. The

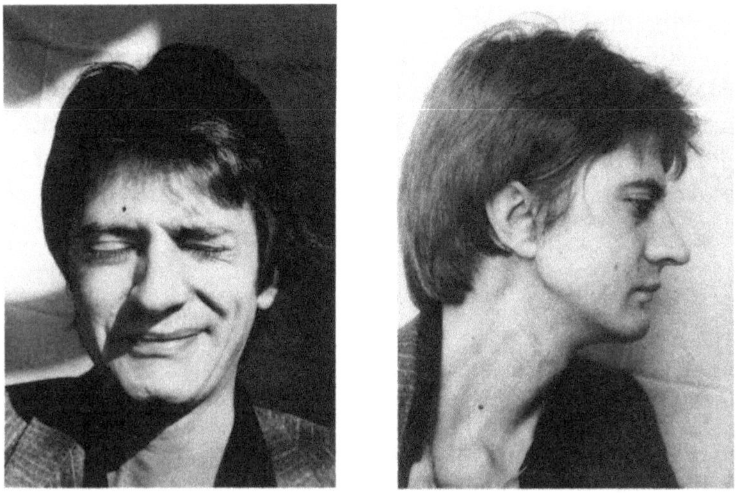

Fig. 6a+b Patient two years postoperatively: His face is quite symmetrical and there is no evidence of a postoperative right-sided facial palsy. There was no further deterioration in the function of the XII nerve which was already impaired preoperatively.

temporal muscle was sutured to the duraplasty which gave additional safety. By these means an excellent sealing off of the cartilaginous portion of the ear was also achieved.

Since the innovation of the soft tube in anesthesia, postoperative tracheotomy is no longer required. Whilst in 1966 Denecke had found it absolutely mandatory, today tracheotomy is to be reserved only for situations where the caudal nerves have to be sacrificed intra-operatively in those patients who had no preoperative malfunction or compensation.

In the case of this 24-year-old male the duration of the operation was 24 hours. A total removal of the tumor could be achieved. The facial palsy, which was evident postoperatively, improved slowly. Two years later, the patient had made a complete recovery (figs. 6a/b). An impairment of the function of the twelfth nerve was detected preoperatively and remained unchanged. Several weeks postoperatively swallowing was undisturbed.

Conclusion

In conclusion we find that even large glomus tumors can be removed, on most of the occasions in one session. Their total removal is emphasized. This has a special bearing for young patients who are generally medically fit otherwise; they have a long life ahead and the importance of a radical removal with simultaneous preservation of the cranial nerves obviously assumes great importance. Preoperative embolization might facilitate the surgical treatment and shorten the operative time. The operative plan can only be carried out by an experienced team of ENT-neurosurgeons who are familiar with micro- and macrosurgical techniques. Modern anesthesia makes it possible for such a lengthy procedure to be well tolerated.

References

[1] Van Baars, F., P. Van den Broek, C. Cremers et al.: Familiar non-chromaffinic paragangliomas (Glomus tumors): Clinical aspects. Laryngoscope **91** (1981) 988-996.
[2] Denecke, H.-J.: Diskussionsbemerkung zu Ungerecht Jahr. tag. d. Verein. Westdt. HNO-Ärzte Bonn 1962. HNO (Berl.) **11** (1963) 95-96.
[3] Denecke, H.-J.: Zur Chirurgie ausgedehnter Glomustumoren im Bereich des Foramen jugulare. Arch. otorhinolaryngol. (NY) **187** (1966) 656-662.
[4] Denecke, H.-J.: Surgery of extensive Glomus jugulare tumors of the ear. Revue de Laryngologie **90** (1969 a) 265-270.
[5] Denecke, H.-J.: Diskussionsbemerkung zu Gejrot und House (1969 b). In: Disorders of the skull base region (C. Hamberger, J. Wersäll, eds.), p. 294. Nobel Symposium 10. Almqvist and Wiksell, Stockholm 1968.
[6] Denecke, H.-J.: Die Chirurgie ausgedehnter Tumoren des Felsenbeins und der Otobasis. Laryng. Rhinol. **57** (1978) 287-290.
[7] Denecke, H.-J.: Operative Korrektur des Schluckaktes und der Stimme bei einseitiger Vaguslähmung. In: Die otorhinolaryngologischen Operationen im Mund- und Halsbereich, (H.-J. Denecke, ed.), p. 678. Springer, Berlin-Heidelberg-New York 1980.
[8] Draf, W., M. Samii: Otorhinolaryngo-neurochirurgische Probleme an der Schädelbasis. Laryng. Rhinol. **56** (1977) 1007.
[9] Kleinsasser, O.: Diskussionsbemerkung zu Ungerecht. Jahr. tag. d. Verein. Westdt. HNO-Ärzte, Bonn 1962, HNO (Berl.) **11** (1963) 95-96.
[10] Kraus, H.: Die neurochirurgisch-rhinologische Zusammenarbeit bei Eingriffen an der Schädelbasis. Mschr. Ohren HK **106** (1972) 16-22.
[11] Müller, H., K. Erdmann, W. Draf: Anästhesiologische und hals-nasen-ohrenchirurgische Aspekte der Langzeitoperationen. Laryng. Rhinol. **58** (1979) 157-161.
[12] Mündnich, K.: Diskussionsbemerkung zu Denecke. Arch. otorhinolaryngol. (NY) **187** (1966) 661.
[13] Parkin, J. L.: Familial multiple glomus tumors and pheochromocytomas. Ann. Otol. **90** (1981) 60-63.
[14] Schlosshauer, B., H.-J. Denecke: Zur chirurgischen Behandlung der Glomus jugulare Tumors. Arch. otorhinolaryngol. (NY) **191** (1968) 738-744.
[15] Spoendlin, H.: Glomustumoren der Schädelbasis. Pract. oto-rhino-laryng. (Basel) **23** (1961) 128-136.
[16] Ungerecht, K.: Zur Chirurgie der Glomus jugulare-Tumoren im Schläfenbein-Schädelbasisbereich. Vortrag Jahr. tag. d. Verein. Westdt. HNO-Ärzte, Bonn 1962, HNO (Berlin) **11** (1963) 95-96.

Rehabilitation of swallowing following paresis of the caudal cranial nerves

W. Ey, H. J. Denecke

Disturbance of deglutition is one of the severest symptoms associated with postoperative or post-traumatic paresis of the caudal cranial nerves. Lesions of the nuclei of the vagus nerve or its intracranial injury are especially associated with difficulties or with impossibility of swallowing. The main problem in these cases is aspiration. It is a serious disorder with potentially life-threatening pulmonary sequelae. We will be more and more confronted with such cases in the future, because the neurosurgeons are developing excellent techniques for intracranial surgery and, with the effective assistance of the anaesthetists, obtain a high percentage of survival of the patients.

In cases with unilateral paresis of the vagus nerve we can consider the problem of rehabilitative surgery of swallowing as having been solved very well, as is demonstrated in the film, but in cases with bilateral vagus paresis we have to deal with many more problems, especially in the high grade aspiration syndrom. The techniques so far employed include tracheostomy with the use of a cuffed tube, laryngotracheal closure procedures, laryngeal diversion procedures or total laryngectomy. For laryngeal closure Habal and Murray [6] described a supraglottic closure procedure, Montgomery [9] did a glottic closure procedure. Lindeman [7] described a laryngeal diversion procedure consisting of division of the trachea with formation of a tracheoesophageal anastomosis by suturing the proximal segment of the trachea to the anterior esophageal wall. The distal segment is used to form a tracheostomy. No reversals were attempted.

Since in the experience of many surgeons the use of a cuffed tube is of limited value for even the temporary control of aspiration, in *our concept* [2, 5] of surgical rehabilitation of swallowing we prefer a plastic tracheostomy (fig. 1). This means the entire tracheal stoma is lined with skin [11]. According to Denecke [3] a pedicle skin flap from the anterior thoracic wall is sutured into the caudal rim of the tracheostomy. It prevents complications such as bleeding and tracheal stenosis. Aspiration is controlled by a so called intratracheal dressing consisting in a Mikulicz-tamponage above the tracheal tube. In addition the tube is wrapped by a gauze strip for further protection of the lower airway. The next very important step in our concept of restoration of deglutition is the so-called cricopharyngeal myotomy (fig. 2). This consists of the division of the pars fundiformis of the cricopharyngeus muscle and of the circular muscle fibers of the cervical esophagus [1, 5, 10]. The next step is the resection of the paralysed pharyngeal wall from the introitus of the esophagus up to the palatine tonsil (figs. 3, 4).

Then the paralysed soft palate is to be corrected by resection of a strip of the mucous membrane from the pharyngopalatine arch and of the pharyngeal wall. After suturing we get an obstruction to the nasopharynx on one side (figs. 5 a–c).

In the region of the glottis there is a big difference for surgical rehabilitation of swallowing in cases of unilateral and in bilateral paresis of the vagus nerve. In cases of unilateral vagus paresis, the glottal repair consists in a cartilage implant into the paralysed vocal cord (fig. 6) and in rotation of the arytenoid cartilage to attain a midline position of the vocal cord. This procedure is done before resection of the pharyngeal wall.

In cases of bilateral paresis of the vagus we also have to do the above described procedures but, in the glottic region we are forced to perform a partial glottic closure. Similar to Montgomery [9] and Strome and Fried [12] the larynx is approached through a midline thyrotomy, the vocal cords and the posterior laryngeal wall are de-epithelised and the glottis is then partially closed with through and through sutures, but, according to Denecke [5], we leave a small fistula in the region of the posterior commissure of the glottis covered with laryngeal mucosa. This fistula enables patients to phonate without any disorder of deglutition. Later on a reversal procedure is possible. Reopening of the laryngeal stenosis can be done by following the rules of plastic surgery of the larynx [4, 5, 8].

References

[1] Denecke, H. J.: Die oto-rhino-laryngologischen Operationen. In: Allgemeine und spezielle Operationslehre von M. Kirschner (N. Guleke, R. Zenker, eds.), vol. V. Springer Verlag, Berlin-Göttingen-Heidelberg 1953.

[2] Denecke, H. J.: Korrektur des Schluckaktes bei einseitiger Pharynx- und Larynxlähmung. HNO (Suppl.) **9** (1961) 351.

[3] Denecke, H. J.: Trachealplastik im Bereich der Halsbasis bei besonderen pathologischen Verhältnissen in der oberen Thoraxapertur. HNO (Suppl.) **23** (1976) 126–128.

[4] Denecke, H. J.: Plastische Korrektur des Schluckaktes und der Stimme bei Vaguslähmung. HNO (Suppl.) **25** (1977) 140–143.

[5] Denecke, H. J.: Die oto-rhino-laryngologischen Operationen im Mund- und Halsbereich. In: Allgemeine und spezielle Operationslehre von M. Kirschner (R. Zenker, G. Heberer, R. Pichlmayr, eds.), vol. V/3. Springer Verlag, Berlin-Heidelberg-New York 1980.

[6] Habal, M. A., J. E. Murray: Surgical treatment of life-endangering chronic aspiration pneumonia. J. plast. Reconstr. Surg. **49** (1972) 305–311.

[7] Lindemann, R. C.: Diverting the paralyzed larynx: A reversible procedure for intractable aspiration. Laryngoscope **85** (1975) 157–180.

[8] Menzel, J., H. J. Denecke: On the pathogenesis, treatment and prognosis of lesions of the vagus nerve. In: The cranial nerves (M. Samii, P. J. Jannetta, eds.). Springer Verlag, Berlin-Heidelberg-New York 1981.

[9] Montgomery, W. W.: Surgery to prevent aspiration. Arch. Otolaryngol. (Chicago) **101** (1975) 679–682.

[10] Seiffert, A.: Zur Behandlung beginnender Hypopharynxdivertikel. Z. Laryng. **23** (1932) 256–258.
[11] Soerensen, J.: Die Mund- und Halsoperationen. Urban & Schwarzenberg, Berlin-Wien 1930.
[12] Strome, M., M. P. Fried: Rehabilitative surgery for aspiration. Arch. Otolaryngol. (Chicago) **109** (1983) 809–811.

List of contributors

Arnold, H., Prof. Dr. med., Klinik für Neurochirurgie Medizinische Hochschule Lübeck, Ratzeburger Allee 160, 2400 Lübeck
Bock, W.J., Prof. Dr. med., Neurochirurgische Klinik der Universität Düsseldorf, Moorenstr. 5, 4000 Düsseldorf
Carini, S., Dr. med., Service de Neurochirurgie B, Centre Hospitalier Universitaire, F-59037 Lille Cedex
Denecke, H.J., Prof. Dr. med., Moltkestr. 20, 6900 Heidelberg
Dimitriadis, A.S., Prof. Dr. med., Otolaryngology Department Head and Neck, Surgery AXE-PA Hospital, Thessaloniki, Griechenland
Draf, W., Prof. Dr. med., Klinik für Hals-Nasen-Ohrenkrankheiten und Plast. Chirurgie, Städtische Kliniken, Pacellialle 4, 6400 Fulda
Estonillo, R.M.D., University Neurosurgical Associates Inc. 230 Lothrop Street, Pittsburgh, Pennsylvania, USA
Ey, W., Prof. Dr. med., Hals-Nasen-Ohren-Klinik, Städt. Kliniken Darmstadt, Heidelberger-Landstr. 379, 6100 Darmstadt-Eberstadt
Frowein, R.A., Prof. Dr. med., Neurochirurgische Universitätsklinik Köln, Joseph-Stelzmann-Str. 9, 5000 Köln
Gerhardt, H.J., Prof. Dr. sc. med., Hals-Nasen-Ohrenklinik der Humboldt-Universität Berlin, Schumannstr. 20–21, DDR-1040 Berlin
Gillissen, J.P.A., Dr. med., Orbital Centre, Department of Ophthalmology AZUA, Academic Medical Centre, Meibergdreef 9, NL- AZ Amsterdam Z.O.
Halves, F., Prof. Dr. med., Neurochirurgische Abt. im Allgemeinkrankenhaus Hamburg-Altona, Paul Ehrlichstr. 1, 2000 Hamburg 50
Heiss, E., Dr. med., Abt. für Neurochirurgie - Chirurgische Klinik - Eberhard-Karls-Universität, Calwer-Str. 7, 7400 Tübingen
Helms, J., Prof. Dr. med., Hals-Nasen-Ohrenklinik der Johannes Gutenberg-Universität Mainz, Langenbeckstr. 1, 6500 Mainz
Herrmann, H.D., Prof. Dr. med., Neurochirurgische Abt. des Universitäts-Krankenhauses Eppendorf, Martinistr. 52, 2000 Hamburg 20
Hinkelbein, W., Dr. med., Strahlenklinik der Universität Freiburg, 7800 Freiburg
Jahnke, K., Prof. Dr. med., Hals-Nasen-Ohrenklinik der Universität Tübingen, Silcherstr. 5, 7400 Tübingen
Jansen, C., Dr. med., Hals-Nasen-Ohren-Abteilung des Städt. Krankenhauses, Winterbeckstr. 1, 5270 Gummersbach
Jomin, M., Dr. med., Service de Neurochirurgie B, Centre Hospitalier Universitaire, F-59037 Lille Cedex
Knosp, E., Dr. med., Neurochirurgische Univ.-Klinik, Allgemeines Krankenhaus der Stadt Wien 9, Alserstr. 4, A-1090 Wien
Knüfermann, H., Priv.-Doz. Dr. med., Städtische Kliniken Kassel, Abt. Strahlentherapie, Mönchbergstr. 41–43, 3500 Kassel
Köning, W., Dr. med., Neurochirurgische Universitätsklinik Köln, Joseph-Stelzmann-Str. 9, 5000 Köln 41
Lang, J., Prof. Dr. med., Anatomisches Institut der Universität Würzburg, Koellikerstr. 6, 8700 Würzburg

Lasjaunias, P., M.D., Hopitaux de Paris Centre Hopitalier de Bicetre, Neuroradiologie, 78, Rue du Général Leclerc, F-94270 Le Kremlin-Bicetre
Lesoin, F., Dr. med., Service de Neurochirurgie B, Centre Hospitalier Regional, Place de Verdun, F-59037 Lille Cedex
Löblich, H.J., Prof. Dr. med., Pathologisches Institut, Knickstr. 5, 3000 Hannover 1
Lozes, G., Dr. med., Service de Neurochirurgie B, Hopital Regional, Place de Verdun, F-59037 Lille Cedex
Manolidis, L., Prof. Dr. med., Otoparyngology Department Head and Neck, Surgery AXEPA Hospital, Thessaloniki, Griechenland
Miles, J.B., M.D., University Department of O.R.L., Royal Liverpool Hospital, Prescot Street, P.O. Box 147 Liverpool L69 3BX
Nover, A., Prof. Dr. med., Augenklinik der Johannes-Gutenberg-Universität Mainz, Langenbeckstr. 1, 6500 Mainz
Pellerin, G., Dr. med., Service de Neurochirurgie B, Hospital Regional, Place de Verdun, F-59037 Lille Cedex
Perneczky, A., Doz. Dr. med., Neurochirurgische Universitätsklinik, Allgemeines Krankenhaus der Stadt Wien 9, Alserstr. 4, A-1090 Wien
Pinedo, H.M., Dr. med., Academisch-Ziekenhuis de Vrije Universiteit, Afdeling Keel-, Neu- en Orziekten, De Boelelaan 117, Postbus 7057 NL- MB-Amsterdam
Reuther, J., Prof. Dr. Dr. med., Klinik u. Poliklinik für Kieferchirurgie der Julius-Maximilian-Universität, Pleicherwall 1, 8700 Würzburg
Richter, W., Prof. Dr. Dr. med., Hals-Nasen-Ohrenklinik der Universität Würzburg, Kopfklinikum, 8700 Würzburg
Rios-Nogales Garces, L., Dr. med., Chir. Klinik der Eberhard-Karls-Universität, Abt. für Neurochirurgie, Calwer-Str. 7, 7400 Tübingen
Rochels, R., Prof. Dr. med., Augenklinik der Johannes-Gutenberg-Universität Mainz, Langenbeckstr. 1, 6500 Mainz
Romeu, J., Dr. med., Hopital Clinic I Provincial de Barcelona, Department of Otorhinolaryngology, Casanova 143, Barcelona 36
Roosen, N., Dr. med., Neurochirurgische Universitätsklinik Düsseldorf, Moorenstr. 5, 4000 Düsseldorf
Samii, M., Prof. Dr. med., Neurochirurgische Klinik im Krankenhaus Nordstadt, Halterhoffstr. 41, 3000 Hannover 1
Schmelzle, R., Prof. Dr. Dr. med., Abt. für Kiefer- u. Gesichtschirurgie der Universität Tübingen, Osianderstr. 2-8, 7400 Tübingen
Schürmann, K., Prof. Dr. med. Dr. h.c., Neurochirurgische Klinik der Johannes-Gutenberg-Universität Mainz, Langenbeckstr. 1, 6500 Mainz
Schwenzer, N., Prof. Dr. Dr. med., Abt. für Kiefer- u. Gesichtschirurgie der Universität Tübingen, Osianderstr. 2-8, 7400 Tübingen
Sekhar, L.N., M.D., Ass. Prof., University Neurosurgical Associates, Inc. Room, 9402 PUH 230 Lothrop Street, Pittsburgh, Pennsylvania 15213
Servato, R., Dr. med., Service de Neurochirurgie B. Hopital Regional, Place de Verdun, F-59037 Lille Cedex
Shaheen, O., M.S., F.R.C.S., ENT-Surgery 97, Harley Street, GB-London WN1DF
Snow, G.B., Prof. Dr. med., Academisch-Ziekenhuis de Vrije Universiteit, Afdeling Keel, Neus- en Oorziekten, De Boelelaan 1117, Postbus 7057, NL-1007 MB Amsterdam
Stell, P.M., Ch.M., F.R.C.S., Department of Oto-Rhino-Laryngology, Royal Liverpool Hospital, Prescot Street, P.O. Box 147, GB-Liverpool L69 3 BX
Strohm, M., Priv.-Doz. Dr. med., Hals-Nasen-Ohrenklinik der Eberhard-Karls-Universität Tübingen, Silcherstr. 5, 7400 Tübingen
Ter Brugge, K.G., M.D., F.R.C.P., Toronto Western Hospital, University Toronto, 399 Bathurst Street, Toronto, Canada

Trassera, J., Prof. Dr. med., Department of Otorhinolaryngology, Hospital Clinic I Provincial de Barcelona, Univ. of Barcelona, Casanova 143, Barcelona 36, Spain
Vermorken, J. B., Dr. med., Academisch-Ziekenhuis de Vrije Universiteit, Afdeling Keel-, Neu- en Orziekten, De Boelelaan 117, Postbus 7057, NL-1007 MB Amsterdam
Vollmer, J. F., Prof. Dr. med., Klinikum der Universität Ulm, Abt. für Thorax- und Gefäßchirurgie, Steinhövelstr. 9, 7900 Ulm
Wannenmacher, M., Prof. Dr. med., Strahlenklinik der Universität Freiburg, 7800 Freiburg
Weidenbecher, M., Prof. Dr. med., Hals-Nasen-Ohrenklinik der Universität Erlangen-Nürnberg, Waldstr. 1, 8520 Erlangen
Wilcke, O., Dr. med., Neurochirurgische Universitätsklinik Köln, Joseph-Stelzmann-Str. 9, 5000 Köln 41

Authors' index

Subject index

Spina bifida – neural tube defects

Basic research, interdisciplinary diagnostics and treatment, results and prognosis

Edited by *D. Voth* and *P. Glees* in collaboration with *J. Lorber*

1986. 17 x 24 cm. XI, 320 pages. With 105 illustrations and 66 tables.
Cloth **DM 148,–** ISBN 3 11 010768 6

This book deals with, in a comprehensive yet concise form, the formal origin of dysrhaphic malformations and at the same time surveys the present standard of knowledge regarding research on its causes and prevention.

The special features of the epidemiology together with the basic research carried out by the Sheffield Working Group, are discussed at length. The problem of both antenatal diagnosis and pregnancy termination with the resulting direct and indirect consequences are treated extensively.

Other chapters deal with operative treatment of dysrhaphic malformations and the complications and results thereof.

Finally, orthopaedic specialists give extensive information on deviations of the spine (which tend to occur frequently) and its necessary therapeutic treatment.

W
DE
G

de Gruyter · Berlin · New York

Bei Fragen zur Produktsicherheit wenden Sie sich bitte an:
If you have any questions regarding product safety,
please contact:

Walter de Gruyter GmbH
Genthiner Straße 13
10785 Berlin
productsafety@degruyterbrill.com